THE THIRD T
THE THIRD

PERPETUA

Kevin Carey

chipmunkapublishing
the mental health publisher

Published by
Chipmunkapublishing
PO Box 6872
Brentwood
Essex CM13 1ZT
United Kingdom

www.chipmunkapublishing.com

Chipmunkapublishing gratefully acknowledge
the support of Arts Council England.

Typeset by Hiltonian Media
www.hiltonian.com

www.perpetua.tv
comments@perpetua.tv

JACK

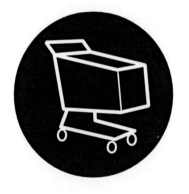

PERPETUA

1

One morning at the beginning of July 2006, in the last year of Tony Blair's Premiership, when reality television was just past its viewing peak, Perpetua, the Special Vessel of God, began her mission, marking the greatest divine intervention in human affairs since Jesus.

There were harassed faces at the CEC morning news conference. As not enough people knew, CEC stood for the Cutting Edge Channel. Initial poor audience figures were getting worse. As the days went by, the edge cut less deeply, less delicately, less unpredictably. CEC was moving ever more rapidly into the mainstream so that its identity was fading. The more it moved the lower its profile and audiences but there was no turning back. CEC was in the grip of the law that gold can turn to dross but dross cannot turn to gold. Each day "CEC" was given new and unflattering meanings in scores of internet blogs and there were rumours that RANT-TV was planning a competition to find the most offensive name.

As with most desperate situations, however, the people squashed into the conference room—less than half the number and size projected in the original business plan—were only interested in their particular tiny piece of the major crisis. It could hardly have been worse: it was early July, a terrible month for news; it was Friday, a terrible day for news; and rain earlier in the week meant that the bulletin would lose its regular slot to a Wimbledon early start.

The BBC was running a major report on melting Himalayan glaciers but CEC could not even afford secondary transmission rights, let alone a reporter of its own. There was a brief discussion on morphing the World Affairs Correspondent (who doubled as the Global Glitz Guru) into a Kanchenjunga backdrop but this was ditched because it was too naff to contemplate seriously. Then there was the usual litany of murders, drug dealings, pronouncements from Junior Ministers, genocides in Africa, suicide bombers in Iraq, Somalia and Afghanistan, lobbyist briefings dressed up as scientific research, financial scandals, local council risk aversion, calls for more public expenditure, calls for a reduction in the "Nanny State", condemnations of central government, condemnations of the "post code lottery", contrived celebrity partnership breakups, football transfer exclusives, killer virus mutants, the completion of major Parliamentary bills and detritus from the morning's ever more desperately warring newspapers.

CEC had somehow managed, in spite of successive waves of "downsizing" and his reluctance to investigate anything, to hold on to Will Dignot, its investigative reporter. The story was that he had been in the wrong place at the wrong time and had discovered that the Chief Accountant had been entertaining his girlfriend on expenses. It was therefore Will's usual policy to stay quiet and hang on to the salary but on this occasion he blushingly honoured a deal and tentatively mentioned that a girl in Grunge Park, South London, was leading a campaign to get people to shop less. He could not have shocked his colleagues more if he had said she was claiming to be God. Will was surprised to hear News Editor Spike Allworthy say that this was a genuine lead item for a Cutting Edge bulletin.

Will had picked up the story by accident. He was crossing the Hypo car park to do his grudging weekly shop when he saw the girl at the main entrance wearing a *god4u* top, standing under a "Shop Less" placard, encouraging people to exercise moderation. The Head of Security just happened to be looking at the outside entrance screen of the customer-protection monitoring system to see if there were any skimpy tops or tight shorts when he observed this unusual behaviour. He turned up the audio feed and when he heard the message he phoned Annie Price, the Store Manager. Unfortunately for Will, he was also picked up by the monitoring system. Annie, who kept an eye on minority TV channels just in case they offered commercial possibilities, recognised him. With the incisive, postmodern analytical grasp that had made her what she wanted other people to think she was, Annie calculated that television coverage of a "Shop Less" message would produce a net rise in sales: a few religious types (steady average bills in the high £80s) would go for token cuts but this would be far outweighed by local media consumers (moderately fluctuating average bills in the mid £90s). The CEC audience was tiny but she only needed 0.5% of the M2500 catchment area (with media-fuelled purchasing in the £130 range) to put her sales figures into solid gain territory. It was worth a shot.

She had to do two things very quickly: stop Will getting away; and stop the woman being sent away by over-zealous, definitely pre-postmodern security staff. As it turned out, neither of these tasks was difficult. She met Will as he was registering for his bar code reader and she flourished a £200 voucher saying he was the random winner of a bar code registration prize. Rapidly checking his record on her hand-held, she found that he knew no more about shopping than investigating: his average bill was £120; his maximum ever, in the week before Christmas, was £165. He bought everything at natural eye level; liked ready meals with gaudy packaging; always fell for special offers in the drinks section even when they increased his spend; and, being a postmodern person himself, paid exorbitantly for his few items of aspirationally labelled organic produce. He would be conveniently detained in the bewildering delights of New World wine for some time.

As for the cause of the stir, Annie introduced herself politely to the girl, showed her ID, said that Hypo welcomed all strains of moderate opinion as long as everyone was free to go about their business and, in a flash of inspiration, asked whether she would like a bigger sign in Hypo livery and typeface but the girl simply smiled, shook her head, and went on talking to a couple of women in designer casuals.

Annie switched monitoring system screens on her hand-held to have a quick check on Will and then watched what her Head of Security was watching. She instructed the system to go on watching him to collect the evidence to fire him for wasting company time. Going back into the store she noted that special offer melons were going too fast so she retained the offer but raised the price. A five minute tour of fruit and veg convinced her that all the salad and fruit were under-priced at the current rate of purchase but that the roots and green veg would never shift unless the price was dropped. Corporate Centre had already raised the standard prices of barbecue meats, bikinis, lager, sun lotion, crisps, paddling pools, ice cream, wasp sting soother, sparkling white wine, garden furniture, sun dresses, bottled water, flip flops, burger buns, ice makers and olives but she had control over perishable goods and special local items. She keyed in an instruction to the store computer which synchronised the price change on the shelf displays, the customer bar code readers, the tills, local and Corporate Centre stock control and management accounts.

Then she saw Will struggling away from check-out with a badly packed trolley which wasn't, she admitted, entirely his fault as the store router forced people to buy their fruit and veg before dumping their wine and beer on top of it. She asked him whether he had enjoyed his shop and he said that he had, eying a cheerful box of end-of-line unpopular and obscure wines designated "De Luxe Exotic Wines of the World". She said she had stayed up late to watch his Naked! series and then suggested—without making an explicit, pre-post-modern connection—by looking at the girl that he had a ready-made scoop and that she would designate him a Premier Home Customer so that he only needed to change his weekly order online and he would have free delivery for a year.

Will asked the girl how long she had been there and how long she intended to go on. She said she would be back tomorrow as Saturday was a big shopping day. He asked her if she minded news coverage and she simply shrugged, sceptically but not aggressively, and went on talking to a man with the biggest trolley on the stand, crammed with beer and TV dinners. Without thinking, Will gave the girl his mobile number.

2

What had started out as a stunning, counter-cultural story turned out to be a lost opportunity. Perpetua started out by saying that the consumer society was morally bankrupt, the sort of thing that people used to say back in the days of Old Labour; it was not so much the words that made the story as the way she looked straight at the camera and really meant it. People should only buy what they really need and give all the rest of their money to poor people. "My mission is to make the poor rejoice and make the rich think about their greed."

Will, vaguely recalling something he had read at school about Robespierre, asked, almost without thinking: "And how are you going to do that?" And that is where it all went wrong. She started talking about dismantling the Christian church which, she said, was beyond reform; something about getting all the congregations to walk out of their buildings and split into "missionary cells", with particular attention on deprived areas. Christian people would want to celebrate together on a grand scale now and again but that did not justify massive, environmentally greedy buildings that stood empty six days of the week; they could hire halls. If the country wanted a whole load of churches as part of its built heritage then the Chancellor should take them over and pay for their upkeep. What had started out as a nice story was turning into a disaster so Will gave the signal for the filming to stop.

Unfortunately, Annie did not watch the whole of the filming. Just after the girl began, saying that the poor would be rewarded, a message came from Corporate Centre saying that rain was heading her way and it was therefore reversing yesterday's price rises and would immediately raise the price of umbrellas, soup, saucepans, sliced bread, video games, sausages, toasters, baked beans, rainwear and processed cheese. Annie went inside and lowered the price of salad and fruit and raised the price of roots and greens with a swingeing rise for the largest potatoes; lunch salad would be replaced by filled jackets.

On her way out she saw a cashier in tense conversation with a customer; the training in steel-hard politeness had obviously kicked in but it was not doing the trick and at this time on Friday the last thing you wanted was lengthening check-out queues. As the price competition between Hypo, Jambo and Lakshmo began to threaten margins, factors like parking, check-out speeds and even lighting and decor began to matter.

The customer—a little old lady, Annie now observed—was saying that she had put a can of beans into her trolley but it had not registered on her bar code reader. The cashier had manually checked the whole trolley and still the beans did not show in the total. Annie told the cashier not to bother, thanked the lady for her honesty, and went on again but it soon became obvious that there was something seriously wrong with the system. Beans were not registering anywhere on the system. They were a well known loss leader but selling them for nothing would cause trouble with the Competition Directorate which was currently undertaking yet another enquiry into price fixing. She texted Corporate Centre which immediately replied that it had picked up the fault in the store's system and it would be dealt with immediately. Meanwhile, word spread and ominous quantities of baked beans appeared on trolleys. Annie told the warehouse not to replenish the rapidly emptying shelves and then had to call the Head of Security because a nasty situation was developing at the whole line of check-outs. Apparently, the system priced up to six tins at zero but for amounts greater than six it charged the standard price. Will looked on, vaguely interested, but could not be bothered with a computer malfunction and left to edit the story.

There was not much editing to do. As the rain advanced from the West, it took out pretty pictures of the Queen at an agricultural show, worthy pictures of the Prime Minister launching a Better Footpaths Task Force, glitzy pictures of Melanie—well, being Melanie—and, of course, Wimbledon and the Test Match at Lords. This meant two things: first, the bulletin was put back in its normal slot which cut down editing time; secondly, there was no competing lead story for a channel of limited means. The only other lead option was a picture of the Culture Secretary on a beach in France in a fetching bikini but not even Spike could find a peg to hang it on.

Things were not much better at the mighty BBC but at least it had super quality melting ice pictures. The *NewSpite* Editor's attention drifted with the ice as this story, for all its pictorial glamour, was old hat. He became increasingly engaged with another screen as Perpetua drifted away from the ethics of consumerism towards Christianity and heritage. There might be an unusual political angle and that is what he needed. Ever since the last Licence settlement the Corporation had been forced to meet public value targets, acting as a broadcasting back-stop, which meant doing anything that the increasingly deregulated sector would not do. On this basis the duopoly was only normatively miserable: the commercial sector resented the BBC but rejoiced in its remit to be tedious; the BBC resented the implication that it could not self-regulate public value but was consoled that only a few jobs had been lost in the last round of Treasury niggardliness.

The Editor rang Radio London and asked for a South London contact. That would be all right as long as the story was co-badged, came the wary reply. A junior reporter was sent off to Hypo but Perpetua refused to talk to the BBC because it was part of the establishment. But the reporter gave just enough away to make Perpetua think it worthwhile to phone Will.

Wearily, as the rain turned yet another July Friday into a depressing anti-climax, Will pondered the barren acres of Fang, his late night chat show. So few people watched it that he might as well have a chat about revolution and socialism with a bit of Christianity thrown in. Fang had long since stopped appealing to the youth who were supposed to watch it as they fell into their scruffy flats with tepid takeaways after a night at the pub; the content and liberalised pub opening hours had blunted Fang, and so his only hope was those too immobile or poor to go out. He had toyed with the idea of calling it Friday Filling but it was too like a modernist joke to be acceptable. He invited Perpetua on to the show and then began to scratch around for other guests. He quickly assembled a short list of revolutionaries from the internet but soon discovered from their abandoned Filipino maids that they had gone to their little farm houses in Tuscany. Finally, he resorted to the architectural angle. He rang the Lambeth Palace Press Office and asked for a bishop. The man said they did not do bishops, they only did the Archbishop. If he wanted a bishop he would have to speak to the Church of England at Church House. When he got past the Friday afternoon voice mails, Chris Smoother treated him with faultless courtesy. Yes, he had seen the Perpetua story and did not think much of it but if he really wanted a bishop it would have to be a Suffragan. Yes, they were real bishops but not like diocesans; they were junior but equal. Will, being postmodern, recognised this as a piece of modernist jargon and ignored it. Did he, asked Smoother, want a heritage bishop or a holy bishop? Will supposed a Bishop could be both but on balance preferred a heritage bishop because he did not think he could keep the discussion under control if it went holy. Quite right, said Smoother, holiness was a very tricky thing best left to experts. Next, Will wondered whether he wanted a humanist, an atheist or an agnostic but, as he didn't know the difference and as he assumed that just about everybody was at least one of these, he got somebody from the National Heritage Directorate instead. Smoother was right; you couldn't keep control of holiness.

3

The show went out at midnight. In its early days Fang had been staged in the atrium of the Paradise Shopping Mall but whether the money ran out before the drug dealers crept in or vice versa was a point that Will had never bothered to investigate. What had once been the Cutting Edge board room was now a studio. When the first guest arrived, Will's spirits sank as Smoother had sent him an Archdeacon—whatever that was—instead of a Bishop. Like most other people, Will assumed that Bishops ran the Church of England, sitting in their cathedrals on Sundays and touring during the week, making decisions about churches, schools and homes, orders of service and the quality of preaching but by the time Archdeacon Varnish had provided a thumbnail sketch of Deans, Archdeacons, Synods, boards, committees, faculties, benefices, freeholds, Churchwardens, ancient rites and "Fresh Expressions", Will could feel himself losing the plot. His spirits rose with the entrance of Aspic from the Heritage Directorate as their frosty greetings showed that he and Varnish clearly knew each other of old and, at the very least, disliked each other intensely. It seemed that every proposal Varnish made for the alteration of a church—and, given his conservative views, such were very few—was blocked by Aspic. It was well known in heritage circles that the Archdeaconery of Patchminster was the most architecturally obsessed, whereas in church circles it was known that it was the most backward in mission.

What annoyed Varnish most was that the Church had to obey the Directorate and pay for the privilege. That might be all very well in the leafy suburbs but slum Deaneries like Grunge Park ran at a terrible loss. The Established Church got no money from the Government but acted as its self-financing heritage agent which meant that money which should have gone on spreading the Gospel went on preserving Victorian fake gothic carving. If the Heritage Directorate wanted to preserve a load of jerry-carved pews it should pay. Will felt the temperature rising with as near to excitement as he ever got but then Perpetua walked in and all three men lost interest in architecture. She said hello and extended her hand to the trio but nobody took it. She turned down wine but accepted a glass of tepid sparkling water. Will asked her whether she had been on television before and she said, with the exception of today, not since she was a baby which did not really count. She had seen Fang once but found it a bit confrontational and shallow.

In the studio Will started by reminding Perpetua of what she had said about her mission to make the poor rejoice by making the rich think about their greed. She had not breathed in before Varnish said this was a wonderful ambition for a young woman, reflecting two thousand years of Christianity.

Aspic retorted that the longer Christianity went on, the wider the inequalities. Varnish said that Jesus was urging benevolence not Marxism and, anyway, without the rich Aspic couldn't have his built heritage and all that art and craftsmanship. Perpetua said that we all had to take the Magnificat literally, not to mention the Sermon on the Mount in Matthew and, even better, the Sermon on the Plain in Luke.

Will sat back as Aspic and Varnish showed every sign of interrupting but she went on: "Jesus My Brother" (emphatic intake of breath by Varnish) "advocated benevolence, people giving to the poor of their own free will; the problem with 'isms' like Marxism is that they force people to do things when the essence of Christianity is freedom, the freedom to be good or evil and to choose good. The Church has become so entangled in property, hierarchy, liturgy, history, dignity, respectability, money, art, aesthetics and, worst of all, morality, that it has forgotten the good news for the poor.

"Most Christians have totally lost contact with the poor. Grunge Park, where I grew up, is almost a Christian-free zone. The Church of England is physically there but not with us; and as the Irish became owner-occupiers and moved out, the Catholic church went with them. It is only in the past few years that some Afro-Caribbean charismatics have brought some cheer and spirituality and the Poles may help the Catholics to make a come-back. We have had a self-confessed Christian Prime Minister and Chancellor for almost ten years but the Anglican Bishops have been so busy fighting about women and gay clergy that they have only received crumbs from the secular table. The thing to do now is for us to abandon our fine churches; just walk out; leave it to the bishops and the lawyers to sort out. Jesus My Brother is needed in housing estates, in mixed rich/poor house groups. If we want to celebrate as a Christian body we can always find somewhere big for a special meeting but the Sunday ritual is over. The Prophets of God Our Parent said love and justice were more important than ritual sacrifices and Jesus My Brother condemned the Sabbath obsession time and again but the Church has ignored My Sister the Holy Spirit. We need to get back to real basics, not the bogus basics of moralising politicians and clerics obsessed with sex. They have taken Biblical references to whoredom literally instead of seeing that they are about idolatry. We all need to concentrate on the basics of finding faith, bringing hope and living love."

Varnish got in first by a fraction of a second: "Churches are an expression of the human aspiration to praise God; liturgy binds and uplifts; in this bewildering world where everybody is so rootless, we need our rituals to keep us anchored, to help us to survive. Churches are symbols of these basic values and it would be irresponsible of the Church to walk away from its heritage. In any case, the General Synod would never approve such a measure."

To his surprise, Aspic was in agreement: "Of course the Church is right to uphold its traditions. I don't happen to agree with Varnish about the purpose of churches. When I was at Oxford I took a great interest in the Pyramids without any inclination to believe what the ancient Egyptians believed. I am as committed to industrial revolution architecture as I am to churches and, anyway, you need not be a Christian to enjoy Mozart's Requiem."

Varnish almost beamed: "So does that mean you will fight for the Christian right to preserve our heritage with the kind of state sponsorship that the arts enjoy?"

Whether Aspic saw the trap or whether he was being benevolent with the taxpayer's money, he replied: "Yes. It's time we re-considered state funding for the Christian heritage. I know that Ministers think that the churches have an important role to play in social cohesion."

Will sighed inwardly at all this consensus and brought the show to a close. Perpetua slipped away as he offered red wine to his two smiling guests. From that day on they were firm friends and political allies.

Annie, exhausted after a terrible day, watched Fang as she picked at her wild Scottish salmon and freshly made apple and celeriac salad, all courtesy of the local farmers' market; she never bought anything in Hypo unless it was a recognised high-value brand. She knew too much about what went into Hypo food to want it to go into her. The beans crisis had only lasted a quarter of an hour but the repercussions went on much longer. A man with a whole trolley load had threatened a cashier. Hundreds of cans that had gone through the check-out were put back on the shelves without registering which meant that other customers, ignorant of the subtleties of the computer failure, took them through again. The system crashed spectacularly and then, equally spectacularly, righted itself as if nothing had happened. Corporate Centre made a huge fuss about anything it did not understand and control; and so Annie had a series of incomprehensible discussions with technicians going over the incident and a rather prickly discussion with the Head of Customer Protection who was in charge of collecting and mining customer purchasing data. The tension only subsided when, by an amazing coincidence, the store check-out and revenue records tallied with stock control. "Thank God," said Annie, without thinking.

Will went into the booth with a glass of warm white wine to review the show. To his horror, he found that the DVD recorder had not been switched on but when he desperately jabbed the play button the programme began. It was all there. "Thank God!" he said.

4

It was six in the morning when Perpetua went to Hypo as this was the time when there would be most shelf stackers but fewest customers. Whether or not she was fulfilling Hypo's diversity policy or hiring those who would be least demanding, Annie had assembled the widest assortment of people.

"Jim," Perpetua said to a Down's Syndrome boy, "take off your Hypo name badge and come and join my mission; we are going to spread good news. And you, Kylie," she said to an obese, spotty, sloppily dressed girl, "come and join me." Then she found: Dexter, an Afro-Caribbean who looked menacing even when he smiled; Jo, a pale, emaciated girl who was definitely on something; Trina, who hadn't spoken for days; and Wayne, who never stopped talking.

On the way out, as she knew she would, she met Annie coming in. "I know you will not mind," she said, "I am taking these friends. Give me today and I will come back and sort out the paperwork." Annie looked puzzled but decided not to protest: this would mean just slightly higher turnover; but nice university students were beginning to swell the ranks; Autumn was a long way off; and Perpetua might yet bring more free PR.

Perpetua led her teenagers into the nearby Paradise Mall coffee bar. She gave Dexter a £20 note and was about to slip out when he said: "How do you know I won't just walk out with this?" "I know", she said and collected a truant, a drug dealer, a joy rider and a bogus Big Issue seller to complete her team. Back in the coffee bar she said: "Our job is to get people to stop being self centred and selfish. We have to do two things: first, remember that there is the all-powerful God Our Parent who loves us; secondly, in recognition of that, we should love each other." "But none of us really believes in God", said Dexter. "I do," said Trina, "it's just all the clutter that I can't take." "Can we have Hindus and Muslims in our gang?" asked Wayne. "Yes, if they want to join," said Perpetua, "but as we are all from Christian families I doubt they will be very interested; but all are welcome. And, by the way, Wayne, this is definitely not a gang, we are an open-ended family. So, to make a start, take off your Hypo badges and all of you put on these". She handed round *god4u* badges and then said: "We are going off for a planning session". Dexter paid the bill, handed the change to Perpetua, who handed it to Andy, the bogus Big Issue seller, and they all went to Perpetua's big, untidy flat. When they arrived she put them all into the living room and said: "It would help if you did not play the music too loud. Find something positive to think about instead of all the stuff about guns, games, football, fashion, rap and rape. Get to know each other and, even more important, take some time to get to know yourselves while I talk to each of you individually to see how we all fit together".

By late afternoon Perpetua had her team. Dexter, well known bully and incipient gangster, was her deputy and the fixer. Trina, brilliant with words but frightened of using the wrong one and frightened of being laughed at for using a long one, was head of public relations. Andy, the bogus Big Issue seller, was the treasurer. Brian, the truant, who had never got on at school because the teachers were too dim, was the natural head of IT. Wayne, the big talker, was put in charge of learning and teaching resources. Jo, who really was on something, was put in charge of organising routines and timetables. Kylie, who needed exercise, was in charge of logistics and moving stuff. Heather, the drug dealer, was health, safety, regulatory affairs, licensing and all sorts of compliance. Jim, it turned out, was a brilliant flute player so he got music, worship and entertainment. That left Bob the joy rider. "We will have to make you legal before we can give you the job you really want."

Perpetua went down to the pilot community television channel and asked if she could put out a message, as part of the local TV opt-out, to all the people of Grunge Park who had been wired up to wean them away from pirate stations. "I know it is really tough living in Grunge Park," she said, "but we have just started a Christian community self-help movement and you can talk to me or any of my people who are wearing *god4u* badges. We will try to help anyone whether they are Christian, from another religion or no religion. God Our Parent wants us to love God and to love each other but we need not get worked up or confrontational about the details."

That evening, for the first time anybody could remember, there were no pirate radio broadcasts. Heather's former associates found that their disposable mobile phones stopped working. It must have been a bad batch. Nobody could explain why all the street lights were working. At the grubby youth club Perpetua and her team moved in and got things organised. Usually there was a three way split between two gangs and those caught in the middle. As usual, there was a great deal of only slightly concealed hostility but after Perpetua had been round and talked to everyone the non-combatants felt comfortable and the two sides confined their rivalry to table tennis. The Youth Club leader, a Toran called Miles, "bussed in" from Excelsior Gardens, was inclined to resent Perpetua's takeover but it was just nice to have an evening without the usual sparring. It was to his credit that he did the work of Jesus even though he hated Grunge Park and counted the days to his weekly visit with dread. "The thing is," said Perpetua, "you should see the positive in these people instead of being frightened of them. They need love not discipline." It was only later that Miles realised that he had been ticked off.

Perpetua told her followers that they would have to go home until they could find a bigger place. She went to see Annie, wearily going through a seemingly endless series of messages from Corporate Centre. "What kind of CVs did you get off those shelf stackers?" asked Perpetua. "We never bother," said Annie. "All we need are any exam passes (and there are not many of them), criminal record and child abuse checks. We have to protect our business and our customers but anything else would be a waste of time and effort. We have weekly snapshot reports on tick sheets." "So you never got to know that Jim is a brilliant flute player or that Dexter has leadership qualities? And, by the way, Trina is an English graduate but she was frightened to put that on her form in case you laughed at her and refused to give her a job. Never mind, a lot of systems are stupid and inflexible. They assume that there is only one Beethoven in a million instead of one on every street corner. It is not your fault. Here is the deal. I will take some of your shelf stackers on a rotation basis and Hypo can benefit from their talents which I identify. That way you will be helping these teenagers to get on in the world." She thought to herself, "I will have followers inside the retail giant."

As she walked home, Perpetua saw a prostitute looking for trade to feed her addiction. "I am not moralising," said Perpetua, "but this life is bad for you. I will take all your worries away. There." And the girl went home not knowing what had happened to her; but she resolved to get help from the parents she had abandoned in shame; and to help herself.

The next time Perpetua went to the youth club, things were not so easy. The dealers, whose trade was being seriously interrupted by the *god4u* people as well as an unexplained technical fault with the mobile phone system and the pirate radio stations, had dropped their prices and brought in additional runners. Addicts and near-addicts were fractious and just wanted another fix. Even the parents of "respectable" teenagers resented this new up-front religion they had heard about from Perpetua's first visit. And reflecting on it, Miles— in spite of his loathing of the place—did not want to lose this Toran outpost. After Perpetua had gone round the room talking to everybody, Jim began to play his flute, Dexter handed round Hypo jumbo coffee-to-go and Kylie handed Perpetua a radio mike. "You have all heard so many times," said Perpetua, "that things will get better. Politicians say it, church leaders say it, Hypo ads say it, drug dealers say it. Everybody says that things will get better but what they mean is it will get better for them if we do as we are told, better for political parties, church sects, supermarket or drug dealer profits. Well I am the real thing. Some of you have known me since we went to Grunge Park Primary together and what I offer is real hope. I am the genuine article." "A jumbo to-go coffee is not exactly the genuine article," somebody shouted. "No," said Perpetua "but I am not here to organise free goods and services and higher welfare payments. In spite of what we are told, more goods and money will not solve our problems. I am here to show us that if we love God Our Parent we will begin to love ourselves, to respect ourselves, to see that we can live full and rewarding lives not based round acquisition or addiction. If we do not like ourselves very much the idea of pleasing ourselves does not make very much sense." At this point Dexter said that there was a group of dealers with knives outside the door. The *god4u* people moved towards Perpetua and the rest filed out, saying to each other that she would get what was coming. It did not pay to rock the boat, and she had always been a bit of a stuck-up madam, even at Grunge Park Primary. Then the lights went out, not only in the club but also in the surrounding streets, and Dexter got all his people into the small kitchen and then forced a back door.

Next day Perpetua texted Dexter to say that her house was being staked out by a couple of local knife carriers, so they should all meet at the Paradise Mall coffee bar. Perpetua walked straight towards the two boys at the mouth of her cul de sac and told them not to be so stupid. They were not really bad and pretending was useless. They dropped their knives at her feet and asked if they could join her group. "No", she said. "Just go and tell everybody else how you have changed and what it means". They weren't very articulate but everybody in Grunge Park noticed.

5

When they had all had a coffee and Andy had paid, Perpetua and the Ten went to the far end of the municipal park and sat on the grass. "First of all," she said, "we need a period of silence to think about how we are going to work together; I will say a prayer and then we will be ready to plan." "What's a prayer?" asked Heather. "It is an admission that we are not totally independent and that we are not exclusively earthly creatures. It is a feeling or a form of words which attempts to bind us together in spirit as well as in action and to bind us to God Our Parent. So it is an individual commitment but it often works inside a corporate framework which recognises that the purpose of institutions like churches is to channel people into a constructive relationship with God. I know that is difficult but the Catch 22 of prayer is that the only way we can grasp what it is is to pray about it".

For the first time in their lives they sat and said nothing for ten minutes and some of them even tried to look into themselves. Jo was having a particular problem as she had not had a fix since early yesterday. She had often told herself she was not really an addict but now she wondered. Wayne also had a serious problem just saying nothing but Dexter, who was never very cerebral, spent the time looking at the others to see that they were concentrating. Then Perpetua said:

"God Our Parent who is everywhere,

in the universe and in us all,

we give ourselves to You as we are Yours;

may we have faith to be worthy of You, Jesus My Brother and My Sister the Spirit

As we hope to be worthy of Your everlasting company.

Help us to love and not to judge.

"I know that is a lot to take in," she said, "but Brian will put it on our home page and will text it into our phones so we can call it up every day." "Are we supposed to pray every day?" asked Bob. "At least once every day, to recognise God Our Parent, to own up to our shortcomings, to give thanks for what is good. It is like training; sometimes it is enjoyable, sometimes not, but we have to do it regularly or we will not be spiritually fit when the crisis comes. I think that is enough difficult ideas for one day. Now, to planning. We need to do two things: first, we must get a bus so that we can move around the country with all our gear; secondly, we should think about a major launch event."

While he was waiting for his driving test Bob trawled the internet for second-hand buses, chose what he wanted and asked Heather to sort out the registration. Then Kylie sourced all the stuff that would need to go into it and when Brian had set up a wireless connection he disappeared for two days to build the *god4u* web site. Meanwhile Trina contacted Will and asked if he could help with the launch event. He thought not but Trina rather pointedly reminded him of his daytime viewing figures which were even worse in high Summer than when CEC was up against Premiership football. Dexter wanted a spectacular with a rap outfit and a load of special effects but Trina said even if they could afford it this was not the way to go. Everything had to be positive and non-threatening, encouraging not bombastic. Dexter complained to Perpetua and she said that the key to the success of the launch would be Jim; she did not want it to be crude or too clever. "Just simple music and a simple message" she said. Heather thought she would have problems with the web casting and DVD rights but CEC was not that particular as long as it kept the linear repeat rights and the options to sell on to news outfits. Jim practised and Jo dreamed of a major tour.

One of the big points of contention was the choreography. Dexter, Trina and Andy wanted Perpetua to launch *god4u* from a platform with an invited audience while the others thought it would be better if Perpetua had a roving mike which would enable her to walk amongst the crowd as she was talking. Brian said that the best thing would be for Perpetua to walk among the crowd but to have her projected onto a big screen so that everybody could see her while she was among them. Trina tried all the major media outlets and the religious press but all she got back was the hope of a feature from the Toxic Times and a commentary from the Petran Stylus which said it was doing a series of "think pieces" on something called "Fresh Expressions of Church".

After the problems with the national media, Jo and Trina thought that going straight into a launch might not be very successful, so they fixed a number of small warm-up events. Perpetua went to a nursing home and got everybody dancing. She went to a special needs school and talked about integration. She organised a meeting with "problem teenagers" and they all smiled and offered to help themselves and each other. She met local traders who offered Summer discounts to pensioners. But the highlight was a late night visit to an Accident and Emergency Department where she gave all arrivals a blessing whereupon they turned round and went home apparently fully fit. Volunteers from local community television stations broadcast and archived these and Trina put together a show reel as a preview to the major event. There were twitches from some national media contacts but each individual incident was put down to local conditions. The connections were not made and the story did not come together but at least there was some good footage for the launch and some local people were organising *god4u* meetings. Dexter told them to follow Perpetua's original strategy and target shelf stackers at Hypo.

It only remained to choose a venue and Perpetua said it should be Excelsior Gardens, an estate of detached houses ringing the Excelsior Golf Club. As a child she had been told that this was the ultimate place, a kind of heaven on earth for those who lived in Grunge Park. Dexter, Andy and Trina had somehow secured the use of the broad lawn between the club house and the 18th Green, overlooked by the hospitality boxes and dominated by a huge display screen. The *god4u* team had brought in a couple of hundred middle class spectators with the promise of a television appearance and CEC sent its combined news and sports team on the basis of the Excelsior's proffered hospitality from which they were pointedly excluded during major tournaments in favour of the BBC and other leading channels.

The link man welcomed everybody and introduced the show reel highlights. These went down very well and for some outlets, once they had been seen in sequence, they were the only point of the event. Trina began to get calls asking for clips of what people called "Miracles". The link man said we were all in for a phenomenal show which would help to define the culture of the age. Most Christian leaders hid in their pulpits and in theological complexities and obscurities but Perpetua was prepared to come out to the people and launch a new kind of Christian message.

So new it was hardly recognisable as Christian.

6

Perpetua said: "We are worthy of God Our Parent and creation on earth and will be worthy to be with God if we: recognise dependency on God and each other; see God in everyone; respect and do not exploit God's creation; celebrate difference; imagine the impact before talking and acting; love and do not judge; put compassion before logic; cry in public; find common ground; stand up for principles firmly but gently; give more than we can afford and take what we are offered; never turn our back—never!

"These are the kind of public principles which we hear about every day but do not observe. These are principles for other people. We always find reasons for not doing what we must do today; it is always tomorrow; it is always the responsibility of someone else. Why are 'They' not doing something about the poor, the environment, the exploitation of women, racial abuse, drug addiction, greed, dog mess, parking, packaging, protest marches, beggars, graffiti, estate agents, trendy vicars, tatoos, cruising, illegal immigrants, violence, obesity, chemical beer, tabloid newspapers, short hair, long hair, short skirts, long skirts, tight jeans, baggy jeans? We always seem to want somebody else to do something about anything we happen not to like.

"Well, if we really care about something badly enough we should do something; but we should tolerate and even try to celebrate most of what we do not like because society is built on tolerance of difference. Without it, society will disintegrate. If we cannot tolerate then we cannot respect; and if we cannot respect we cannot trust; and if we cannot trust society is finished.

"Every winter we condemn the commercialisation of the birth of Jesus My Brother but we spend more and more every year; the louder we complain about materialism the greater our self indulgence. We say that the gifts are to celebrate the birth of My Brother but they are a form of social competition; even our generosity in providing goods for the poor in developing countries can be a form of showing off; goodness of this kind is dangerous. We should give some time to the poor nearby as well as sending chickens to Africa; and, most of all, we should not condemn our children to lives of greed by raising and meeting their expectations in their first few celebrations of My Brother's birth. Forget Father Christmas and remember the Child of Christmas.

"We have built society on competition because, we say, it is natural. What makes us think, even if it is proper to behave on the basis of our individual preferences and on the basis of personal advantage, that we will gain? When we say it is natural to be selfish, is this just a convenient theory to support our selfishness? In any case, there would be no roads without collaboration and then what good would there be in big, shiny cars. The real problem with collaboration which is, rather than private property, central to God's will, is that it usually benefits the rich who resent it and puts burdens on the poor who submit to it.

"As competition in the world becomes more fierce we all become more stressed and think that consuming more goods and services will handle the stress. They do not. They just suppress the inner turmoil. We are not basically bad at all but we escape from our better selves, we hide ourselves from the truth with holidays, cars, clothes, houses, drugs, booze, contrived lust, hypochondria, pointless games," (frown from Trina) "Soap opera, opera, sport, curtains, carpets, drills, dolls, toy meals on big plates. We talk about very little else. Our entertainment glitters with 'beautiful people' and things; but have we ever wondered who pays the price for our beauty and things? For all the documentary television we watch, have we ever really seen a gold mine or a sweat shop? Do we really think that it is good enough for Hypo to sign up to a vague ethical policy? Does this free us from all responsibility? Nearer to home, have we ever imagined how cleaners, hospital porters or waiters survive? Have we ever found out whether our restaurant tips go to the waiters and those who wash up or whether they are just pocketed by the management?

"What do we think we are really worth? How do we compare the stress of a management life at £200,000 a year with our office cleaner's life at £9,000 per year? When we say that we are paid for expertise and for responsibility, how do we know how this compares with others on lower pay? It is not so much the behaviour that is wicked (though it is bad enough), but our refusal to be honest with ourselves and see the consequences for others of the lives we lead, all the time telling ourselves and each other what hard lives we lead. The wealth and exploitation are bad enough; the lies are worse; the indifference is worst of all. Yet if I say that we must care and never be indifferent, I do not mean that we should judge other people; what do we know about causality and motivation? We pretend that we know why people kill, why people are addicted, why people abandon their spouses, why people don't like us, why society breaks down; and worse, we think we know why individual people do desperate things. But we do not know. In a world more crammed with information than it ever has been, in a world with more graduates than there ever have been but, most of all, in a world where almost everybody has access to the teaching of Jesus My Brother, we spend our time reading and thinking about trivia which persuades us how difficult it is for us to be good and how easy it is for everybody else to be evil. We frame our certificates and read rubbish, we talk of community and make divisions between ourselves and the more deprived, we take the moral high ground and abandon those less fortunate than ourselves to the low ground. When we say that people are immoral what we are mostly saying is that they are different; their weaknesses are simply different from our weaknesses, their strengths different from our strengths. And every time we attack difference and every time we rank uniformity over difference we damage our society. If God Our Parent had wanted us to be all the same we can be sure that that is how we would have been created.

"On this basis, of our deliberately distorted understanding of the world, we presume to judge when only our creator can judge. Only God knows what is in the hearts of people; only God knows about the complexity of motive; only God knows about the minutiae of causation. We were put on this earth by God to love and not to judge; to love of our own free will not because we are forced by convention or pressure. This would all be bad enough if I were standing next to Jesus My Brother when he said similar things two thousand years ago: but we know about the Incarnation; we know about the Crucifixion; we know about the Resurrection; and we are no better. If anything, given what we could know and could do, we are worse. I know Jesus talked about how difficult it was for the rich to be with God but that was supposed to be a warning and an encouragement not an excuse to stay away.

"So what have we learned from Jesus My Brother? Have we learned anything about humble birth, about good news for the poor, about sacrifice, about the triumph of good over evil? Do we suppose that the main point of the life of Jesus was to be the founder of churches which are now at loggerheads with each other? Do we suppose it really matters whether there is such a thing as the Holy Trinity?"

At this point she got a sharp, warning look from Trina who mouthed: "Stay concrete; stay off theology."

Perpetua went on: "I know this is a lot to take in but above all I want us to remember that principles are not abstract things that we can choose to pick up or put down; and they are not something for other people to adopt. We do not choose principles the way we choose a car; and we should not believe that because we have a very big car we are exempt from principles. As God's creatures, created to love God and each other, when we do not do this we are moving away from our natural state, the thing we were created for, and that is why we are so stressed and why we try to escape. Do we really think that God would expect us to do anything for which we have not been given resources? It is time to stop running away from ourselves and God; it is time to come home to God and to ourselves".

What they went home to was private but, without buckets or bowls being rattled, they left thousands of pounds with Andy.

7

Press coverage of the Excelsior event would have been non-existent had it not been for a picture of Perpetua surrounded by her inner circle. "That," said Sneer, the News Editor of the Toxic Times, "is a classic piece of political correctness that should make us a good story. All that girl needs is a blind Indian and a Chink cripple to score a full house. We'll run that!" But there was an immediate objection, not to Sneer's language nor even to his news proposal, but to the underlying strategy. "Look," said Prussic, the Deputy Editor, "we're currently running a campaign against Archbishop Hawthorne of Canterbury and covering the accusation that we're racist by using Archbishop Mwanga of York as our battering ram. Put this girl's 'refreshing approach' to Christianity alongside Mwanga tomorrow morning as a way of bashing Hawthorne and then we'll have a whole day to work out an angle of attack against politically correct, opportunist Perpetua and her rabble." "But," said Dowte, a new recruit from Oxford, "that would be inconsistent". "Don't be stupid!" shouted Sneer. "That's the kind of crap you get at university but it doesn't hold in real life. We are always attacking politicians for being inconsistent but we couldn't sell papers if *we* weren't. We make people discontented and then suggest solutions; we lengthen and shorten hospital waiting lists; we support and then attack people; we condemn the 'nanny state' and 'post code lotteries' on alternate days; we want everything to be perfectly controlled from the centre and locally controlled at the same time. And nobody knows more than us about the power of genuine and bogus medical research for making people alternately desperate and euphoric. It's good for circulation because our kind of people only feel really involved in society when they're grumbling about it or superior to it. Either people spot our cynicism and they don't mind or, more likely, they don't spot it. Our only two consistent, over-riding principles are hating lefties and making people unhappy".

Trina was shocked when the TT arrived next morning. Perpetua had gone missing straight after yesterday's event, saying something about the need to pray alone. It was a classic Sneer two-birds-with-one-stone story. The page 5 headline screamed:

NEW BLOW FOR TIMID PRIMATE

In a blistering attack on the Archbishop of Canterbury yesterday, new broom Perpetua said that the conventional church had failed to turn back the tide of greed and materialism. Speaking at an upbeat *god4u* launch event at the exclusive Excelsior Golf Club, the firebrand leader said that the church should return to its traditional values instead of espousing trendy, politically correct causes. In a carefully worded attack on the Church of England establishment and particularly its beleaguered leader, Archbishop Hawthorne, she said he is increasingly seen as part of the problem not the solution for a church in crisis.

Dowte looked at the story and went to Perpetua's full text on the internet, winced, and then reported for his short course on fiddling expenses.

When Perpetua got back to the bus she winced too. "Look Trina, it is not your fault. These people have lied about what I said and there is therefore every reason to believe they will go on lying. We have to remember that there is nothing we can do about this. They exist for the sole purpose of destroying idealism and encouraging discontent and greed." Perpetua was right in particular as well as in general. Stirred by the chance of being famous, Miles rang the TT to describe the last meeting at the youth club. If he had reached Dowte nothing might have come of it but Sneer happened to be walking past the News Desk phone when Miles was put through. Being an experienced photographic analyst who knew what he wanted, Sneer got straight to the point: "You are a Toran, right? Have you noticed that Wayne is a queer? Have you further noticed that Jo is on something? Much worse though, we've been digging around and we've found that Perpetua's a credulous fool: Dexter's got a criminal record for assault; Beth is a known drug dealer; and we haven't been able to track down Andy yet but we soon will." Overhearing this litany, Dowte muttered that it was the job of Christians to work with and save sinners but Sneer and Miles were against him. Gangs of perverts and crooks masquerading as Christians could not be tolerated. Sneer received a call of apparently mild protest from Smoother at Church House who said that Hawthorne was in good spirits and nobody minded a bit of knockabout; but he hit a raw nerve when he implied that the TT was a tabloid and another when he said the PM's Appointments Secretary was not inclined to reward those who attacked the Church to which Her Majesty was so devoted. Meanwhile, Miles went up the Toran ladder to its most hard-line Suffragan Bishop and the story was nicely tied up before the afternoon conference to sort out the pages: "I propose," said Sneer, pleased with another "two birds" effort, "that we run with 'Thugs Pose as PC God Squad'. This gives us two stories. We can depict these people as thugs but we can also attack the PC selection which makes it twice as good."

The story ran:

> In a move of breathtaking audacity, firebrand Perpetua, in a plot to sideline traditional Christianity, has recruited a gang of thugs and perverts to travel the country de-stabilising homely parish congregations.

In a stark warning, the influential Toran Bishop of Castlegate, said: "Careless liberalism has allowed all kinds of undesirable elements to get a foothold inside the church but the Perpetua threat is much more dangerous because her gang are posing as Torans."

A highly respected Grunge Park Christian youth organiser added: "As soon as the gang arrived I knew there was something nasty about them. They just took over our club and I was worried that they would try to recruit gays or sell drugs under cover of being Christian."

A Church House spokesman said: "We are grateful for the TT's courage in uncovering this threat to down-to-earth, mainstream Christian witness."

Perpetua's chief fixer, Dexter, who has a criminal record, threatened the TT with retaliation if it went on investigating the gang. In a move seen by influential observers as a cowardly climbdown, Perpetua has gone into hiding.

It was the worst day of Trina's life. She felt she had let Perpetua down and been naive. Dexter was indeed threatening to find Sneer's car and slash its tyres but he had not been approached by a reporter. The others were edgy and miserable. Perpetua texted Kylie and she got them all into the bus, told Brian to switch off the wireless connections and told Bob to drive to a deserted spot where they could keep some silence, pray together and then talk constructively. *god4u* was going to get nothing from the media; it needed God.

8

"It is going to be like this all the time", said Perpetua. "For most people, particularly those who do not think much about it, Christianity is not about communication with God Our Parent at all; instead it is about the exercise of social control; and for some people who think about it a great deal, it is about exercising a very narrow kind of social control focused on sexual behaviour. What people like the TT regret is not the decline in worship of God Our Parent, they regret the inability of Vicars to enforce uniformity. The sadness is that Torans and Petrans both want to enforce goodness through force, through law and rules, when their task and ours is to persuade people through our love that they should choose to love of their own free will. When two people behave well, one under threat, the other voluntarily, the outcome looks the same but that is only the human outcome. The spiritual outcome is radically different. Torans and Petrans are not bringing people into God's fold, they are whipping them in and guarding the doors, making Christianity into a prison. It is quite obvious from what Jesus My Brother said that the most important attribute of Christianity is love; love regardless of behaviour, background or outlook. Look at us; most of us got into trouble or became depressed because of a lack of love. The modern individualist approach describes this problem as a lack of 'self esteem' but this is secondary. How can we esteem ourselves if nobody loves us? Our purpose as God's children is to be so clean in ourselves that the love of God can pass through us to shine on other people. The pure light of grace, refracted through human material, breaks into the diverse colours of human virtue and kindness.

"We have got very muddled, too, about churches. They exist as frameworks for the collective celebration and mutual support of individual believers. A church does not believe anything; individuals believe but faith can only survive in a difficult world if we all help each other.

"Now I want to talk about God Our Parent, Jesus My Brother and this world so that we can think and pray during August to prepare for our work.

"There was a great entrepreneur, the Great Founder, who gave all that he had to a mighty foundation but the trustees forgot the original aims of the foundation and squandered the money, took the Founder's picture off the wall and put up pictures of themselves. Much worse, they re-wrote the Founder's mission statement so that only their own kind could benefit from the Foundation. So the Founder's son, a man of immense vision, re-constituted the Foundation and made its benefits open to the whole world. Again the Trustees began to re-write the mission statement, narrowing those qualified to benefit. 2,000 years on, I am the one appointed by the Founder and Jesus My Brother to remind the world that what it was given was a foundation of love not of rule, a foundation of hope not of fear, a foundation of trust not of judgment, a foundation of generosity not of contracts.

"When Jesus My Brother preached the Word of God at least he was only speaking to worshippers who had gone astray. Today most of the people who need our love have been shut out of the Foundation for so long that simply reforming it from inside is not enough. What we will hear is that it is the fault of those who are outside that they are excluded. But there should not be an outside and an inside. It is like this: ancient builders were fascinated by enclosing space to protect them from the heat and cold, so they developed architecture to create ever bigger buildings. When Jesus visited the earth he talked about points of love that would radiate outwards from people to people. But His followers went back to architecture, mental as well as physical, and they built brick walls and stone walls and book walls and jargon walls and rule walls; and they presumed to divide the good from the bad, and those who were thought bad stayed away, and in every generation more people were defined as bad, so the good dwindled in number inside their big, empty buildings, inside their walls of brick, stone, books, jargon and rules.

"I have come to help us once again to turn worshippers into points of light to radiate the love of God; we are moving, networked points. We do not need the safety of walls of any kind; if we love God and leave ourselves open to the light of Our Sister The Spirit, we will not need to be defensive and protective. We will have the confidence to take the good news of God to all people and not mind if some of them are not the kind of people we like. The less we like them, the more we need to love them.

"As for us, we who have been at odds with society, we who have suffered and, yes, sinned, we know better than most people what it is to be rejected and it is our special mission to speak to the rejected. It is so difficult to preach love to the rich and powerful but the poor will respond. Remember what it was like when we felt a hint of love.

"The way to look at it is this: there was a group of people who enjoyed every earthly thing, and now and again they would organise a welfare camp for the poor. They would build a temporary settlement outside town in summer or commandeer a massive warehouse in winter. They would pay people to bring in all kinds of food, clowns, chiropodists, sleeping bags, benefits analysts, second hand clothes, drama instructors, first aid kits, counsellors, books, preachers, toiletry packs, dentists and fancy hats; and the poor were brought in and given all these things but the benefactors never turned up. So the poor always went away sad and turned to their old ways. One day, a lady who had once been very poor but had won the lottery became a member of the welfare committee; and when the camp took place she went down there and cooked in a fancy hat and sang along with the choruses and handed out small bits of money and took notes on little things that might be done. And next year she went back with a few like minded friends; and as the years went by, the number of her friends grew and the number of people needing to come to the welfare camp fell.

"We are not to discount the rich; we must never go on appearances and we should never make generalisations. Work with anybody who is prepared to share our values; but concentrate on those who need love most; and concentrate on those who find it most difficult to understand what love is. If they sneer at us we must not give up. We might need to bring a colleague to help or see if another member of our family is more effective. We are not the same and must not be jealous of the talents of others. The benefit of such great diversity amongst all children is that it gives God Our Parent so many different ways of projecting love to creation."

All through August Perpetua taught the *god4u* family with times of intense discussion, times of prayer and of worship. The family grew in faith but Perpetua constantly reminded it of how fragile that faith would be under attack. As the end of the month approached she sent workers all over the country and kept the Ten for a final retreat. The Spirit was on the move.

9

Annie Price returned from her holiday at the Club Copulata ready for the long run-up to the Festive Season. An automated analysis of October/December sales for the previous three years at Corporate Centre had established forthcoming stock requirements and in June she had indented for some local needs, largely to cater for the Afro-Caribbean community. The corporate decor palettes had arrived together with the festive music pack. The floor-space reallocation drawings and timetable were almost complete and so, after a somewhat routine briefing with her senior staff, it was cascade time. Almost immediately, however, there was a problem. The warehouse staff, scanning the list of special products, lodged a list of objections: there were no Christian Christmas cards; the Advent Calendars were full of chocolate and robins but no Scripture quotes and drawings; the Advent and Christmas wreaths were full of holly and mistletoe but had no candles; the Christmas tree decorations were all baubles and candy but no little sheep or kings; the Christmas books were all secular, and the Christmas music contained no carols. Word was passed to the shelf stackers, five of whom, unknown to Annie, had just returned from Perpetua's August getaway. They came together for mutual support to Annie's office. They did not mind the secular Christmas—after all, the Christians had nicked it from the Pagans so the Pagans nicking it back was fair enough—and they would happily stack shelves with Father Christmases, reindeer, mince pies, tree lights, trifle sponges, Christmas ale, Bing Crosby re-treads, chestnuts, tinsel, crackers, garish coloured plastic trees, snowmen, fairies, brandy butter, champagne, turkeys, Christmas pudding, silly socks, port, Morecambe & Wise DVDs, Stilton in jars and any number of naff presents and they would not mind doing some of it to Winter Wonderland, Jingle Bells, White Christmas and even Rudolf the Red-Nosed Reindeer, as long as there were some Christian goods, the playing of Christmas carols and specific recognition of Christmas in the special store decor plan. They would find a team of volunteers to build a massive crib near the trolley stand and would put up a couple of smaller cribs inside.

Annie played for time; she would consider what they had to say. What she actually did was to read the Corporate Centre Manual section on special events and festivals and check the files of the five protesters. The Manual was simple enough:

> We live in a multi-cultural society where it is important not
> to offend significant customer groups; Christian festivals such as
> Christmas and Easter might give offence to Muslims, Hindus, Jews
> and atheists; but Muslim festivals like Eid, Hindu festivals like Di-

vali, Jewish Festivals like Hanukah and atheist festivals like Remembrance Day are not likely to give equal offence to Christians.

Annie did some quick mental calculations about the relative economic
value of cribs, firecrackers, 7-branched candlesticks, crescents, ornate daggers,
Crucifixes, prayer mats, Stars of David, turbans, Halal meat, kosher meat, turkeys, Buddhas, Ganeshes, Patkas, prayer beads and hot cross buns and decided
that, on balance, whatever the religious sensitivities, Corporate Centre was
mad. She then turned to the files and found, on the basis of weekly snapshot
reports, that all five had progressed since Perpetua had proposed her rotation.
Perpetua! Of course! The shelf stacker rotation.

Next morning Annie said that she would convene the Hypo Community
Forum but they had already thought of that. It contained a Rabbi, a Mullah,
a Guru, a Sikh priest, a policeman, a member of the local Amenity Society, a
representative from the Social Action Directorate, two District Councillors
and, of course, an enforcer from the Directorate of Health and Safety and two
community representatives (marked "obstructive busybodies" in the confidential notes) but no specifically Christian representative. They would just have to
overcome the anomaly that store people should not be on the Forum; two of
them would represent the Christians until Annie could find a Vicar; and Annie,
on the spur of the moment, asked Perpetua.

By the time the meeting came round it was hardly necessary. All the religious representatives said they supported the store's celebration of Christmas along with their own festivals. The Manual was rubbish. How did ignorant
atheists know what upset religious people? What upset religious people was
ignorant atheists. However, what made the meeting totally redundant was the
surge of support for the "Put Christ Into Christmas" campaign organised by
the shelf stackers throughout the Hypo chain. Picking up from Perpetua's first
broadcast, and work in the early part of the August retreat, Perpetua's people
had formed missionary cells each with a mixture of rich and poor people. The
rich did the talking and threatened boycotts; the poor did the shouting and
threatened sit-ins. god4u shelf stackers had become strong in nineteen stores
so far and the curve was getting steeper, and even though they were in a tiny
minority of stores the risk of a shelf-stacking crisis in December was unthinkable, given the competition. If they fired the current stackers the new intake
might be even more militant. The only consolation was that spies in Lakshmo
and Jambo reported similar trends.

Dowte came on the phone. Was it true that Hypo had changed corporate
policy on the Festive Season? Annie would get back to him. Corporate Centre
was, as usual, completely tied up in its own complexity, trying to work out
whether the policy change would be of net benefit after the emergency de-

signing and despatching of new decor packs and last-minute Christian stock. In the end it put out a simple statement which most of the press, even the TT, in love with retail and its advertising revenue, glossed more or less sedulously verbatim:

HYPO FRONTS RETRO XMAS DRIVE

> In a move to gain competitive edge in the cut-throat grocery world, Hypo is heading back to the Crib. Blessed by other religious leaders, the move was greeted by an upbeat Archbishop Hawthorne who thought this might be the turning of the tide. Observers say Lakshmo and Jambo are bound to follow.
>
> The *god4u* campaign to "Put Christ Into Christmas" has been a startling tactical success but there are worries it will lead to further demands from religious militants.

Trina felt almost pleased but that was not quite the end of the story. Sneer, caught between attacking Hawthorne or Perpetua, worked out another "two birds" story and typed the following into the news pool:

THUGS BLACKMAIL FOR CRIB

Archbishop Hawthorne was duped by Perpetua's gang of thugs into welcoming Hypo's change of policy on Christmas. This was forced on management by *god4u* infiltrators who blackmailed the store chain into a policy change which observers say will cost shareholders millions and result in price rises for hard-pressed customers.

The story went through the usual sub-editing process and was assigned to Page Seven. Nobody noticed until the late night re-write for the Final Edition that something very strange had happened to the story in the early editions:

KIDS GOODWILL FOR CRIB

> Archbishop Hawthorne was buoyed by Perpetua's *god4u* family, welcoming Hypo's change of policy on Christmas. This was approved by management who respected staff and community feeling. Observers say this should produce extra growth of 1%.

Sneer was speechless and immediately suspected Dowte. Trina and Smoother were puzzled. Perpetua was silent.

10

Jo and Kylie were putting together the final details of the September tour. Jim was composing some new music for the worship DVD/CD and Trina was having her usual trouble with Perpetua. "It does not matter what we say, it will be twisted. At least if we stick to worship nobody can touch us." "But you said you could open the eyes of the most hardened unbelievers, didn't you? Well, it's about time you did something." "I am not ready." "If you don't do something to capitalise on the Hypo success we will be out of business. We need something like the events on the show reel tour but more spectacular." "But I am not ready yet."

Perpetua relented. The tour began with the same kind of venues as the show reel tour but everything was escalated: old people in a home started looking after the staff; special needs children paired with 'normal' peers to help them with homework; teenagers volunteered for community service while waiting for job placements; and in a spectacular move from which the media were barred (to Trina's great regret), Perpetua emptied a complete long-term stay ward. Within five minutes all the patients were gone, Perpetua was on the road and officials were left with a problem. This was solved when they interrogated the computer records of those who had left: details of procedures, improvement and discharge were all complete; targets had been exceeded and the beds stood ready for some early new admissions. The PR angle was promising but puzzling. Hospital CEO Mrs Ali Falling decided to keep a low profile. If the year-end targets were met nobody would want details of a ward with a 100% turnaround in a day.

Trina's annoyance was modified by the steadily rising profile of Perpetua on those occasions when she allowed media coverage of her activities. The open-air worship sessions had started out as rather pathetic, with a few people coming along out of curiosity, mainly to listen to Jim's music which he had been working on with Brian; but word got round and people left feeling much better than when they arrived. There was new hope among the deprived. Drug dealers, first restive at the fall-off in trade, were giving it up; prostitutes, first fretting over the reduction in the number of their clients, were finding that they could afford to give up once their dependence disappeared. The numbers grew. There was nothing sensational happening and the changed expressions as people left did not tell the story well enough for television; but the tide of anecdotal material was huge, in blogs and free newspapers, on community radio and local television. The established media were still cautious but the word was getting out in more than 200 languages to a global audience.

Inevitably the worship gatherings attracted the attention of the Health and Safety Directorate which called Heather in for a compulsory "friendly chat". Community medical workers became restive as their charges brought back unwanted medicines. The drug rehabilitation unit worried that it would have to be shut when it had taken years to get it established. People felt disoriented without the normal accompaniment of danger, distress and down-at-heelness. Having nothing to grumble about brought its own stresses.

At the worship, Perpetua's message was always the same. Human beings are God's creatures, made so that we can choose to love God. Because we are creatures we are not self-sufficient. We know we have to look outside ourselves for completeness and some of that happens with family, friends and loved ones but even then we feel there is a gap. There is no point trying to fill it with alcohol, drugs, cars, holidays, casual sex and so on because we know deep in our hearts that these are like ramming Polyfilla into a gaping hole. Her Sister the Spirit was trying to find all of God's children but it had to be two-way; we all had to try to find God Our Parent not so that we could have treacle poured all over us; we were not babies who needed that kind of parenting. God will help us to make ourselves whole.

The problem with churches, said Perpetua, is that they are not committed to giving people the means to love God, they want to hold on to the means so that we have to use the church as an agent. The Christian church is not a supplier; it should be a channel through which all are members of the One God; as long as people exclude themselves from the church or are excluded from it, it is flawed, incomplete. How would we feel if there was a local celebration and some of us felt intimidated and did not dare to go into the hall and others were kept out by the committee? Yes, we know how we would feel because it has happened to us and the celebration committee is the church. This angered the Torans and the Petrans equally, the Torans because they did not believe in individual self-determination and the Petrans because they did not believe in letting everybody in. In spite of their supposed differences since the Reformation, the Torans and the Petrans were very similar. Miles and Father O'Helly had enjoyed the stiffest of ecumenical relations (nobody in Grunge Park could work out whether Father Bill was Anglican or Catholic) but, had they thought about it instead of clinging to historical cliches, they would have found much mutual comfort. As it was, Perpetua's final worship of the tour, back in Grunge Park, brought them together in mutual anger and recognition. The institutional church was being undermined and all Christians, whatever their differences, needed to stand together. Miles told O'Helly about the history of the *god4u* gang as far as he had heard it from Sneer, and O'Helly, who did not need much artifice to conceal his homosexuality from Miles, advised a joint assault. The TT, though instinctively anti-Catholic in a tradition going back to the Spanish Armada and reinforced by the huge wave of mid 19th Century Irish immigration, would be prepared to overlook the point if the target was good enough. It was. The target was Wayne.

But somehow Sneer's plans got into Dowte's computer and somehow he found himself texting Trina.

Perpetua agreed with the rapidly maturing Trina that whatever she said would make no difference to the campaign against Wayne but there could be no delay. There was a serious internal reason; Dexter was heavily anti-gay and had been put through an intensive period of prayer and learning by Perpetua to get him sorted out. If there were problems within the family it was easy to see what tensions there were in the wider world.

The event was much easier to organise than any other kind of religious occasion because the central point was sex. Perpetua had already made major statements on justice, ecology, crime and consumerism but the big one had been missing. CEC was happy to broadcast a late night show. *Scanties*, the most notorious Grunge Park night spot, was reluctant to help as nobody would pay the full entrance and then be forced to listen to a speech; but the combination of a grant from Andy, free entrance, and the chance to be on television guaranteed co-operation and a full house. The club would also get favourable coverage and Hypo had agreed to sponsor the drink and some food.

For the press, the opportunity to take pictures of Perpetua surrounded by almost naked teenagers was too good to miss, a point which did not escape Miles and Father O'Helly.

11

Perpetua said: "Since I began my Mission on behalf of God Our Parent, Jesus My Brother and My Sister The Spirit, I have tried to talk about the really important issues such as the need to recognise the purpose of God as our loving parent and the purpose of humanity as creatures made in love to love God and each other freely. Because of that, I have talked about the importance of social justice, of good news for the poor, of love of creation, of love of those who repent. Only in understanding—not just intellectually but in our hearts—that we were created in love to love, can we recognise our purpose. This is the only way we will find any true peace.

For a start, we must commit ourselves to seeing God in everyone. It is not for us to say that God loves this person but not that person; that God has stayed with this person but abandoned that person. Whatever we do, God loves all of us; and, in reflecting that, as creatures of God, we should love everyone. And the more difficult we find it to love certain kinds of people, the more we must try. In a society where people are so obsessed with choice, we cannot pick and choose who we love, who is our neighbour. The more difficult it is, the harder we must try.

"Our world is so obsessed with sex that I cannot avoid dealing with it specifically; but I can only do that inside this framework about love. If we do not understand the basics of God and humanity, the rules we make about sex are empty.

"One more piece of framework has to be put in place before I can begin. Christians who say they know what God wants can be right in general terms. They can say, as I have said, that God loves us and wants us freely to love God. That is clear enough. But when Christians say they know how God works, they are wrong. All this theology that we have put together in 2,000 years is approximate, it is no more than guess work, it is elaborate, striving and sometimes beautiful metaphor and, the attribute we forget the most, it is provisional. I have seen people in church solemnly saying the Creed and not understanding a word of it; and there is no reason why they should. It might have made sense to forth and fifth century Greeks but it makes no sense to us now. When people say they know what God is or what God wants in detail they are wrong; and being more definite in what they say certainly does not make what they say any more definite.

"So when Christians say they know how we are to behave in order to love God and each other they are profoundly wrong. What matters is the basic motivation of a person in thought and action and the nature of that motivation is known fully only to God; quite often it is not even known very clearly to the person. People who presume to judge according to outcomes—end products—are totally out of order. Christians who keep on telling us they know what the Bible tells us about this and about that, down to the last detail, seem not to have noticed that Jesus My Brother told them not to judge other people; and the same Christians who seem to love St. Paul more than My Brother ignore him when he wrote that people have different gifts and what really matters is that the Christian Church should find room for everyone.

"Finally, just to get one more piece of introduction off my chest, Jesus said that it was the purpose of His Disciples and their successors to serve; I cannot say that I see all that much service in this relentless judgment."

Miles felt comfortable. To his credit, Father O'Helly shuffled slightly. In contrast to the audience which was utterly attentive, Will fidgeted nervously, wondering how he had ever agreed to the broadcast. Annie, helping with the drinks, wondered when Perpetua would get serious.

"So, to begin at the beginning. God created the world but no human knows how or when. God's Chosen People, the Jews, told two different stories to help them focus on God as Creator and as Our Parent. In the first, women and men were created at the same time, in the second woman was born of man. Not surprisingly, after the age of matriarchy when agriculture and warfare put men into earthly power, they settled on the second story. How can anyone think that God created women inferior to men? Where did they get this weird idea of 'male headship' from? Well, it fitted in with society about 1000 years before the birth of Jesus My Brother and it was still pretty widespread when St. Paul was writing; but there are pronouncements on major issues in the Bible which we have properly accepted as redundant such as slavery, treating women as property, genocide, infanticide, capital punishment through communal stoning, so why this, now? The answer is all about power: the power to rule; the power to judge; the power to exclude; the power to self glorify.

"The idea that certain jobs are reserved for women or men is outdated. Women and men in general might bring different kinds of gifts to a task but different women and different men bring different gifts. Surely we are too mature to generalise, to say that just because one sex generates eggs and the other fertilises them, this has massive consequences for what people do outside child generation.

"There may come a time—it is quite possible, given the advances in medical science—when the world will only need a couple of men for every 100 women; at that time the idea of 'Male Headship' will be absurd. But we cannot make sensible social rules for then right now. What we must do in the light of what we know about God's will is to make rules for a fair society and at the moment that means equality between the sexes. In the meantime, clergy would do well to learn some biology instead of sounding off from a knowledge vacuum about sexuality. God Our Parent gave us brains so that we could intelligently respond to The Word; if he had wanted a domineering, brute force response he would not have bothered with brains."

Father O'Helly shuffled uncomfortably and tried to catch Miles' eye but he was looking the other way. He had been deeply shaken by what Perpetua said but whether it was anger or revelation he could not work out. Part of him wanted to push through the crowd for fresh air but part of him was totally held. Will saw some hope. Annie served drinks during a short break, watching Hypo ads for silk thongs, viagra, singles holidays, phallic cars, dating services and oblivion.

12

During the interval Perpetua walked round the room explaining quietly to small groups of teenagers why enjoyment was only one part of life, that love was much more important; and how she had been sent, as God's Sacred Vessel, a sacred space, to give people room to love.

"Now let us focus more closely on human relationships. Their central purpose is love. At root, what matters when we form relationships with people is that we love them more than we love ourselves; the idea of a relationship is not that we create room for us to expand our sphere of operations, our ego, our libido, but that we create the means by which the beloved has more room to grow. Making room for ourselves by invading others is a misuse of power, it is exploitation.

"Some of those relationships, as I have said, create space for others; some create a deepening of human understanding; some create children. It is strange in our over-populated world to insist that every relationship should create children and that if it does not it is not valid. Here we are back with motive. The issue with birth control is not the pill or the condom, it is why we use them. If we control birth so that we can enjoy sex without commitment and go on consuming ever more resources then that is greedy; but if we control birth so that we can show love to another and also be more responsible parents and give more of our resources to the poor then that is generous.

"Coming to you, here and now, I suppose your big questions are about sex outside marriage. It is definitely not a sin for two people to agree to have sex; the sin lies in the exploitation of one person by another. The use of power, money, status and emotional blackmail are just as much forms of rape as using alcohol, drugs or physical force; and this exploitation goes on inside as well as outside of marriages. Jews and Christians have promoted marriage because it was needed when populations were fragile and property relations difficult; but the great flaw in marriage has always been the implicit idea that women are inferior to men. With a relatively stable population and a welfare system, the social forms of committed relationships are bound to change. As loving creatures we are naturally inclined to form loving relationships but it would be very strange if the forms had not changed between hunter gatherers and now. Honest motive and faithfulness of purpose are required in every generation but they are not always shown in the same way. Likewise, going back to my comment on biology, there was a time when polygamy was widely practised by the Chosen People (or, rather, the chosen men) but it seems much less appropriate now. Conversely, the Chosen People frowned on gay relationships but that censure is not appropriate now. It is difficult to see, given the state of our evolution, how anybody can say that homosexual relationships are not part of God Our Parent's creation.

"However, this is not the end of it. It is so important that we form relationships with people on the basis of love, of creating space for the 'beloved other' to grow, but we are corporate creatures; so any relationship will only survive the difficulties of our highly competitive world and highly competitive, God-given genes, if it is supported by a community. Most important of all, however, is that we should seek God's special blessing and protection on those things we value most; so if we say we most value our love for somebody then it is natural that we should call for God's protection. My criticism of relationships outside marriage is, then, that they are not committed consciously to God. As creatures we should commit all our relationships to God but in the case of those to which we give an exclusive purpose it is important to provide an exclusive framework. Traditionally this is called 'Marriage'. But what matters is what it is, not what we call it. If that committed relationship involves children then it is even more important that it is committed to God. Further, because we all know how difficult it is to stay faithful in a single marriage—for the simple reason that we all live longer than we did in the time of Jesus My Brother—it is irresponsible as well as irreverent to fail to ask God Our Parent, Jesus My Brother and My Sister The Spirit for their special support. Furthermore, one of the things I hear most often from people of our generation is that we do not know anything about God. Well it is true that our parents showed very little regard for God and that they were caught up in the selfish but shallow dream of perfect happiness through greed, a vice turned into a public virtue by politicians, but that is no excuse. If we want to know how to up our score for a certain computer game, we find out; if we want to improve our technique so that we can persuade somebody to have sex with us, we find out; if we want to avoid paying for intellectual property by illegal downloading, we find out; if we want to know what kind of sensation we get from certain drugs, we find out. Our choice of short term relationships, computer games, theft and drug abuse is choice; it has not been forced on the most highly informed society that has ever lived. We can choose God or we can choose to ignore God; but it is our choice; that choice is why we are here.

"So, we must never fool ourselves. When we say that we can have a relationship without a special commitment, the chances are that this will be selfish; and if we form a long-term relationship without committing it to God, we are just making things more difficult for ourselves than they need to be. In that sense, and in that sense only, long-term commitments outside marriage are sinful, because sin is a deliberate act of distancing ourselves from God. This is why it is so sad that Christians think they know how to judge between one kind of relationship and another, excluding some and accepting others, when God Our

Parent wants all relationships committed as a matter of free choice.

"It is easy to draw contrasts, in a society so rich in the literature of experience, between two gay people in a lifelong, constructive relationship which brings them closer to God and a long-term heterosexual relationship where the man treats his wife like a slave so that she lives in utter misery. Meanwhile, as he treats his wife like a slave, as a lesser person than himself, defying God's law, he presumes to say that the relationship between the two gays is inferior to his relationship. Without knowing what happens inside their house he says that what happens in his own house is superior to what happens in theirs. What he sees as a good Christian marriage she sees as a desperate degradation in which she is bullied and raped. At last she inherits some money from her mother, enough to free her from economic imprisonment; and she runs away; and he says that divorce is against the will of God. Can he really mean that his cruelty can forever exercise a veto over her having a new, loving relationship to help restore her shattered life?

"We must never get that far. Whether we begin a relationship in lust, economic cynicism or a craving for power, it will not go well. The young, who should know better by learning from the mistakes of their elders, make the same mistakes; their elders, who should know themselves better, judge themselves favourably in comparison with the young.

"I love you all. Above all else, love one another; and mean it!"

Perpetua's speech was listened to in complete silence but once she had finished the conversation was animated. Dexter got into a discussion with a group of gays in one corner; Heather and Jo talked to some former drug users; Wayne asked Father O'Helly why he was so publicly anti-gay when it was easy to see that he was gay himself; it took one to know one! Annie felt proud of the kids who had started out as her shelf stackers, as if it had something to do with her.

Miles finally dragged himself out of the door to liaise with Sneer who had made an inside deal with a couple of 'friendly' policemen to raid *Scanties* while Perpetua was still there but his phone wouldn't work and he went back in, relieved.

13

The media response to the sex sermon was low key. They had worked themselves into a frenzy through two days of build-up but, as usual, they were not very interested in what people actually said, only in speculation about what they were going to say. Only Morning Money, accustomed to detail and complexity, seemed to understand what had been said; the rest found the story too much trouble. Will was disappointed by the speech because he thought it had not done much for audience ratings but, in fact, it had out-performed rival channels such as Soft Centre and Hard Rock on that Friday night; and the payments for downloads of the speech steadily rose over the weekend. The religious press was outraged by the attack on the Creed, a point which united the Torans and Petrans although they had their quite separate concerns with other aspects; but they soon grew tired of the Creed and resumed their sexual slanging match quoting Perpetua out of context in spite of universal access to her whole text.

Sneer, frustrated in his attempt to call in the police, published a piece with an outraged response from the Bishop of Castlegate but the story had run its course. For whatever reason, the Wayne campaign petered out.

As the bundles of morning papers were taken in, Perpetua handed her bags to Kylie at the side of the bus. She was about to disappear from the media for almost six weeks. The plan was to visit Stumpy Knoll, a grim housing estate up in the North, far away from metropolitan attention.

Just before she left, Perpetua caught Miles and O'Helly in the Paradise Cafe as they chewed sulkily and suspiciously over the previous evening. "I wanted to say a few things that it would not be fair to say in public," she said. "For a start, Father, why are you so publicly anti-gay when you are gay yourself? And why are you so anti-women when it is the women's movement in the church that has been brave enough to provide most of the support for gay clergy? At least Miles is straightforward; he says that neither gays nor women can be clergy; but you say women cannot and then stay silent about gays. The least you could do, father, is to repay your debts to the women for their support of gay clergy. I know you say there should not be a trade-off but the Nicene Creed was a trade-off about Jesus My Brother; next to that these sexual matters are small things. Since when was Christian doctrine a thing of purity? It is simply a way of helping people to formulate ideas that give them encouragement to seek God. As for you, Miles, stop smirking. Where do you suppose your doctrine came from? Well, a lot of it came from Parliament which was not all that bothered about God; it was very bothered about the personal acquisition of wealth and avoiding royal decapitation. Since then Protestant Doctrine has even failed to acquire the Catholic veneer of selflessness and objectivity; it is simply a matter of powerful and self-opinionated males fighting it out.

"How do you ever expect to bring the poor and benighted back to God if you persist with this 'Male headship' argument? The only people who get anything done in sink estates like this are powerful, determined women; and you go in there and tell them they are second to their menfolk who have impregnated them and fled. They see the expansion in the number of women nurses, women teachers, women doctors, women social workers, women lawyers; and you tell them that there is no room for women priests. They see violent, so-called 'red-blooded' males who rape them and carry guns and knives; and then they see quiet, self-effacing gay blokes; and you tell them that the violent ones are natural and the quiet ones are unnatural.

"But I give you this, Miles. I know you hate being here; you try to hide it but your fear is visible; but you are here. So to that extent you are offering a sacrifice to God. As for you, O'Helly, seven years in theological college seems to have done you no good at all; but, like Miles, at least you have stuck at it through some very tough times, almost blackmailed and outed by a parishioner who hated all Catholic gays because he wrongly thought they were all child abusers. You should be ashamed of yourself for not supporting Wayne.

"The thing that neither of you seems to be able to grasp is that people who have no relationship with God are not foolish enough to think that they can get help in starting a relationship from a church indulging in a never-ending, ill tempered, obsessive seminar on sex and gender. When the church is more interested in the church than it is in God you cannot expect to bring people to God; and, less importantly, you cannot expect to bring people to the church.

"If only you could see that what unites you is the sacrifice and the heartache, the fact that you do what you do for the love of God. If you could only make that sacrifice count by transforming it into love rather than censure. Your existence is not justified according to how orthodox you are or the people you attract to worship; your existence is justified according to how effectively you communicate the idea of the centrality of God's love to people who are lonely and who quite naturally feel a hollow at their centre. Do you think that they really have children in their early teens, or take drugs, or smash up bus shelters, as an act of defiance, as a public mark of self-assertion? But this is sad, attention-getting escapism. It is just a different, less elegant form of escapism than keeping a mistress, getting drunk on vintage champagne and driving recklessly in open-topped cars.

"The best thing you can possibly do is to support each other instead of fighting. Each of you has different but important insights into the will of God, obscure though it is to humans. If we combine the Catholic interest in rigour and the Protestant enthusiasm for the cause, we might still have a chance.

The other thing you could do is find nice partners; both of you. See you in Advent!"

As Perpetua went out, Dexter came in. "God moves in mysterious ways," he said. "So he does," said Father O'Helly, looking deeply suspicious. "Don't worry," said Dexter, "I'm just here with friends to get you organised in time for Christmas."

Miles and O'Helly were not sure whether they would organise with Dexter or against him; either way, this lack of freedom to make up God as they went along was deeply distressing.

What if God was not as like yourself as you thought he was?

14

It was the final Friday of half-term in Stumpy Knoll and the usual knots of truants at the Cedars Shopping Mall was supplemented by hordes of bored teenagers who had seen all there was to be seen and spent more than there was to be spent. So bored were they that Perpetua and her newly gathered *god4u* family aroused a little interest and Jim's playing attracted an increasing following. Led by the group, hundreds followed Perpetua out of town, texting others as they went, so that by late morning there were a couple of thousand people listening to Jim and generally waiting for something to happen.

Brian soon had everything hooked up so that Jim's flute and backing track were nicely integrated. Then Perpetua began:

"I am unable to guess what we thought we were coming out here for, perhaps just some music in the open air, but it seems to me that we need to think about ourselves a bit. All the reports I have read and the comments I have heard since I arrived here at Stumpy Knoll say that you suffer from multiple deprivation, a lack of stimulation and abnormally high levels of addiction and criminality with a tendency, reports add, for people to fall into a state of permanent victimhood.

"Well, granted, the poor have had a raw deal from society but what is new? The rich expect us to behave better than they behave themselves. They look down on us and then are horrified when we look down on other people. The difference is that their exercise of moral superiority is usually more manipulative than ours. None of us should look down on anyone. We are all creatures of God. I know the idea of God is a difficult one, that many of us have hardly heard of God, even as a theory, so let me say a bit about that.

"We may not have heard about God but God has heard about us. First of all, God is not an idea like well-being or peace. Secondly, God is not a crazy creator who makes things for fun. As Einstein said, God does not throw dice. Neither is God a clock maker who wound the world up and let it go. Neither is God simply an explanation for how things are that we can choose to believe in or not. This last point is important because for hundreds of years now God has not been marketed as the source of all love, God has been marketed as one of a number of explanations for why we are here now and, on the whole, that explanation has lost out to much more down-to-earth ideas from science. This has led us to believe that science can answer every question; but it has failed. It has no way of answering questions like: why is there something rather than nothing; why do we try to reach beyond ourselves; and why are we all so sad?

"You may wonder why I am saying all of this to you. It is because I respect your ability to understand difficult ideas and talking to you like this is an expression of trust. If we treat each other like adults we will more readily behave like adults. Still, I know that many people here are distressed about the here and now, so what can we do to make ourselves feel better? There are some researched answers to these kinds of questions but they usually end up talking about money and access to goods and services. I am not discounting money. The Government and the rich will give the poor anything but money. They say it will not help if they 'throw' money at a problem. True, they should come closer and put it in our hands rather than throwing it from a distance; but the real combination for change is justice and love.

"God is love; the universal, all encompassing 'person' that is the source of love. God feels like the day you wake up in the morning and know that everything is perfect and that it will go on being perfect, the complete clarity of the air, the sharpness of the atmosphere, the detail of every blade of grass, every dew drop on every petal; every set of reflections in glass; and the smell of the perfect breakfast, fresh bread and coffee, is only a hint of a flavour compared with what it really tastes like. Most reality is a poor shadow of our imagination, our fantasy, but God is the opposite. God is infinitely better than anything we can imagine.

"God is the massive relief when we have been frightened and find that we are safe; the lights coming on after a storm; the fog clearing after a terrible muddle. Yet these, too, are only indicators. All of these ideas push us towards the central ideas: that we are loved; that we are not alone; that there is hope; that we can reach levels beyond our imagining; that we can reach these levels through a combination of our searching and our listening, of moving and staying still.

"We cannot live if we think we have to do everything; but neither can we live if we think we can do nothing. Here we are, caught between these two wildly unrealistic ideas, everything and nothing. We are neither everything nor are we nothing; we are something; and what makes us what we are is being part of God's universal goodness.

"But God is also trouble, not because things only work if they are painful (not all medicine tastes nasty) but because standing up for God in a hostile world is trouble; because asking difficult questions is trouble; because doing something different is trouble. I hear all this stuff about rebellious teenagers but when any of us wants to do something different the rest close us down. Sometimes saying anything in a lazy culture is trouble. When we ignore God it is more than hard, it is empty.

"I can see why we are all put off by the dark churches with their heavy doors; they look more like fortresses than havens. I can see why we find Christian leaders forbidding; I can see why our experience at school has left us hostile to books like the Bible. But we can find our way to God through our own route as long as we keep in touch with others. It is like climbing a steep rock face and being on a rope, doing what we have to do but in tune with the others in the party. As long as we work together and stick together and work to be respected according to what we do, it is possible to find a new way of living. God is beautiful, God is elegance and trouble, God is Grace and conflict. But right at the centre God is constant, like a nucleus. We can learn to see God in everybody, particularly people we dislike; but it is equally important to listen for God. And, if anything, listening is more difficult than doing."

At this point Trina and Dexter both indicated that people were getting restless. Perpetua signalled to Jim to play and asked if anybody had any food or drink to share. They looked at the crowd and there was only the odd can of soft drink.

"Ask if I can share a drink," said Perpetua, and a can was brought to her. She bowed her head and said: "God Our Parent, Jesus My Brother, My Sister the Spirit, help me now to show these people the glory of God." She handed the can back to Dexter who noticed it was sealed. She dug down into her bag and produced a small burger in a heat-proof wrap; and then another can; and another burger. The supply went on and on with the occasional break for a vegi-burger and a sugar-free drink. There was even a gluten-free wrap; but mostly it was just small cans and small burgers.

The crowd didn't really notice what was going on but the Ten did, and wanted to ask questions. "Later," said Perpetua. "We will have tomorrow for prayer and discussion before Sunday worship."

"Was that what they call a miracle?" asked Kylie. "Yes," said Perpetua, "but it is best not to think about it too much. Those young people hardly noticed what happened but when they think about it they will wonder where the food and drink came from. You know it was a miracle but these things do not take place to prove how powerful God is; they happen to show how God wants us to be close. The kids will think about what happened and then the memory will fade; for us it cannot fade. In spite of the press, what has happened so far has been easy. All that is going to change."

With each bulging black bin liner that went into the bus, the Ten became more puzzled and, for once, could not wait for their time alone to begin. They went to a rather dilapidated former youth hostel on the moors.

"Jesus My Brother used to talk about the Kingdom of Heaven but that is a difficult idea today; too much baggage about kingdoms and too much fanciful art about heaven. Let us start by dividing God from heaven; God is not heaven; being with God, a real, knowable, all-loving person, is heaven. We are in heaven when we are in a state of rapture with somebody and that somebody is God. Christians have said from the beginning: 'thy Kingdom come on earth as it is in heaven'; but that is not going to happen; it cannot happen because being on earth means that we are in a state of imperfection, of waiting. But we can do two important things: first, we can make every relationship as close as we can to God's relationship with us; secondly, we can pray to God and listen for God so that we are strengthened and encouraged by little glimpses of heaven. Jesus used to talk about heaven in stories but we need new stories. Heaven is the place where all conflicts have been generously resolved; where the poor finally enjoy ease; where the striving attain rest; where the broken are mended; and, above all, where the lonely are embraced; and everyone is loved.

"You can think of it this way. There was a man who was kind to everyone and, unusually, he grew very rich. The more money he made, the more he gave away; and the more he gave away the more he made. He had a beautiful wife who loved him as he loved her; their children were happy and constructive and always came home at major family occasions like Christmas and Easter. He loved music and read many books which filled him with rich and strange thoughts. After his beautiful home the place he loved best was his local, rather scruffy church. He had offered to pay for its complete renovation or to build a new one; but in the end he liked it the way it was. He said his prayers and, on the basis of wanting to lead a balanced life, he even polished some of the choir stalls. And still, when he died, he was completely overawed by the beauty of being with God for which his wonderful life on earth had not prepared him.

"And there was a girl who could sing and dance. And for some reason her voice did not crack nor her limbs tire as she got older. She felt the beauty of the music and actions flowing through her; and wherever she went people smiled at her. And yet this was nothing to the music and dancing in heaven; and nothing to the smiles she saw there.

"And if the rich and accomplished cannot imagine heaven, how much more wonderful will it be for the poor and broken. We who are looked down upon and deprived, who never even get into the queue for the best things of life, will find our natural place in heaven. You could think of a starving man who eats an unending dinner, or a slave labourer who sits at her ease; or an orphan who has parents to run to; or a blind man that sees his wife. But none of this would be close; and yet, the further we are from heaven on earth the nearer we are to heaven.

"Now this is the point of what happened yesterday. A miracle is not a piece of magic; I did not wave a wand and make something happen. A miracle is God's way of allowing people on earth to see a little more than usual of the power of love. Miracles are not to make us gasp, they are to soften our hearts. Jesus My Brother performed many miracles but almost all of them were for the poor and the broken, the sick and the disabled. But not only for them. He performed miracles for those who, in spite of their worldly power and wealth, managed to hang on to their commitment to God. So in loving the poor we must not forget the troubles of the rich. But I came to bring God to the poor and the desolate, the helpless and the hopeless. The churches have tried to do this but they have seriously failed. They have lost touch with their own poor and take refuge in the distant poor. It is our job to re-connect Christians with their downtrodden sisters and brothers."

Then Perpetua outlined the campaign plans for Christmas.

15

Perpetua had decided to go to Stumpy Knoll because it had recently suffered from tension between the white and Muslim communities. She was invited to preach at a usually badly-attended evening service but word had got round the church was packed. As she stood, in a moment of silence, in the pulpit, somebody shouted: "Keep our country Christian!" "One day," said Perpetua, "two tough guys in white vans were involved in a minor accident on the main road a few miles outside Stumpy Knoll. They jumped out of their vans and started punching each other. One of them was knocked bleeding to the ground and the other one drove away at high speed, leaving his victim lying between his van and the road in full sight of the traffic. An off-duty paramedic drove past but did not want to get involved in case of troublesome insurance claims. An officer of Neighbourhood Safety drove past but he could not become involved because he had an important meeting scheduled with the police. A Curate drove past but he was too frightened to become involved; he was worried that the victim might be carrying a knife. He looked like a very unpleasant customer; it was probably his own fault anyway. Then a Muslim taxi driver stopped at the scene. He saw the National Front badges on the man's clothing and the swastika tattoo on the back of his right hand. But he got a cloth and cleared away the grime and blood from his wounds and bound them up with a couple of clean rags. He hauled him awkwardly into the back of his taxi, sent a message to Control and headed for the A&E Department. When they got there, the man was abusive but the Muslim and a couple of Filipino nurses managed to calm him down. They dressed his wounds and discharged him. The young man, still confused, moaned about his fate and hurled abuse at the Muslim. The taxi driver took him to the nearest Wayfarer Lodge and offered a swipe of his credit card as surety. The Manager, who disliked the look of both of them equally, bridled but, in the end, still grumbling, agreed to take the man. Next day, the victim, feeling a lot stronger, threatened the Manager with violence if he refused to give him the cash for a taxi against the credit card the Muslim had left. He phoned and asked for a white taxi driver and was re-united with his vehicle and drove away. The Muslim paid the bill and said nothing.

"And again: not long ago, a rich man offered to build a community centre for Stumpy Knoll. The Catholics said it had to have a religious orientation. The Protestants said it had to have a different religious orientation. The Muslims said they needed their own space free of contaminating influences and they could not—in spite of equal rights legislation—allow women to be included. The rich man, who was very patient, realised that the groups would not immediately talk to each other face to face, so he set up an email list to seek more detailed views. When he collated all the replies, he found that his proposed centre should exclude: Christians, Muslims, Hindus, fascists, people with a criminal record, vandals, teenagers, people who weren't 'respectable', women, and men. People were so afraid of each other that they did not want to share any space. The rich man recognised that there were different traditions but he was anxious not to give up the project. So he built a circular centre with separate rooms round the edge, shaped like wedges of cheese with the point chopped off, for each of the groups; but he established core facilities in the centre, lit by a huge skylight, that everybody had to share. 'You can be what you like,' he said, 'in your wedges. I disagree with the way you want to do things but I am not prepared to use my wealth to impose my own views. If you want to sneak past each other in the central area without greeting each other then I will be very sad.'

"At first, the different groups were very suspicious of each other but after a while they held joint discussions in the central area and discovered that while they could not share full meals together, they could manage juice and tea. As they learned more, their suspicions declined. There were classes on different religions and different cooking traditions. Sometimes the women from different groups met together; and sometimes even the men would share a game of backgammon or dominoes. At first they grumbled because the rich man had not built different 'centres' at different points on the Knoll but after a while they began to look out for each other. It was never easy and it was never comfortable but their common decency overcame the prejudices of their leaders.

"So," said Perpetua, "who are the terrorists and who is our neighbour? Do we want to feed alone on our misery or do we want to share our misery so that it can be turned into comfort? Do we want to sit in our houses watching different, narrow television channels and Internet sites, or do we want to learn from each other? Do we want to live in fear of everybody who is different or do we want to learn to live with them so that everybody is more comfortable? Try to work out what we have in common and what is different? We are not so different as our prejudices would lead us to believe. I am sorry to say that Christians must take a lot of responsibility for this, whether it is militant Torans and Petrans or timid Medians.

"But to return to the story. After a while, some of the more thoughtful people began to notice something very curious. Tension eased between the different groups such as the whites and the Muslims but the disagreements persisted within the different groups; each group had a spectrum of opinion from fundamentalist to liberal. The fundamentalists tried to impose restrictive rules but the liberals stubbornly maintained their hold on the central area and would not allow it to be commandeered by militants from the wedges. They often suffered great hurt, mostly from their own people; but they stayed where they were. As time went by, the number of militants shrank and the use of the central area increased. When things got difficult there was a temporary outcry for separate centres for the different groups but it never lasted long. This was not a perfect world; there was always tension; there was always a need for peace makers and peace keepers but everybody felt safer."

The congregation was very subdued when Perpetua had finished and, after the closing hymn, people went away quietly, feeling ashamed. During the next few days Perpetua visited as many of them as she could to bring comfort and to help them become more constructive. People got used to Perpetua and her stories. They were prepared to tolerate her because she brought good luck. Crime and drug abuse went down, people who had been sick for months got better. Volunteer groups began to spring up without the hectoring of Community Leaders. A Community Radio station was set up in The Cedars and the drug-centred pirate station disappeared.

The extremists watched and waited. Once Perpetua left, everything would get back to its familiar, competitive way. All this love was dangerous; only power was reliable. But somebody had got hold of her mobile number and there were frightening messages from pay-as-you-go phones. The Knoll didn't need her to wreck the delicate balance between criminals and enforcers, addicts and rehab workers, poverty and Government grants. After a few days the senders began to receive strange messages on their mobiles such as: "Turn the phone on turn hate off", "Love is communication" and "Smile get better". The hate messages soon stopped.

16

It was the first Saturday in December, only 23 shopping days to Christmas. Annie's shelf stackers and warehouse staff had kept their word. Once the Christian consignments arrived they had worked harder and more cheerfully than she could remember to get everything in place. The mighty crib had been built the previous evening with some of her former staff, such as Dexter, coming back to help. When she inspected the work she said: "But where's the baby? I thought that was the whole point." "No," they said, "he won't be coming until Christmas." "But this is Christmas, isn't it?" "No. This is Advent, the period when we wait, when Mary and Joseph are travelling to Bethlehem. We can put the shepherds off here to the left and the Wise Men even further off here to the right; but everybody's waiting."

Because it was Saturday, Corporate Centre's Crib Policy couldn't be updated, so Annie agreed to a notice, combining pragmatism with sales, which read: "We apologise to all customers who are expecting the crib to contain a baby but it will not be born until Christmas Day. For further details, consult our Christian book and Advent Calendar collections. We are sorry if the lack of a baby causes any of our customers distress."

She need not have worried. Had she known, Annie might have used the term "Biblical" (as of locusts) to describe the way in which Christian items were swept from the shelves. There had been an increasing habit of late for Christmas shoppers to wait until the last minute to buy what they needed but these people wanted their Advent Calendars in Advent; they wanted their baby-empty cribs now; they wanted to get their Bethlehem star cards sent now; and they planned to play carols for the next four weeks. By the end of the day a pattern had been identified by Corporate Centre which went into emergency procedures. Sweat shops all over the planet were switched from Spring bunnies, Hobbits, squirrels, Booby Dolls, giraffes, soldiers, vampire bats, fairies, hedgehogs, robots, ballerinas, elephants, spoof politicians and wombats to produce extra crib sets. Print runs were re-scheduled, pre-Christmas bogus sale lines were delayed, airline freight allocations were secured at inflated prices. Far away, workers bargained for "Infidel money" because they were forced to produce idols. There had been nothing like this since England got through to the semi-final of the Galactic Cup after a fluke goal scored after the Brazilians wrongly thought they had heard the final whistle. Annie eyed the figures with mixed feelings as the Corporate Centre consolidated report came through. Would this mean a fall-off in conventional sales which would not make up for the extra effort and expense? "No," said Perpetua, appearing unannounced, "these new Christians will buy goods up to the last penny, more than ever before, and give things away to the needy. We are planning a special event next week. Poor people, particularly those affected by the recent rioting, will put in bids for the things they really need and rich people will buy things and match them with the bids." "But what if the poor people put in a bid for alcohol and cigarettes?" "Well, we will not exactly welcome that but it is not right to offer to give unconditionally and then start making rules. After all, you might, for a variety of reasons, object to fatty food, mini skirts, soldier toys, booze, beauty products, cigarettes, sexy underwear, sugar, party costumes, beef, violent video games, pork, crackers, chocolate and crisps but I doubt you would want a Christmas entirely devoted to turkey, sprouts, potatoes, board games and socks."

All through the next week Brian worked his way down the Excelsior mailing list, securing promises. He arranged to pick up bids through a text-messaging service and Andy balanced the books using an on-line pricing service. Whenever Hypo prices were higher than Jambo or Lakshmo he let Annie know. Heather sorted out all the issues with Trading Standards, insurance and, of course, the Health and Safety Directorate and Kylie sorted out the logistics of getting all the goods into a sequence, matching the bids with the wrapped items. Reluctantly, Annie used her database to email customers to car pool, leaving 1/3 of the car park empty for the exchange.

There were two innovations: first, Perpetua said that donors should not give their own gifts but should give a representative gift so that nobody knew who had given what; and secondly, recipients were to receive a representative gift and then deposit it where the actual recipient could pick it up quietly any time between now and Christmas. This meant that recipients did not have to demonstrate before everybody else what they really needed. Perpetua said they were all to celebrate giving, not the giver, and to give comfort and not embarrassment to the recipient. The donors were somewhat put out and the recipients mistrustful but everything went very well; and Will got an upbeat piece for the early evening news. You were allowed to broadcast good news stories on Saturdays in the run-up to Christmas.

After the Grunge Park Trial the scheme was to roll out nationwide a week later. Experts, in places far more widespread than the TT, forecast that the anonymity rule would ruin Perpetua's good intentions. This did not happen but there was strange problem to be solved. As the enthusiasm of the donors rose, the bids of the recipients fell. Where Grunge Park asked for 2 dozen light ale, Stumpy Knoll was satisfied with a dozen. "No problem!" said Perpetua. "There are so many people who are too timid, frightened, isolated or frail even to ask for things. We can spend the next ten days using the bus to get things to the people who need things most. And we will have to organise volunteer transport for other towns and cities. Traders and deliverers are fully occupied at the moment but we ought to be able to get some help from farmers."

Annie could not believe the figures as they came in. Generosity was producing better sales than selfishness. Last-minute advertising was switched from "Treat yourself this Christmas" to "Treat a neighbour this Christmas". It felt like the first Christmas she had ever known, only spoiled by a note from the shelf stackers who said they would be finishing at 1700 in time for local Crib Services. One day they would go too far but, for the time being, the Christmas (or was it the Advent?) spirit reigned.

17

Paradise Lodge, the home for the elderly at the back of the shopping mall car park, had not seen better days; even by the standards of its time, the era of civic architectural brutalism, it was grim. People had forgotten whether the erratic behaviour of the inmates or the barbaric behaviour of the addicts outside had made window bars necessary but only rust would ever remove them. The main difference between Paradise Lodge and Parkwood, the local prison, was that people came out of prison alive. The two institutions were in grim competition: every time budgets forced standards down at Paradise Lodge, Parkwood argued that prisoners could not be treated better than aged gentlefolk, so it cut its rations. Every time budgets forced standards down at Parkwood, Paradise argued that what was good enough for healthy middle-aged men was certainly good enough for a frail, predominantly female, population, gentlefolk or not.

Perpetua had been into Parkwood and while she was inspecting the kitchen block she lifted a giant pan lid and asked about the grey mush which, she was told, was meat sauce for pasta. She then lifted all the other pan lids in turn before inspecting the dry stores. Half an hour later, nobody could take in what was happening. When the inmates removed the lids from the pans they were filled with rich, steaming meat sauce and soft, fresh pasta. There was crisp salad in the large, chipped enamel bowls, freshly squeezed juice in the jugs and an unbelievable array of fruit and cakes. In an unusual, spontaneous act of co-operation, the officers and inmates shared out all the food (as there was more than enough to go round) and, without even mentioning it, everybody decided that silence was the best policy, as any report of events would confuse Regional officials. One of the inmates, however, did tell his mother who faithfully visited him every Thursday what had happened and, as she was a kitchen worker at Paradise Lodge, the story quickly got round.

There was, therefore, an air of expectation when Perpetua made her visit. As it happened, her visit was scheduled to coincide with the Christmas lunch and she had agreed to provide music for the carols. But the budget was so low that the prospects were not good: the turkey was grey, the sprouts yellow, the potatoes marbled with blue, the parsnips brown, the stuffing sickly pink, the pudding an odd shade of orange, the crackers limp, the fruit drink weak and the tree lop-sided. While Jim drew the residents into a circle and encouraged them to sing carols, Perpetua went into the kitchen to help serve the drinks and came back with a trayful of ugly glasses full of sweet or dry sherry which immediately livened up proceedings. As the singing became more hearty Perpetua wandered round the room and then spent some time alone in the kitchen. When the meal was served the turkey was golden brown with a firm, rich creamy breast; the sprouts were a deep but lively green; the potatoes were crisp and solid; the parsnips were caramelised; the stuffing was moist and brown with flecks of herb, mushroom and bacon; the rich, dark pudding glistened under its recent brandy dousing and it was accompanied by a huge Stilton; the dusty wine bottles all bore forbiddingly obscure labels; the crackers cracked and the tree stood to attention. It all seemed so natural that nobody commented when Dexter carried in a tray of many shaped and coloured bottles. Never had Paradise Lodge heard such lusty singing and never had the poor old people enjoyed themselves so much since the imagined golden age when they lived in their own homes. As with Parkwood, everybody, without discussion, thought it best for the Council not to hear of the wonders that had taken place but one of the care staff was married to a van driver for the local free paper and a story appeared saying that Perpetua had found an anonymous benefactor for the Lodge Christmas lunch; but there was no investigation of the spectacular quality of the cooking. Bill Midway, Vicar of St. Simple the Lesser and Chaplain to both institutions among many others, made some kind of connection between the two lunches but he said nothing.

On the Thursday before Christmas Perpetua went to the children's ward at the hospital. She told the children stories about her Auntie Mary and the donkey and the stable. She went round every bed and before she left it was noticeable that some children looked much better. She went into the Sister's office and said: "Look, the children will be better in time for Christmas which means that those with a home can go. We will need emergency paperwork for the three with no known home." The Sister looked uncertain but Perpetua said she would get Heather to sort it out. Following a familiar pattern, everybody thought it wisest not to make too much official fuss. The doctors worked immensely hard all afternoon checking whether the children were ready to be discharged from hospital. The patient records uncannily matched the improved conditions of the children. Targets would be met, budgets could be cut and new admissions would begin early in the new year. Everybody was puzzled but nobody would talk.

Then she took the Ten away for their final pre-Christmas quiet day. "It is so lovely that God Our Parent is breaking through into the world to bring comfort to those who are in prison, in homes and in hospitals. The papers will talk about some of the children experiencing miracle cures but, as usual, they will not have a clue what they are writing about. The world we live in and the special world of God Our Parent are much more porous than most people think; if we pray and listen we can break into God's world and if we open our hearts and pray God can move into the place where our heart is open and break into our world. God always makes space for us and so we must make space for God; that is why I was sent as a Sacred Vessel, providing space that the world can inhabit.

"Before too long people will begin to put some of the pieces of our mission together. This is the end of our peaceful time. We have been able to work quietly but it cannot last. Pray for strength at Christmas so that we can face the trials of the new year. I will be a celebrity and then I will be torn apart. I will be accused of all kinds of nasty offences and driven out of society. You will be dragged down along with me but My Sister the Spirit will never leave you."

Dexter warned O'Helly and Miles that there would be a big event at Christmas. Naturally, they said that they had their own people to take care of; but they would keep an eye out. They decided not to co-operate with Dexter who was, they told themselves, all mouth.

18

The shelf stackers at Hypo worked intensively right up until their 1700 deadline; there would be enough stock for the rest of Christmas Eve and they had promised to be back two hours earlier than required on Boxing Day. They gathered round the massive crib by the main entrance, together with some senior staff including Annie; even the checkout staff were represented. Perpetua settled the animals, pushed the shepherds nearer to the entrance, turned the kings in the right direction for the last stage of their journey; and then she slowly and fondly lowered Jesus Her Brother into the manger. She said a prayer for peace in the land where he had walked and taught; and she prayed for the poor and the lonely. Annie gave her a voucher and she gave Annie a Christmas story DVD.

Meanwhile, Will was making final arrangements to broadcast Perpetua's midnight service from Grunge Park Civic Centre. He had been reluctant but, as Perpetua said, he did not have much ammunition against comedy repeats, blockbuster movies and celebs getting drunk on air. CEC was still uncertain whether Perpetua was a star just bubbling under or whether it was wasting its time on her but Christmas was notoriously bad for minor channels, even with growing audience fragmentation and a move away from the majors.

By eleven o'clock those who were attending St. Simple the Lesser's Midnight Mass were enjoying carols round the font and the new freedom from drunks resulting from more liberal licensing hours. Perpetua and the Ten spread across the area, going into the pubs, clubs, bars, burger joints and takeaways, gathering people for the Civic Centre. "Don't gulp; bring the bottle with you. It's all right to bring food as long as it's in something," said Trina. Dexter and Andy had gone on a special run gathering the homeless and the helpless, shivering addicts and rough sleepers, scattering them amongst the festive crowd so that they would have people to care for them.

Will watched almost with satisfaction as the the huge Civic Centre hall, usually only seen on election nights, became crammed with the oddest assortment of people who did not look, even to Will's inexperienced eye, like worshippers as they held onto beer cans, wine bottles, kebabs, crisps, bags of chips and all kinds of strange, stomach-churning items which made up a lurid kaleidoscope.

As midnight pipped at BBC Broadcast Centre, the suave Giles Proud was in a state of near hysteria. He had sat at the output verification screen to check the first shots of the live coverage from London Minster but instead of seeing the decorously arranged choir, a breath away from Silent Night, he saw a rough sleeper with a can of Export, sitting on the floor. He could not come to terms with what he was seeing; he could find no explanation. The Continuity Studio Manager froze.

The worship started with a couple of carols, led by Jim and the backing track; and then some local children acted the story of the birth of Jesus in the traditional words and the traditional manner. The only thing that had changed since Perpetua acted at Grunge Park Primary was the use of the Nativity Play as a vehicle for parental competition. There were designer tea towel head dresses and rustic gear; many of the angels were displaying prominent fashion logos; there had obviously been fierce competition in the camel and King sectors so that the camels looked bought rather than made and the Kings seemed to have adapted their gear from Harry Potter costumes. There was little of the humble worker or the sage. Then Perpetua read the story from Luke before going on to the last verses of the Crucifixion in the same Gospel. People were visibly shocked and upset.

By this time, with a skeleton staff, Giles realised he could do nothing; he did not know why BBC1 was picking up the CEC feed and why he could not switch to the Minster.

Perpetua said: "Tonight we are celebrating the birth of Jesus My Brother. We were all pleased and excited when the Nativity Play was being performed and we enjoyed the comfortingly familiar words of Luke. We all like to celebrate the birth of a baby but when we are trying to understand somebody's life we should not stop there. Most life stories do not spend very long on the birth and early childhood; so why are we so interested in Jesus the baby? I think that most of us hardly know any more; it is a holiday celebrating a birthday which means giving presents.

"But the whole point of celebrating this birth is celebrating this life; you cannot celebrate a life if there is no birth but it is the life that counts. God Our Parent loves us so much that Jesus My Brother came to re-unite all creatures with the Creator; because he was God and human he was showing us that there is something of God in all humans. But we killed him. We only liked the miracles he performed but not what he said; and when he threatened the old ways, the authorities, on behalf of all of us, killed him. And when he suffered, we all crowned him with thorns and drove nails into his hands and feet; and we are still crowning him with thorns and driving nails into his hands and feet. Or, just as bad, we sit and watch while other people, on our behalf, crown him with thorns and drive nails into his hands and feet."

Somebody began to cry and Trina gestured frantically (off camera) to Perpetua. "We know all of this in a vague sort of way, like a distant story, like Sooty, Francis Drake, Star Trek, William the Conqueror, Sherlock Holmes, The Seven Dwarfs, we have a vague idea about Jesus My Brother; and we do so like to celebrate a birthday. But Christmas is useless without Easter. How many of us will be here to celebrate the death and rebirth of Jesus My Brother? We would not be celebrating his birth at all if He had not died and if He had not then been re-born on Easter Day. But the point of Jesus being re-born at Easter is that He is here with us now. He is with us in the street, He is with us here as we meet; and in a few moments He will be here with us in a special way when we share a makeshift meal together."

Fortunately, there was only a skeleton switchboard staff and the barrage of red lights began to fade. But even in a vast building that was almost empty the story spread. Perpetua was on every UK channel; and, as the minutes went by, World Service reported coverage in Canada and the USA.

All over the land, clergy were hurrying home from their own late night services to grab a few hours' sleep after a long day and before an early start. O'Helly was miserable even though his dwindling congregation had not been a surprise. Pouring himself rather too much whiskey, he slumped in his chair in front of the television. Pouring himself the smallest of brandies, Varnish recognised the voice on the television left on in the kitchen. "So," said Perpetua, "in a few moments Jesus will be here with us in a special way when we share a makeshift meal together." Something about the word "makeshift" caught Varnish's attention; there was nothing makeshift about the Eucharist. He took his brandy into the kitchen. A fragile old man and a tiny girl were making their way to the table where Perpetua stood; all it contained was a Cross, a glass bowl and a large glass jug. The girl handed a large bag of crisps to Perpetua who carefully shook them into the bowl. The man gave her two large cans of Export lager which she poured into the jug. O'Helly had a horrible feeling that he knew what was going to happen next. *god4u* stewards were mingling with the crowd, handing crisps and cans to some of the people who were empty-handed so that everybody was within reach of food and drink. "Now hold what you have carefully and still and make sure everybody is holding on to something or somebody with something; everybody must have a physical part in this preparation.

"On the night that Jesus My Brother was condemned to death by the whole human race, he took bread and wine and made Himself present in them through the blessing of My Sister The Spirit; and in all the ages since His re-birth, Christians have taken bread and wine and have done the same. Here and now, in that succession, I bring myself, as God's Sacred Vessel, and Jesus My Brother, through the power of my Sister The Spirit, to you in a special way through the food and drink which we all hold together and which we will soon share. These crisps and all the food you hold are my body and the body of Jesus My Brother; this beer and all the drink which you hold are my blood and the blood of Jesus My Brother; Our full presence in these offerings is accomplished within the love of God Our Parent and in the power of My Sister the Spirit. In these gifts God is one. The whole of the world's people from the beginning to the end of time are gathered with us here in these offerings, represented by the Christian Church all over the world."

With a wrench, Varnish realised that Perpetua had extended the "Sacred Elements" beyond bread and wine; and she was not ordained! Did that make it better or worse? She bent down to the tiny crib below the table and picked up the baby. She raised the baby and the cross so that all could see and then tied them loosely together with a thread of gold and a thread of crimson and then laid them on the straw, the cross almost completely concealed by the baby.

Perpetua gave beer and crisps from the altar to the Ten and to other people nearby while rough sleepers gave food to the rich and the rich gave wine to office cleaners. Blacks gave food to whites; Indians gave drink to Slavs. As the food and drink were finished and containers, bags, cans and bottles were collected, there was hugging and crying.

O'Helly winced at the physical contact. "Now that we have gained new life from Jesus My Brother, we will listen to the beginning and end of the story again." So she read Luke's account of the birth, ending with the shepherds, and the story of the Crucifixion from the trial to the tomb. "You cannot sing the carols and mean it unless you have Easter in your hearts." She took the infant tied to the cross out of the crib and the crowd, stewarded by the Ten, came to the front to kiss the baby and the wood. The Civic Centre faded out with no credits.

Giles, who was now in Continuity Control, watched the Channel logo appear without any intervention from the Studio Manager. "Hit the button for the next programme," he said "and we can re-schedule while it's playing." The enquiry would be extensive and unpleasant but it would be worse if normality was not restored as soon as possible.

Varnish thought that normality would never be resumed. He was right.

19

Bill Midway had broken the habit of a lifetime and asked Perpetua to preach on Christmas morning. He always enjoyed giving his familiar sermon in front of a full congregation which knew what to expect and would be disappointed if it got anything new.

She began: "We are here to celebrate the birth of Jesus My Brother. But you cannot do that in here: first, Jesus My Brother is not here, he is among the poor who never come in here; secondly, he only lives in the crib for a few weeks but he hangs on the cross forever amidst the oppressed. But the Church is stuck in the birth and has forgotten how to understand suffering. For the Christian church in most places, suffering is only an idea."

Bill was extremely restless, his hard-earned sense of fairness seriously challenged, but Trina squeezed his hand and whispered that it would be all right in the end. "Thirdly, this should not be a club with an over-priced roof, all about money and fund raising and architects and Faculties and heritage. The only way to meet Jesus My Brother is to walk out of here."

At this point Bill, summoning every last ounce of courage—after years of restraint, after years of Bishops, Suffragans, Deans, Archdeacons, Synods, Councils and Committees; after blizzards of Measures, Regulations, Directives and Faculties; after unmet appeals, targets, contributions and balances; after demoralising fêtes, coffee mornings, jumble sales and talent nights—rushed towards Perpetua. Trina thought this was trouble but Bill put his arm round Perpetua's shoulders.

"In conclusion," she said, "we will celebrate the presence of Jesus My Brother here with us now and then we will celebrate this special day with a special event."

Bill went through the Eucharist unfussily and briskly and, at the end, Perpetua went back into the pulpit. "I know you love this beautiful old church but we need to love Jesus more. Jesus My Brother came to bring good news to the poor and that is what we are going to do now. What Jesus wants us to do today will not take long. We will form ourselves into groups of three or four with people we do not know very well. As we go out, we will receive a tiny replica of My Infant Brother and a tiny cross. We will take these to the address on the package and promise that we will return to the same house this coming Sunday morning.

Many people avoided the distribution point at the back of the church and went quietly out of the side door. It was the hard core of regulars, Bill noted, who were most anxious to get involved. They were deeply conservative but they had been moved. The occasional church attenders had not been able to tune in. One of the Churchwardens began to get angry but his colleague calmed him down; nothing was compulsory but the church was more important than a church. Bill wanted to go out immediately with his people to show a good example but Perpetua asked him to stay behind. "It is going to be very difficult for you later on, Bill, so do your grieving properly now. You will come back often enough but it will never be home again. Look into every corner, remember little details, thank God for the way that the two of you have shared this lovely building; and get some strength to face the bleakness of Grunge Park; and although that will be difficult enough, the wrath of your superiors will be much worse. The powerless grumble, the powerful grind."

As he locked the door, Bill was indescribably sad, not cut but infused with regret. Every earthly thing that he had loved was in his church; but he knew he was called upon to make a sacrifice because what he really loved was his saviour Jesus Christ. He had known for a long time that this day would come. He had not known how or when; but in the interminable hours of committees, fund raising and structural discussions, in the hundreds of stock sermons and slowly revolving rotas, in the inexorable struggle to stem numerical decline, he had known that a time would come when God would break through. He had even prayed for it; and so he could not hold back now.

His mind was taken off himself by the angry shouts of O'Helly. Dexter had made short work of his tiny, deeply committed, congregation, which was now joining Bill's parishioners.

Early the next morning Perpetua went with Andy to see the shelf stackers at Hypo and bought up all the unsold separate crib kings. Wayne loaded cartons of materials into the bus while Bob and Kylie went through the supplies check list. Unnoticed, the bus headed out of Grunge Park.

"Yesterday we reached the point of no return. We have to strengthen ourselves because when we get back we will meet very great hostility. You will be put under pressure and I will be vilified. By Easter I will have been eliminated but I will then make myself known to you and the whole world." "You mean you are going to be killed?" asked Brian. "Yes." "But this is a law abiding country," he said, incredulous. "Up to a point. Next week I am going to send you out, on the Feast Day of the Epiphany, to make God known in all the major cities of this land. What you saw me do at Grunge Park, you will each be doing in a different place. You will be helped by our network in Hypo and other superstores; accept their help. Speak to the people. Ignore hostility from people, the media and the established Christian church. Work with those who will honestly work with you, be careful of those who have their own agenda. If something seems honest to you, say it, because My Sister the Spirit will be with you; but if you are not sure, say nothing, text Trina."

Two weeks after Christmas Day, on the Sunday on which the Feast of the

Epiphany was celebrated, each of the Ten led a congregation out of a major church. Each small group delivered a parcel containing three kings to a house in a run-down area, promising to return the following Sunday. Most clergy, deeply attached to their churches, people and way of life, but also with a recognition that the poor were not receiving the good news of Jesus, were left flat-footed. They did not know whether they wanted this "Fresh Expression" to fail or succeed. Varnish, on the other hand, was very definite. Perpetua had to be stopped and he would go to any lengths to stop her.

20

In the first instance, nobody thought that the Christmas midnight broadcasting mystery had anything to do with religion. Senior BBC engineers were called in from their cold turkey to give their opinions. The Directorate for Independent Media (DIM) was on holiday. Will received a succession of calls from his MD, alternately angry that CEC was being accused of incompetence and pleased with all the coverage. The BBC archly reported on itself as if it were an alien body. As an advocate of open government and the public's right to know, it would be instituting an internal enquiry. In the fierce sales advertising war Hypo claimed that its television channel selectors were more reliable. The TT morning news conference, populated by the mediocre and the hung over (with the exception of Sneer who was neither), canvassed a spectacular variety of conspiracy theories: Tony Blair had blocked infrastructural investment to punish hostile media; the BBC had staged the mix-up to show that it needed a higher Licence Fee settlement; revolutionary hackers had subverted the system; Al-Qaida was conducting global media manipulation trials; the fast food industry had bribed networking engineers in a promotional coup; not even the extra terrestrial was excluded. Dowte, still not entirely contaminated, wondered whether the switch had some supernatural significance but Sneer was hostile until he received a call from Smoother. He was in Bethlehem as head of a Christians For Peace In Palestine delegation whose major purpose was to condemn the security wall and the Israelis and provide support for Palestinians. He had not seen the CEC broadcast but he had seen the Internet clips and in his view this was a deliberate attempt by non-accountable congregationalists to subvert the traditions of the Christian church. He had also heard that the Perpetua gang had strong-armed their way into a church and evicted the Vicar and his congregation. It was unnecessary to contact Hawthorne who would only cloud the issue with his endless subordinate clauses.

Everybody was bored with Christmas but news was thin so Sneer dumped all the conspiracy theories and sided with Dowte. Technically, it wasn't a "two birds" story but it was near enough:

PERPETUA GANG CHURCH COUP

In a breathtakingly audacious Christmas coup, Perpetua and her self-proclaimed gang-church hacked into the national broadcasting system. Her Black Mass, using crisps and beer instead of bread and wine, wiped all other programmes off air. Brandishing a cross and a figure of the Infant Jesus, she ritually strangled the baby, bound it to the cross and tossed it into the crib.

On Christmas morning the gang forced its way into St. Simple the Lesser, a venerable church in Grunge Park, and evicted the congregation. Following her usual practice, Perpetua and her gang fled from the scene of their crimes.

A spokesman for the Church of England said that this was an assault on two thousand years of traditional Christianity. It was also an attempt to downgrade our cultural heritage. Christians, he said, "are proud to be the chief financiers and curators of our built heritage. That is what Jesus would expect of us."

Following his usual policy of evasion, Archbishop Hawthorne of Canterbury refused to comment. Number 10 refused to comment even though the crumbling broadcasting infrastructure is yet another example of a Blair broken promise.

A spokesman for the Catholic Church said: "Although Anglicans have ruined their own Christian authenticity by getting entangled with women and gays, we extend fraternal sympathy to them. This is the result of trendy liberalism. We hope that they will learn the lesson and become more strict."

On the following Monday the conspiracy theories had all been abandoned in favour of a frontal attack on Perpetua:

GANG CHURCH TARGETS FAITHFUL

HAWTHORNE FLOUNDERS AS GANG CHURCH STRIKES

DISSIDENTS THREATEN CHURCH HERITAGE

G4U THUGS SET 1K CHURCHES TARGET

HERITAGE FUNDING CRISIS TRIGGERS TAX FEARS

TOURISM SLUMP FEARED AS THUGS TARGET CHURCHES

As this was a matter of extreme urgency, the Church of England's CEO, Newman Cranmer, intended to call a crisis meeting for the following Wednesday but Smoother forced his hand. Events in Iraq, the weather and a massive outcry over allegedly racist comments on a reality television show might provide the Church with some time to react but Church/media relations were volatile.

Cranmer had two immediate problems. First, there was a strong move by Torans in the Church of England, led by Steve Digger under the banner of "Fresh Expressions" to plant worship groups outside the familiar parish model; but most people were clear that the Church needed to retain control of such initiatives. Perpetua was making explicit what had been implicit; did the Church want to keep the Torans under the banner of "Fresh Expressions" or would it be better off without them? Secondly, the Varnish lobby that saw Christian witness bound up with heritage and culture was immensely powerful but costly. In many ways Digger's strategy was a response to the crippling Varnish policy; or, put the other way round, although Varnish hated Digger's "Fresh Expressions" he knew that he needed Digger's income stream. Torans were better at getting money and Petrans were better at spending it. It was an unsustainable formula. On balance, the Church needed Toran enthusiasm to survive but it should not be allowed to threaten the parish structure and the hierarchy within the Church. Perpetua's worship was a blatant, though grotesque, act of "Lay Presidency"—an ordinary person posing as a Priest—which many Torans supported but the saving grace was that she was a woman. Torans had promoted the fascinating paradox that Presidency was not important but that women could not preside, thus downgrading even further their public regard for women. At least Petrans, who opposed women as priests, thought being a priest was important.

Smoother's advice was that the central issue was not the built heritage nor the direct issue of Presidency but church authority over clergy, ritual and buildings. Digger would go on digging, Varnish would go on varnishing, Cranmer would go on juggling and formulating but a church without authority stretching back to Christ himself was not a church. Only saintly, unrealistic people like Hawthorne were interested in theology. The public, particularly those who never went to church, needed to know where they were. There were hundreds of beautiful ancient churches but a rapidly declining number of church goers to maintain them. This meant that without the buildings the Church would disappear.

Hawthorne and Perpetua would both have to be marginalised.

21

The Christian press reaction was predictable. Miles, reading his *Fortress*, was thrilled with the drama of a self-proclaimed lay President at an impromptu Eucharist; and he was even more uplifted by a leading-out from a traditional church. This is what the Torans really wanted. Bishops were a barrier to Christian growth. If the people of God thought that somebody was right to minister then that should be that; and if that ministry meant abandoning traditional structures, so be it.

Except that nobody from the Toran stronghold had nominated nor checked Perpetua for orthodoxy. Nor would they have because, whatever her spiritual qualities, she was a woman. The *Fortress* did not so much weigh as shout its way through these contradictions before concluding that: "No matter how effective Perpetua may be at spreading the Word of God (and there is still very little evidence), that word must be inevitably tarnished by she who proclaims it. Ultimately, a project to preach the Bible in an unbiblical way is doomed."

Varnish, reading *Church and State*, could not hope for so much emotional stirring and intellectual excitement. The C&S cautiously welcomed the outreach to the poor and needy but, like the *Fortress* but in more subdued tones, queried the orthodoxy of the situation, noting that "Fresh Expressions" should not threaten the parish structure and should be under strict episcopal control: "It is for the Bishops to determine how 'Fresh Expressions' should supplement, not replace, the traditional parish structure. If the authority of Bishops is broken over the issue of clerical appointments then the Church of England will disintegrate, an outcome which many Torans seem covertly to desire; but such a disintegrated church would not be worth capturing, rendering a Toran victory Pyrrhic while inflicting a huge blow to traditional, duly-constituted Christianity. There is a fundamental contradiction which Torans refuse to face between their adherence to what is Biblical in ethics and what is equally Biblical in ecclesiology. The Petrans, on the other hand, are indifferent, almost hostile, to 'Fresh Expressions' and seem prepared to indulge in the liturgy of Pope Pius XII with their face turned firmly towards the high altar and away from the unchurched. Sadly," it noted, "the moderately liberal leadership of the Church is being squeezed by conflicting Petran and Toran agendas".

Only the Orthodox Petran *Stylus* got to the heart of the issue in a leader whose analysis was as cool as its advocacy was hot. O'Helly, bred in this thermal paradox, felt himself totally grounded in what he read:

"A careful analysis of the worship event led by Perpetua on Christmas night reveals three issues of significance to the Orthodox Petran Church and to the wider Christian community which are in theoretical ascending order but practical descending order of importance: the elements of Eucharistic sacrifice, the status of the self appointed celebrant and the nature of the Godhead.

"First, by acting as she did, Perpetua claims that the Sacramental Elements need not be bread and wine. This might scandalise many Petrans but it is not beyond the bounds of possibility to imagine a situation where such practises might take place. Should a group of believers, stranded on a desert island with a priest, be denied the comfort of the body and blood of our Lord Jesus Christ simply because bread and wine are absent? Might not corn cakes and pineapple juice do just as well? Surely the significance of bread was its cheapness and universality and of wine its freedom from contamination. Secondly, and more contentiously, Perpetua has asserted the right of female Presidency. The arguments on this subject are too well rehearsed to require further airing but it should be remarked that the issue in this case is complicated by her claim of Presidency without the authority of a Bishop. In spite of the legitimate questions which Perpetua's self-proclaimed ministry raises for us all, it cannot be denied that her egregiously uncanonical behaviour is the result of a fatal weakness in Anglican discipline—encouraged by such Toran Bishops as Castlegate—which was bound to result in blatant defiance. This can only further endanger ecumenical dialogue. Thirdly, and most outlandishly, a careful examination of the text would seem to indicate that Perpetua is making a claim to a share in the Godhead."

O'Helly felt a deep recognition as this is what had struck him so forcibly when he watched her.

"It is one thing for each of us to claim childhood in God and brotherhood in Christ—a relationship enjoyed in a peculiarly intense manner by Priests at the Sacrificial Altar—but quite another to imply that her relationship is in some way unique. What she says may simply be hyperbolic or careless; and perhaps by writing in this way we have accorded what she says an exaggerated degree of importance. Nonetheless, she should subject herself to detailed doctrinal scrutiny in the cause of creative theological dialogue."

At their routine Ecumenical Partnership meeting, Miles and O'Helly fenced cautiously over the Perpetua issue until Bill arrived when they made things as uncomfortable as possible for him. As usual, the meeting got nowhere: Miles hated social action but he persevered; O'Helly hated social action and oscillated; and Bill loved social action but was frightened of those who needed it. He tried to explain the potential of house groups for bringing the poor back to Christ but, for their remarkably similar reasons, Miles and O'Helly froze him into silence. There were ways of enforcing orthodoxy through church membership but it was much more difficult to control the selection of participants and material for house groups. When Bill left they agreed that Varnish would have to be urged to take strong action over his dereliction of duty.

The weekend secular press was incapable of following the theological nuances of schism and sacrifice but it recognised that an already weakened church was under further threat; and it had begun to sense that Perpetua was a celebrity who could be built up and, at a convenient moment, knocked down.

"How do I come out of this?" she asked the Ten. Most of them stayed quiet but Dexter said: "I don't understand the details but you are God in the way that Jesus was God." "You could not have known that," Perpetua replied, "unless God Our Parent had caused My Sister the Spirit to speak to your inmost heart. This idea is not easy but I am a special manifestation, a Sacred Vessel, of God on earth; and for that I will soon be ridiculed and humiliated and killed. It was meant to be from the beginning. As with Jesus My Brother, the world cannot bear to see perfect goodness; it wants to see goodness tarnished so that all those who strive for goodness end up resembling the wicked." "But," said Dexter, "we will ensure that you will come to no harm. We all have friends from the old days, before we met you, who will see that you are properly protected. We can always put pressure on church leaders and the media; we have our ways." "You must not say that or I will send you away," said Perpetua. "When I called you to follow me I was calling you to a new life. You will let me down when I am in trouble but my life will save you and God's Spirit, my Sister, will guide you. Before then, we need to bring God's message to the people." "Yes," said Trina. "So far the media have had it all their own way, it's time for you to appear on *Fighting Talk* where you can speak for yourself." "I cannot say that I like the title of the programme," said Perpetua, "but I suppose I have no real choice."

The *Fighting Talk* rules were simple. Each participant was allowed to pre-record a statement of up to 1200 words without knowledge of the other statements. After the statements were broadcast, each participant could respond and then there was a free-for-all.

22

The Toran statement:

Although we welcome the freshness which Perpetua has brought to the Christian life of our community, she has destroyed her credibility by over-reaching herself. If she had been content to promote the Word of God within the proper discipline and under the supervision of a Biblically authentic Christian tradition, she might have done some good but instead she is a source of discredit to God's Word.

The Bible, as the Word of God, is the only authority on which Christianity is based, regardless of personal preference, structures of power and authority, social and economic trends, fashion and fad. It states unequivocally, as the will of the one true and living God, that women are to exercise no authority in the Christian church. This God-given command overrides any claims of human equality or justice.

Likewise, the Bible forbids any form of homosexual practice. This is an unmitigated evil which all Christians must unequivocally condemn.

It is therefore deeply regrettable that a woman with undoubted Christian commitment and powers of persuasion has ruined her claim to be heard by usurping authority in Christ's church and by knowingly allowing a self-confessed homosexual person to be one of her inner circle. We are also aware that she has gathered a large following, many of whom live openly sinful lives, contrary to the Word of God. Her lurid lifestyle and that of her followers has brought shame upon all the people of God. Regardless of any words or deeds which she might have delivered in support of the poor and downcast, these have been completely discredited by her claim that the good she does is of herself. No good ever comes from any human being; it is only through Christ's death that we are saved.

Scripture is clear that God will show no mercy to those who are blatantly in error and seek to perpetuate their wickedness: the destruction of Sodom and Gomorrah and the subsequent annihilation of Israel itself show the lengths to which God will go to punish His unfaithful people. As we stand on the brink of global disaster and moral disintegration, we are forced to admit that our own wickedness has brought this about. Only a firm Toran stand against the subversion of right religion can save the world from destruction. Perpetua is a symbol of the beguiling power of false prophets, the serpent in our midst who would tempt us into an easy acceptance of our current state as one which accords with

God's Word. She is a perpetrator of the liberal sleight of hand which makes the world in its own image and then claims Biblical authority for what it selfishly wants.

Yet the crisis which we face is not simply one of general tendencies. By her conduct, Perpetua raises the central issue for the Christian church today: how can it impose the authority of Scripture upon a society, including much of the Christian community, that has sold out to liberal decadence? For two thousand years Christians have fought against paganism and idolatry, against loose morals and disobedience to the requirements of Scripture, but the new challenge does not come from the blatantly idolatrous but from those who call themselves Christians.

We therefore declare our intention to maintain the authority of Scripture above the careless liberalisation of the Church of England. It is our intention to work within the Church to maintain the true faith not only within established structures but also through "Fresh Expressions" and if the Church authorities seek to prevent us through bureaucratic obfuscation, we will resist. We, as the true adherents of Scripture, retain the right to appoint to the Christian Ministry any person we find fit for that purpose, regardless of the obstructive conduct of Bishops. Only as a last resort will we abandon unrepentant Anglicanism to its fate.

We have been driven to the verge of despair by the Church's approval of the ordination of women to the Christian ministry in spite of the clarity of Scripture on this issue, and we will continue to oppose the compounding of this error in the proposition to appoint women to positions of Episcopal oversight. In spite of the collective view of the Anglican Communion on the sinfulness of homosexuality, we grievously regret the Church's failure to expel that large number of its ministers who openly tolerate this practice and we, even more vehemently, condemn the failure of the Church to expel that large number of its ministers known to be homosexual. This is the result of an underlying tendency to regard all points of view as equally valid, regardless of Scripture, to equate the flawed social justice of this corrupt world with the divine decrees contained in the Bible, and to relegate sexual matters in a sexually obsessed society from a position of moral primacy to one of indifference.

It is totally unacceptable that we who are faithful to God's Word should be expected to betray that faithfulness by colluding with its enemies; this is why we refuse to share the Lord's Supper with those who blatantly contradict the will of God; but we wish to emphasise that this adherence to Scripture in no way abridges our deep compassion for sinners. We are prepared to welcome all those who sincerely repent into the fold and to work with them to strengthen and maintain their commitment to the Word. The Church of England is in sore need of a collective and sustained act of repentance, to recognise its terrible betrayal, and to renounce its errors.

The Church of England, and its liberal allies, particularly in North America, is institutionally corrupt.

The Church has therefore reached a crisis because it has allowed intellectual and social fashion to override its traditional tenets. Because its leaders no longer respect Scripture, it is not surprising that many Christians are bewildered and are often tempted to abandon the Word of God altogether. We therefore propose that there should be a proper check on all activities within the Church of England.

First, all those who are in any formal position within the Church of England must be re-licensed on the basis of their acceptance of full Scriptural authority

Secondly, those seeking ordination must submit themselves to the most rigourous test of orthodoxy, strengthened by regular refresher training

Thirdly, likewise, those licensed to preach must observe the purest degree of orthodoxy and commitment to Scriptural authority, submitting drafts of their sermons to duly appointed overseers

Fourthly, all those who provide Christian instruction must agree to submit to orthodoxy monitoring

Fifthly, we propose a commission to sanction authentic Christian books and other materials

Finally, we are reminded by Perpetua's initiative, that house groups which claim to promote the Word of God should adhere strictly to manuals and other material which fully accord with the traditional Christian commitment to Biblical authority.

We are extremely reluctant to bring financial pressure to bear on the Church in order to ensure the passage of these measures, but we will do so in obedience to Scripture if we are given no alternative. We reserve the right to withdraw financial support from a corrupt Church and to secede from it with all our rightful assets.

23

The Anglican Statement:

We, as the rightfully constituted successors of the Apostles and in full membership of the one, true, Catholic and Apostolic Church, declare and affirm that, through the authority vested in us by Jesus Christ, manifest in the traditions and practises of the Church established, no true and orderly Christian witness may be properly observed without the exercise of duly constituted episcopal oversight which embodies the tradition of the Church in all its fullness, together with the consent of the people of God expressed by the Crown in Parliament in Episcopal leadership and Synodical governance.

While welcoming the impetus which the somewhat impromptu and colourful witness of Perpetua has given to the Christian cause, we profoundly regret her failure to submit, as a self-avowed Member of the Church of England, to its due authority. As a fully formed Christian institution whose witness is based upon the foundations of Scripture, tradition, reason and experience, we re-affirm our continuing commitment to embrace a diversity of theological perspectives; but what we cannot tolerate is ecclesiological indiscipline.

As a Church committed to diversity, we deeply regret any attempts to drive us into entrenched positions on the two issues which currently most engage us, human sexuality and the position of women in the ordained ministry. Whereas there are those within the Church who hold that the homosexual state is part of God's creation, the consensus is that it is a manifestation of flawed and sinful man and that, as such, although we will always extend a welcome to homosexual people as children of God and sinners like ourselves, and will always exercise compassion for their condition, we cannot agree with that liberal minority. Likewise, although there is a minority within the Church which holds that the Ministry of women is contrary to Holy Scripture, we affirm our understanding of God's Word that the time was right to admit women to the Ordained Ministry and that their acceptance as Bishops is not contrary to Scripture.

These issues have been exhaustively discussed by the Church of England and by the Anglican Communion and we are committed to continuing the dialogue with those who are disaffected:

First, we will listen to homosexual people to understand their experience and to see how as a Church we can better meet their needs within the context of our overall theological understanding

Secondly, we uphold the Church's traditional teaching on the the unique institution of Christian marriage (notwithstanding our recognition that many of us fall short and that divorce is a visible sign of our human weakness)

Thirdly, we will continue to respect and to acknowledge as true Anglicans all those who disagree with our position concerning the role of women in ordained ministry.

A further issue which has not commanded so much attention as those which relate to sexuality and gender is that of "Lay Presidency" which was asserted publicly by Perpetua at her Christmas Night worship. This relaxation of the Eucharistic tradition has been proposed, and even practised, in parts of the Anglican Communion in contravention of a generally recognised doctrinal consensus, paradoxically by parties only too anxious to claim the inviolability of that consensus in matters where they are in a majority. Perpetua therefore finds herself siding with extremists on "Lay Presidency" while opposing them over matters of sexuality and gender; she may soon be faced with a painful choice.

This state of affairs only reinforces our emphasis on ecclesiological integrity and discipline. Notwithstanding our traditionally generous and mutually respectful theological stance, we cannot tolerate ecclesiological laxity. The Church of England, as part of the Anglican Communion and the Church Catholic, is based firmly upon the centrality of the Apostolic Succession concretely expressed in the Episcopacy as the apex of the threefold order of Bishops, Priests and Deacons. We therefore deeply regret Perpetua's taking upon herself, without due authorisation, a degree of spiritual authority and oversight, and we equally regret her undisguised attempt to overturn the parochial tradition of the Church by resorting to an unauthorised "Fresh Expression". It has been fully understood from the beginning of this new movement that it is to supplement, to plant anew, but not to supplant, the traditional structure of the Established Church. We fully acknowledge the witness and commitment expressed by many lay people in the founding and leading of informal study and prayer groups in their homes and we would not accept the proposal being forwarded by Torans that such groups should be strictly supervised by the clergy; however, such groups are but an adjunct to the broader corporate witness of a clerically led Church and cannot be a substitute for the regular observance of duly authorised worship.

By this we do not wish it to be understood that we are in any way against the continuing growth of "Fresh Expressions". It may well be that such initiatives must inevitably prosper through new forms of worship which are less rigourous in pursuing our Scriptural and Sacramental traditions but we are ever mindful that the Holy Spirit will bring God's Grace to all his people in a variety of ways which do not necessarily reflect the full richness of the tradition and practice of the Established Church. We are therefore fully committed to this new movement in spite of what may appear to be its shortcomings.

Mindful of the need to bring the Word of God to the un-churched and to combat materialism and poverty —which are two sides of the same coin—we would not wish to find ourselves in a confrontational position with a person of goodwill such as Perpetua. We only ask that she should submit herself to the guid-ance of her Bishop who will endeavour to assist her in discern-ing, should she genuinely have been called, her true vocation. We also call upon the Rector of St. Simple the Lesser to abandon his adventurousness in support of Perpetua and likewise to submit himself to the authority of the Bishop.

It is the mission of the Established Church as a curator of our indivisible religious and cultural heritage to preserve a pres-ence in every town and village in the land through prayer and through the physical presence of a consecrated church; that is why we underline the necessity for any "Fresh Expression" to be anchored in the religious and cultural traditions of our land. We deeply regret that, as the Church Established, we do not enjoy such endowment from the State as that to which we feel entitled as custodians of an ever more costly heritage estate supported by an ever dwindling Church Membership but we accept this as one aspect of our Christian witness, as our sacrificial contribution to a land whose fibre is coarsening under the immense pressures of egotistical materialism.

Finally, we express our concern that, as noted earlier, Per-petua's intemperate actions have, perhaps unwittingly, stirred up those very forces of intolerance that she would wish to be stilled. It is only in steady continuity of witness and purpose that true reform can be accomplished; the Church, like its precious build-ings, is always in need of careful and iterative refurbishment but will suffer irreparably from over zealous renovation.

24

The Orthodox Petran Statement:

We, the one, true, Orthodox Petran and Apostolic Church, solemnly declare that in spite of her current prominence, the claims of Perpetua are insignificant in themselves, being advanced by a lay woman. Nonetheless, we are bound, as a matter of public interest, to clarify the issues which her actions have raised so that there is no misunderstanding of the theological issues which she has raised, issues of faith and order which necessarily concern all faithful people.

First, and least important, Perpetua implicitly claims to fulfil a priestly function. There are three fundamental reasons why she is grossly in error in this respect:

- No woman can hold any ordained office within the Holy Catholic and Apostolic Church of which the Orthodox Petran Church is the true core. This practice is without foundation, contrary to Holy Scripture and to the venerable traditions of the Church dating back to the witness of the Apostles. All women who presume to enact any Ministry, Sacramental or otherwise, are impostors.
- Any person who claims to minister within the Church without due Episcopal authority is an impostor. Only those in the direct Apostolic Succession, concretely enshrined in the See of Peter, may properly ordain Priests and Deacons to perform such functions, Sacramental and otherwise, as are permitted by Canon Law.
- Bishops in the Anglican Communion are not encompassed in the Apostolic Succession as their predecessors broke from the embrace of the See of Peter; it therefore follows that their Priests and Deacons are not duly ordained as Ministers of the Church.

Secondly, Perpetua asserts that the Sacred Elements in the Sacrament of the Eucharist need not be bread and wine. In a spirit of speculative exuberance there are some within the Church who have suggested that the Elements are a matter of indifference; that there are circumstances in which other substances might be substituted. There is no precedent for this suggestion and both Scripture and Tradition affirm the centrality of bread and wine as the inalienable Elements of the Sacrifice of the Mass.

Thirdly, and most preposterously of all, Perpetua claims to be part of the Godhead, thus denying its Triune nature and committing an act of unmitigated blasphemy. No matter how schismatic groups have differed from Mother Church none has denied the integrity of the ancient creeds and their enshrinement of the Trinitarian doctrine. Yet Perpetua's claim is not that there might, in theory, be a different understanding of the Godhead, but that she is an integral part of that Godhead. No doubt we are all children of our Creator and brothers and sisters of the Redeemer—and no doubt duly ordained priests enjoy a special brotherhood with Christ when offering the sacrifice of His body and blood in the Mass—but these relationships are of a different order from that enjoyed by the Economy of Grace in the Trinity to a part of which Perpetua outrageously stakes her claim. There are those who hold the view that all theology is provisional as well as being metaphorical and that, therefore, it can be re-formulated in much the same way as physics, encompassed by succeeding paradigms, but this position is untenable, calling into question the guidance of the Spirit. It is inconceivable that Holy Church should attempt to improve upon the inestimably valuable work of our predecessors at Chalcedon and Nicaea. What hope could there be for the faithful if their well loved and understood articles of faith were reconstituted to satisfy the airy speculations of theologians who are playing with fire? Some know to their cost that at some point they must make a choice between their dangerous fancies and the demands of orthodoxy.

Beside these issues, some of those raised by Christian commentators are trivial and easily dealt with. The most prominent of these is Perpetua's known espousal of a homosexual man as part of her entourage. We recognise the superficial attraction of the proposition that it is the duty of Christian leaders to minister to the sinful but that is quite different from providing such sinners with a degree of legitimacy which would seem to condone their sinfulness; at no point has Perpetua ever publicly condemned her associate. Less important yet, but still worthy of attention, is the claim by some that Perpetua is attempting to fragment the Church of England by encouraging its congregations to abandon their traditional worship and share the good news in house groups with the unchurched. This is so misguided as hardly to require refutation but, for the record, tradition bears out the common understanding that there can be no salvation outside the properly constituted authority of the Church Catholic and Apostolic whose core is the Orthodox Petran Church. Those who seek to be saved in the isolation of their own homes, deprived of the duly constituted Sacraments and cut off from the guidance of their priests, will struggle indeed for any sense of the saving Grace of Our Lord Jesus Christ, for only through the Church can He be found. The history of heresy, primarily amongst those churches which call themselves Protestant or Reformed, is one of progressive fragmentation as their individually centred strategies fail. There was a dangerous moment when many in the Church misunderstood the generosity of spirit in Vatican II, believing that it had in some way legitimised heresy, that it had accorded some legitimacy to Protestant and Reformed sects, but this error has been steadily countered during the past four decades so that Vatican II can now properly be put into its orthodox perspective. Only Schismatics seeking a bogus legitimacy within the ambit of Mother Church could possibly misunderstand the repeated calls to orthodoxy by successive Bishops of Rome.

In a spirit of ecumenical brotherhood exercised under the extreme provocation of an Anglican Communion careering out of control, we offer some simple advice which we hope will be taken in the constructive spirit in which it is given:

- First, it is only by adhering to doctrinal, as well as ecclesiological, orthodoxy that discipline can be restored and schism overcome.
- Secondly, the current liberal freedom extended to its members by the Anglican Communion is a false freedom compared with that enjoyed within the Orthodox Petran haven of the Catholic Church.
- Thirdly, although there are some on the Toran wing of the Anglican Communion who appear to make common cause with Mother Church, their persistent dilution of the Sacramentality of the Christian mission is a major contributor to the rot which threatens the very foundations of English Christianity; a "fresh expression" without principle, Scripture or the Sacraments is not an expression worth delivering or hearing.

Finally, we remain committed to ecumenical dialogue as long as this does not compromise our fundamental integrity. With all the generosity of Our Saviour we will welcome with open arms those who have repented and wish to be re-united within the one true church. Perpetua is a warning against Schism which should lead to a renewed and serious attempt to reconcile the Church of England to its rightful place as the beloved and obedient child of Peter. The alternative, of further disintegration, will delay that reunion for which all true Christians must pray.

25

Perpetua's Statement:

The creation of the universe by God Our Parent was an act of pure love which made all of us so that we could freely choose to love God Our Parent. There is no other purpose in creation that is not subsidiary to and an enablement of that love; even the Angels in all their purity cannot choose to love but can only do the will of God as messengers of the truth.

Yes, love grows wild as the plant that is not cultivated grows coarse; so God's chosen people ran wild and became coarse; and in spite of the warnings of the Prophets, God's people could not be brought back to honour Creation by returning God's love. They, who had started out with a cruel code, enshrined it in a myriad complicated laws which substituted law for love.

And so as love grew wild, Our Parent sent Jesus My Brother down to earth, in another act of perfect love, to live as a human being and as God, two attributes fused in one being. And, as creatures made to choose, we chose not to love this man and then to turn on Him; and he died for all of us in an act of perfect love so that we might understand the lengths to which Our God will go to show that we are encompassed in divine love.

And on the third day after his death on the cross Our Lord, Jesus My Brother, came back to earth, the perfect embodiment of the triumph of love and the confirmation of the irreversible offer of salvation to all. And when He had gone to join God Our Parent, they sent My Sister the Holy Spirit to live with all of us; and in the power of the Spirit, Paul explained how love is superior to the law, how love, in the Spirit, infuses the inheritance which Jesus left to us, embodied in the flawed but beloved Gospels and living daily in the hearts of all who love My Brother, individually as supplicants and collectively in His imperfect Church which attempts to witness to the triumph of love.

Yet love grows wild and love grows coarse and the ground in which it attempts to flourish is made ever more alien by our choice to elevate vanities over love: there are the vanities of hierarchy, structure and power, brought into the Church to mimic the vanities and cruelties of earthly power; there is the vanity of orthodoxy which puts doctrine above love; there is the vanity which puts the Sacred words of Scripture above love. Scripture is God's warning of how humans may so easily fall from love; it is the book of love not the book of law. And yet it is used to judge where only God can judge, not to affirm which is the purpose of humanity in creation.

There is the vanity of earthly possessions, so often condemned in Scripture and by the Church and yet never overthrown by those who proclaim the purity and beauty of the lilies of the field. Those poor aspirations of the oppressed to live unhindered are nothing to the palaces of the princes of state and church; not just palaces of stone but of authority and oppression; palaces that presume to judge, that presume to regulate, that measure love as if it were grain or gold.

I have come down from God Our Parent to proclaim that love which has not so much grown wild or coarse but which is being suffocated by sophistication. Our poor Chosen People were misled but they were never indifferent; their law was in defiance of love but it was misplaced not indifferent. Now God's creatures made to choose between loving and not loving have found a new way; they have abandoned the obligation to choose. They do not understand that doing nothing, that turning away, is a choice in itself. There are many who live in nominally Christian lands who are never given the opportunity consciously to choose the love for which they were created.

I have come to renew the power of love, to free God's offer of love, made irreversible in His Resurrection, from the grasp of the powerful, from the tyranny of judgment, from the oppression of condescension, from the cowardice of plenty. Like Jesus My Brother I have come to bring good news to the poor, to save sinners, to warn the rich against complacency. I have come to dismantle the barriers that the occupants have erected against the wanderers, against the poor, against the illiterate, against the oppressed, against those who are different, against women. I have come to proclaim the full communion of all people with Jesus My Brother, an indivisible communion not graded according to secular or priestly rank; the humblest worshipper who dare not walk forward from the shadow at the back of the church is no less the Sister or Brother of Jesus than the Priest who offers the Sacrifice of the body and blood of Jesus. That communion with God Our Parent and with Jesus is only distinguished in degree by the love we choose to give to God. As I came from God to proclaim afresh the Gospel of love in succession to Jesus My Brother, my love is perfect like the love of Jesus.

The Church is struggling but sadly misdirected. It is not my purpose to condemn but to show the better way. Love of place is a deep consolation but it has overshadowed the sacrifice of love; the love of place has overtaken the love of God. Instead of enhancing the channel between God and worshippers, the place has become an obstacle, the worship an escape from the direct call of Jesus My Brother. I am so sad when I see how hard the people work to raise funds for the organ, the roof and the re-ordering; they are doing what they think is right, led by those who have put themselves in authority. There is a time to build and a time to travel; and we have spent too much time building and not enough time travelling.

How disfigured is the Church locked in unceasing civil war to wrest a greater share of dwindling power and authority to exercise them over the lives of their sisters and brothers instead of loving unconditionally.

Love can grow wild and coarse and it can grow strangely in this alien soil; but we can still choose love, fulfilling the purposes of creation. To love unconditionally is not to fill space but to clear it, to leave room for the other. The true love of God Our Parent is that which leaves space for the love of our creator to grow in all of us; if we love God and make space, that space will be filled with God's love. This has often been described by clever people as a mystery; it is not a mystery, it is the common reciprocity of creative love between creator and creature.

We shall have to be brave to proclaim the primacy of love; and I shall be killed like Jesus My Brother; but love will prevail.

In spite of her very different emphasis from the other presenters, and in spite of her forecast of her own death, the first question to Perpetua was on the subject of homosexuality: everybody understood the primacy of love but that did not mean that anybody could call anything love; you could not equally call married love and homosexual love the same thing.

"Remember," said Perpetua, "that human love is only a shadow, a metaphor for divine love. Only God Our Parent knows how people individually and collectively choose to love; all you have to go on is the human activity which you see and define. So you can make classifications of human love of which you variously approve but that has nothing to do with divine love; this is intellectual arrogance, it is worship of words.

"How can you question what God Our Parent chose to create? You say that homosexual love is unnatural as if the natural was yours to define. You say that homosexual love is against the will of God but all you have for evidence is the Biblical text which you refuse to see as a series of metaphors. But even at a mundane level you do not know whether homosexuality is natural because none of you knows anything about human biology, demographics and fertility."

Then Sneer asked: "If you have members of your gang who are clearly criminals, how can you talk about an ordered society?"

"I have never talked about an ordered society," said Perpetua. "That is your obsession. I am not the least bit interested in an ordered society. If you read your Bible which I am sure you do not, you would know that divine justice is very different from human justice. In a world of creatures made to choose—who often, inevitably, choose wrongly—there is a need for human institutions to dispense human justice, imperfect justice for imperfect humans. But the love of God is beyond justice and I will love all my followers as children of God and as my sisters and brothers. If anyone has evidence to bring my followers before the powers of earthly justice, that is up to them."

"You claim," said a Petran, "to know the will of God but how do you know that you are not simply expressing your own personal opinion?"

"I have a rather simple, isomorphic rule," said Perpetua. "If I can recognise what we say and do in terms of what Jesus My Brother said or did, then I think, using the human language metaphors, we are as close as we can get. I do not see the persecution of gay people, the denial of the equality of women, the construction of the Creed, the assertion of Papal or Toran power, as mapping onto what we know of the life of Jesus My Brother. His culture might not have approved of certain things, such as the economic equality of women or, for that matter, an organisation which broke away from Judaism, but we keep confusing what we see on the one hand with purpose and motive on the other; we cannot know how to de-code God's purpose nor human motive."

"We know", said Varnish, "that Jesus founded a church but you are tearing people away from it."

"We know that Jesus wanted his Apostles to continue the work which he started, to preach the love of God shown in incarnation, death and resurrection but Jesus was not specific about the form although he thought the church should be corporate and mutually supportive, living under the guidance of Our Sister the Spirit. But he was not particular about form. I am calling for house groups and there is a long tradition in the Christian church of trying to get back to ancient practises of which house groups are the most ancient. It is not me that has to make a case for house groups where bread is broken by loyal and devout but not theologically trained people; it is you that has to make a case for huge, physical churches and a clerical hierarchy which, in the name of my Sister the Spirit, excludes people from serving God when they say they have a calling and which, until recently, automatically excluded all women from serving even though the mother of Jesus My Brother served God Our Parent with her womb and with her whole, perfect life."

"But," said a Toran, angrily, "you are denying what is so clear in the Bible about women and homosexuals."

"There is no time when all Christians have been unanimous about every aspect and verse of the Bible; but there are some simple points: first, we cannot take all the Bible literally because there are bits that contradict, like the death of Saul; even you know that. Secondly, we reserve the right to change what the

Bible means on issues like slavery and divorce; even you do that. Thirdly, even if the Bible is right about moral issues, we are usually presented, in an imperfect world, with a conflict of different requirements and we have to choose; even you have to choose. Say it is correct to think that Paul—and I do not think this is so—condemns loving gay couples, as opposed to gay prostitutes, then how do we balance that against Paul's call for Christian unity at almost any price? Are we saying that the gay price is too high compared with other considerations such as the need to preach Christ's love throughout a hostile or indifferent world? Are we really saying that it is our right to decide that what God wants in particular, which is the subject of dispute within the Church, is more important than what God wants in general, which is not in dispute? One of your answers, I know, is that Scripture is indivisible and that, therefore, all its requirements are equal. If you think that, you clearly have not read the minutely ranked requirements of the Law."

A woman asked: "How am I supposed to feel when my Priestly calling has been rejected because I'm a woman?"

"I am very, very sorry; this is a terrible kind of tyranny where people presume to judge who has been called. Who might not be a good pastor or counsellor is one thing, but who might and might not be called by God is quite another. One of the most damaging ideas in the New Testament is that the Church is the Bride of Jesus My Brother. Because the church is the creation of Jesus, it is therefore inferior to the Godhead that created it; so, by inference, Paul says, women are inferior to men. The image has stuck fast, it has suited the male church. Follow me."

Most of the Christian questioners had very different views but they shared one vehemently; this woman would have to be stopped.

26

Annie's Hypo was on the crest of a wave: Christmas sales figures were the best ever and had risen faster than those at Jambo and Lakshmo; there had been a special commendation from Corporate Centre for the niche religious Christmas sales and the consumer feedback on the store decorations and music; the crib had gained good press coverage; and industrial relations could not have been better, with Perpetua's people dampening down the hotheads and always ready with constructive suggestions. Annie surveyed the higher than targeted figures for items brought in specially for the January sales and indulged in a brief fantasy about how she would spend her executive bonus.

The shelf stackers came to discuss special arrangements for the Easter stock. It would be just like it had been at Christmas, they suggested. No it would not, thought Annie, vaguely recalling something of the prelude to Easter. What did they have in mind? No Easter Eggs or hot cross buns until the Monday before Easter; a special stand for crosses and crucifixes; another stand for Holy Week and Easter books; appropriate Holy Week and Easter music throughout the store; a Calvary display outside the main door; and no opening on Good Friday.

It had been easy enough to accommodate the Christmas requests but this was unreasonable. It was all right to have Nativity books, cribs and Christmas carols with simple peasant folk, animals and kings, and the baby was an obvious winner; but Lent books, dirges, crosses and a blood-spattered man dying an agonising death, that was quite a different matter. Violence was all right as long as it stayed firmly in the DVD sector.

Granted, the religious goods had added a dimension to sales but the idea of Lent was to reduce consumption and the whole point of Holy Week was to take away the feel-good factor. Jesus hanging on a cross outside the main door was hardly an incentive. The embargo on buns and eggs was also not practical; the Easter eggs were already in the warehouse and the hot cross bun contract for a month's supply had just been signed. As for Good Friday closing, this was impossible; it was one of the best days of the year and this year it would mark the official launch of garden furniture, barbecues, lager lite, ornate plant pots, sparkling wine, the Slight Summer clothes range, slow melt ice cream, solar panels, canoe kits, ice makers, golf umbrellas, punch sets, Mediterranean fantasy, rose bushes and sun screen.

The shelf stackers, determined but sad, refused to negotiate. Christmas was important but Easter was even more important. But Annie had no room for manoeuvre, even at a local level. Silently, they removed their store overalls to reveal their *god4u* badges, neatly folded them and put them in a tidy stack on a table in the corner. Each of them thanked Annie and said goodbye; they would meet again. The Corporate Centre pattern analyser soon showed that the same thing was happening everywhere. Late January was a bad time to get replacements and the management contingency plan would have to be implemented. Late that afternoon the Jambo and Lakshmo figures began to emerge; by the end of the day there was hardly a shelf stacker in the country. The news was full of ordinary people talking about the importance of Easter, how we tolerated Christmas because of the commercialism but that Easter had been down-played because it was too up-front religious. Christmas belonged to everyone but Easter, Ramadan and Divali had particular significance; everybody was prepared to allow Muslims and Hindus to celebrate their festivals but there was a prejudice against Christians in a land where the Queen was the head of the Established Church. A succession of clerics were shown in various degrees of embarrassment; they had clearly not been briefed to talk about Holy Week and Easter. Perpetua was on all channels saying that her next big project was to bring Easter back to God's people. After "Put Christ Into Christmas" it was "Put yourselves into Easter."

Annie, working late on the emergency stacking rota, called Will who said that CEC was dropping its association with Perpetua because retail advertising was too important to risk. Will phoned Sneer to say that the advertisers had been leaning heavily on CEC.

Sneer's dilemma was that although the TT was in favour of the free market it was running a campaign against the power of the supermarket triopoly; and it was in favour of Christianity but running a campaign against Hawthorne and Perpetua. As this was a problem in logic rather than news values, Dowte was called in. He suggested:

G4U GANGS ROCK MEGAMARTS

In a surprise move yesterday that rocked the megamart trio headed by Hypo, g4u gang leaders called a shelf stacker strike. The gangs, which have built up a stranglehold labour monopoly, have called for compulsory Easter observance.

A Church of England spokesman said: "It is scandalous that the name of Jesus should be invoked in an industrial dispute. This is not a theocratic state; people don't want Easter stuffed down their throats."

Experts have warned that in a tight labour market megamart prices are set to rise, punishing weak and greedy management.

Gang leader Perpetua is threatening to bring the country to a standstill on Good Friday to draw attention to the day when Christians believe Jesus was killed. Church leaders are nervous that this might mean even more rapidly falling congregations and a rise in the emotional temperature. "Good Friday is really dangerous if handled the wrong way," said a senior Orthodox Petran cleric. "You have to be careful not to let emotions get out of hand. That is why we have such solemn ritual to keep everything under control."

Sneer thought that he spotted at least four birds. Dowte was earning his keep at last.

Shelf stackers converged on Grunge Park from all over the country. Perpetua hired the Civic Centre for a half-day commissioning ceremony, telling her followers to go back to their communities and strengthen their house groups.

"Do not worry about making a living. If people want what you are offering they will find ways of supporting you. Remember that the idea is to combine rich and poor people into single groups so that the poor can be supported in their worldly needs and the rich can be supported in their spiritual needs. Never forget that heaven was made for the poor and that the rich will find it difficult to find their way to God. We all feel sorry for the poor because of what we see; but we must feel sorry for the rich for what we do not see. The happier they look the more they are in danger. Help them to be brothers and sisters of Jesus My Brother.

"Never argue with people. You are not theologians; you are messengers of the word of God; people will know you for what you are. Wherever people are, whatever their background and culture, people always know goodness when they see it; and love must shine out from you. Nothing else matters."

27

Perpetua rented a top floor flat in Grunge Park for a couple of months which she shared with Trina and Kylie. Dexter, Andy, Wayne and Jim rented a flat lower down in the same block and the others were all nearby.

The initial effect of their mission had soon worn off. The gangs were roaming, the dealers were dealing, the pimps were prowling and the pirate stations were bawling.

"There is no quick fix," said Perpetua. "When we came here first I was just performing some acts of kindness by relieving suffering. This needs trust and trust is based on the recognition of love in the person we are looking at. Love is a first and second person thing; it is I love you and it is you love me; it is not I love him or she loves them; that is just a report. Taxes are not love; not even charitable donations are love. Giving things to people is not love and it might be the opposite. If you give a poor person money, advice, even cigarettes or a bottle of beer, it does not automatically build trust. It might build gratitude or dependence but that is hardly the basis of trust. When we give people space so that they can wander ever more widely from the place to which they are chained, then they begin to trust themselves and they begin to be familiar with space; and fear is replaced by trust. Then, one day, they even dare to think they could do without the chain."

Word soon got round that Perpetua was holding daily sessions on self esteem, trust and love. Most people thought this was just more sentimental rubbish and some of the long-term unemployed boys went round to disrupt the sessions. They found when they got there that the atmosphere was strange and that they could not use their customary tactics; nobody shouted back or threatened. Kylie moved furniture about to make things comfortable, Jo encouraged old contacts to get involved, Wayne prepared study sheets and slides and Heather won her battles with the Council, Health and Safety Directorate and a host of special initiative Directorates that threatened to sue Perpetua for conducting unauthorised teaching sessions in a special zone.

In the afternoons Perpetua went round to visit the elderly and the sick, mums who were reluctant to come out with their babies and those who were too frightened to go anywhere. At night she went round the estate with some of the Ten, calming anger, giving hope, curing pain, combating fear.

One day a heroin addict asked for help. "I had a terrible childhood. My parents were alcoholics and they were violent towards each other and me. The only way I could escape was through taking drugs." "Yes," said Perpetua, "but it is all over now. We cannot mine love from the past that is not there and we cannot fill in the space that was empty but we can find freedom in new space.

Drugs are a poor escape; but God is not an escape at all. We always need to look at ourselves but we also need to look at other people, straight into their eyes. Try it with me; now.

"I will cure your addiction but that is only the beginning. You must stop thinking of yourself as the victim of your parents' violence and think of yourself as a child of God Our Parent who is worthy because of that parentage, who is loved by God, who is entitled to the same concern, respect and love as everybody else; and who was made to love. But we cannot love people if we refuse to look straight at them. Imagine how difficult it is for a blind girl who is unable to look into the eyes of a man whose eyes say he loves her. If we look, we will see God Our Parent in all his children and, before long, we will feel Our Parent flood back into us. Nobody can do that for you; I can only create the basic condition to make it easier for you. I have shortened the distance between you and God Our Parent, which is a way of saying that I have forgiven your sins, but only you can then choose to go forward or go backwards."

In many ways the most difficult task was integrating the people who came from outside to join the weekly house groups. They had so many strange ideas about people who were poor or addicted. The mistake they most often made was to think that they could solve the problems that people faced instead of giving them space and confidence to solve their own problems. They found it difficult to look at people; they clutched their handbags and wallets, kept looking round, starting at the creak of a door. They sipped tea as if it were poison. In a way which Perpetua had expected, it was those who had been thought to need help that did the helping. Those who had been brave to leave the comfort of their Sunday worship found that the broken were sometimes better at offering their brokenness than the supposedly whole were at offering their wholeness.

"One of the dangers, as you know, is becoming sentimental," said Perpetua to a social worker. "There is bad and good in everyone but the bad and good in the people of Grunge Park is just more obvious than that in the people of Excelsior Gardens; they are less bothered about rules because they have never known what most of them are; but they do know that if people come into your house you offer them something. And they realise that many of their guests are having a real struggle. They see it in professional workers, politicians coming to canvass, the occasional clergyman. They are not sure whether it is them or the visitors who are the source of the embarrassment."

Perpetua went to a different house group every day, led the worship, gave a little talk and then said the sacred words, usually over bread and wine. She knew that using other food and drink would upset some people; and she had made her point. It did not need to be made all the time.

Some of the local therapists picketed the entrance to the flats. They said

Perpetua was stealing their trade. "Come in and see," she said. "You tell people that other people cannot heal them, and that is right. You tell people that they can heal themselves; that is half right. I tell people that if they put themselves in the presence of God Our Parent the combined effort of God and human can heal."

Many people felt better after direct contact with Perpetua but the greatest impact was made by g4u-TV which broadcast Perpetua's talks and Jim's music. House groups from all over the country were transmitted live and Bill Midway was a frequent contributor. Uptake across the community multiplex and the internet was better than the CEC reach and it allowed the various groups to keep in touch. Everything was calm but Perpetua kept warning of hard times to come.

She went into all the dark places of needles and knives, broken glass and broken lives; and she listened to all those who came to her and sought out all those who did not come. They all wanted a cure and she cured them; but she said that was only the beginning. News of her work seeped through social services specialists up to the media. But every time one story appeared there was a call for something more spectacular; there was an inflation of expectation. One day soon it would be time to flip the image from wonder worker to wicked witch. Sneer who had, by coincidence, begun to see Smoother regularly, knew that it was only a matter of time; and timing.

28

One evening Perpetua took Dexter, Trina, Andy and Kylie into central London. They went down a featureless street to a grey, metal door. Perpetua entered a pin code and, inside, they ascended in the lift to the top of the tallest building in the city where there was a massive bundle of communications equipment. She took them into the technical suite next to the board room and switched on a processor and a huge flat screen.

"I am Moses," said a small man with a weak voice. "Under the power and guidance of God Our Parent I led the Chosen People out of the misery of alienation. God performed mighty wonders in Egypt, when we were escaping and while we waited for the time to enter our new land. The people were never satisfied but God never gave them up."

"I am Samuel," said a brisk young man in strange clothes. "I urged the people to worship God but all they wanted was an earthly king. Look what good it did them! As if any king has ever done any good for longer than it suits him personally."

"We are Isaiah," said a trio of men, one obviously a farmer, one an official and one a mad-looking guru. "We spent all our lives warning against the evil of material things and the need to turn to God; but nobody took any notice. It was so difficult striking the balance between warning and promising, it wore us all out; but in the end it was the promising that won out".

The screen went blank, the four shuffled slightly, then the screen went unbearably bright so that they had to close their eyes. "It is all right now," said Perpetua.

"I am that promise," said Jesus. "I came from God Our Parent to be the human aspect of God, to live with the creatures made to love. I was killed by the world to save the world; I absorbed in my pain and death all the wrong choices, all the freedom not to love that was, is and will be."

At this point Dexter made a lunge towards the record button on the player but Perpetua put out a silent hand.

"Humans needed to know, in a concrete way, rather than in the difficult abstractions of the Old Testament, that God is not an idea that explains the universe but that God transcends human life. I was killed and came back to life and then returned to God Our Parent. I sent Our Sister the Spirit to give strength to those who carried the message of God's love all over the world but they, poor children, understood brick more readily than spirit, rule more readily than freedom, judgment more readily than love and, in trying to come closer, forgot what Paul told them and put philosophy before faith. They somehow believed that the one God was three and could only be three and that God had made a rule that I was the only human existence of God that would ever come to the planet earth. It is obvious that earth people do not know on what other planets God has lived in physical form and to what pain and suffering those physical forms have been subjected. Christians have invented the idea of a 'full and final sacrifice', telling God that there are to be no more interventions; it was full but it was not final. The finality has made it easier for Christians to understand my life, to find a paradigm for theology; but one of the essential points about God is that the reality is impossible for human beings to grasp, so in trying to get nearer through logic they have got further away.

"Perpetua lives directly in my footsteps as the latest earthly manifestation of God. But even this is a mystery beyond words. Christians say that they are all children of God and that I am a special Son of God Our Parent but they do not know what is the same in my sonship and what is different from theirs. Likewise, Perpetua is a special Daughter of God Our Parent in the way that I am a special Son; but humans cannot separate the children of God into a hierarchy; it does not work. Perpetua is God's Sacred Vessel, sent to give space to the world but fated to be filled with its wickedness and misery.

"When Paul asked for foolishness he meant the submission to God without calculation; but humans were made to calculate. The important choice is between calculation and submission, between individual gain and universal love. The Greeks, like Icarus, like the builders of Babel, wanted a God they could subdue, make subject to the limited language they were given by God. So proud are theologians of the formulation, they forget that in matters pertaining to God, speech is metaphor. The Greeks did not really know what they were talking about when they wrote the Creeds so it is hardly surprising that people today do not have a clue. The idea of God is difficult but it is not complex. A person needs no learning to weep at the foot of my cross. The theology is not an opening up but a closing down; it is a human assertion of intellectual power and not just power over the ill educated but, worst of all, power over me, God Our Parent, Our Sister the Spirit.

"Often Christians talk about divine judgment as if they know what it is and how it will fall. They do not see that earthly judgment is completely different from divine judgment. They claim to speak for God Our Parent and for me. This is the worship of words and not of The Word. It is intellectual idolatry, it is the wickedness of rationalism. Above all, theology is a risk, a venture on the cusp of possibility and disaster.

"Listen to My Sister Perpetua and do not make the same mistakes when you listen to Her that my people made when they listened to me. I know you will be unfaithful to Her as you were to me; I know you will deny Her as you denied me; I know you will kill Her as you killed me. These are the inevitable consequences of the freedom to love; that in weakness we will use freedom destructively. But do not compound individual weakness by forging it into a structure of denial, a structure of theology and calculation, a structure of power and exclusion. Renew my Church in foolishness and love."

The screen went unbearably bright again and then went blank. After a while Dexter said: "It would have been good to record this for the others." "No," said Perpetua. "This was for you to know and for you to remember in the dark days when you realise what you have done; then you will need to realise what I have done. There will be a right time to explain but it is not now."

They left without another word, following in the footsteps of Perpetua, Sister of Jesus, Daughter of God.

29

One night in February Perpetua and her closest followers went into the Hollow, the most dangerous sector of Grunge Park. Heather had warned the police, who said this was a particularly hazardous thing to do because they were not "free to intervene" and strongly advised against it.

Perpetua said: "I have come to lead you out of here. You are all trying to escape from cruelty, violence and poverty and all that you do for escape is to inflict cruelty, violence and poverty on somebody else. It is so difficult to break this chain of cruelty, ugliness and poverty but God our Parent can do this." "So why did he drop us into this to begin with?" asked one of the gang. "God did not drop you into this; imperfect human nature means that people make all kinds of wrong choices. God says that what we have to do is to play the hand we have been dealt. The worse the hand, the more help we will get. This is a promise. When God flickers through our brain for a split second, all we have to do is to make it stick there for just a second longer. That is a beginning." "Why did my mum die of cancer, then?" asked another. "Because we can never live in freedom if there is no hardship. The problem for us is not the general idea of freedom and hardship but the way it strikes particular people and leaves others unhurt. We are often struck by how the wicked seem to thrive while the good seem to suffer. God knows why. Individual suffering is bound up with God's purpose for us but we do not know how. We can pray that it is taken away, as Jesus My Brother prayed before His death, but it is really a prayer for the strength we have already been promised; it is not really a prayer to change something. Now and again God does actively intervene and changes something without a human explanation; but mostly we are who we are with our joy and suffering and with God's great strength with us. These are difficult answers; but we all depend on other people to behave well and frequently they disappoint but you cannot blame God for that; and the problems get worse when people respond to bad behaviour with bad behaviour. It means that people end up not being able to trust each other. If we react to a lie by telling a lie we stop trusting other people but then they stop trusting us."

Perpetua knew she was right but felt uncomfortable. Human language just could not handle the relationship between God's love and earthly suffering. All she could do was to tell her listeners that whatever their sufferings they would be healed and whatever their wrongs they had been forgiven. She put her hands on the head of some people, hugged others, looked straight into the eyes of her listeners and made sure they looked straight into hers. With the help of God she could cure earthly sicknesses like addiction and she could give people hope but she knew that humanity cannot know the deep meaning of suffering. The small crowd went away quietly. Next day Perpetua received a threatening text telling her to stay out of Grunge Park affairs.

On Ash Wednesday she held the worship in Fallen Arches, the biggest fast food restaurant in Grunge Park but there was only bread and water on offer. She said: "This is the first day of Lent, the traditional time for turning back to God and getting ready for the death and Resurrection of Jesus My Brother. It is a time to remember some truths about ourselves: we are the richest people in history but we live amidst poverty and deprivation; luxury lives alongside degradation; we use force to control society instead of bringing love to grow society; we know more about medicine but live amongst sickness; we know more about damage to the earth but we go on damaging; we know more about the human psyche but allow child abuse and cruelty to travel down the generations; we know more about causality but resort to harsh criminal justice; we are rich and breed poverty; we are sophisticated and breed coarseness; we are safe and breed insecurity; we are clever and breed ignorance; we are powerful and breed cruelty.

"There will be no escape for the rich. We condemn and imprison the poor; we brand sickness as criminality; we punish the powerless for our own neglect. After two thousand years of time to reflect on the life, death and Resurrection of Jesus My Brother, we are still denying His message of love.

"Let me warn us all: turning to God is not a matter of throwing a few coins at the poor; it is not even a matter of giving a percentage of our wealth to those who need it; to turn back to God we have to give more than we can really afford. The richer we are, the more difficult it is. It is like everybody having to go through a very narrow space to get to a wonderful land; the more we are carrying, the more we have to drop before we can get through. The more we understand the human condition, the more responsibility we have to assuage the wrong, not by asserting our learning and being superior but by gently leading those who have gone astray. It is like explaining to the sick why a difficult operation will make them better and that they need not be afraid. They have no need of the fancy Latin and Greek words for what is going to happen; they need to trust our learning to go forward to what will help them. And, most of all, the better we know the way to that land, the more time we have to spend leading other people there; knowing God brings huge responsibility. Those who have had a glimpse of that wonderful land must share it with all their powers; it is like a traveller who returns from a long journey and takes responsibility for explaining as clearly and powerfully as she can what she has seen so that her travels are a source of richness to everybody not something she hoards exclusively or sells to a newspaper.

"We who are here now are rich and clever and many of us have travelled and enjoyed a glimpse of that wonderful land for which we use the word God or Heaven; but we have forgotten it because we are carried away by all kinds of distractions and indifferences. It is almost as if we are ashamed of what we have seen. Lent is the time to clear away the distractions and stretch out towards God."

The people came forward to Perpetua and she made a sign of the Cross on their foreheads with the traditional oil and ash and she gave each of them a set of *god4u* calling cards: "Remember that you are dust and to dust you will return but let Jesus live in you so that you can carry him to a stranger where He would be".

She blessed the bread and water, called on God Our Parent, Jesus Her Brother and Her Sister the Spirit to bring God to the people in these simple gifts.

Some people from the traditional churches were there and some from the house groups but many who went home, determined to change their selfish lives, had never heard of Jesus except for vague memories of the Christmas story; if they had ever known Easter, they had forgotten it.

30

Sneer, oblivious of Lent and of Perpetua's influence on the unchurched, decided to launch his major attack on the day after Ash Wednesday. The attack was unfounded but no less effective for that:

GOD4U GANG TARGETS CHURCH

In a move of breathtaking audacity Perpetua and her *god4u* followers plan to wipe out the traditional Christian churches and replace them with gangland religion made up of cells all headed by her own thugs.

Church of England sources have expressed concern that she is destroying the traditional fabric of Christianity, emptying the churches and dismantling parish organisation. Crisis talks are scheduled for later this week but insiders are not optimistic. There are rumours that Archbishop Hawthorne has some sympathies with Perpetua and there have been calls for his resignation and replacement by the more forthright Mwanga.

In spite of difficult relations between Anglicans and Orthodox Petrans the Pope has supported the Church by excommunicating Perpetua. In a gesture of unprecedented solidarity the Pontiff said that churches might disagree about difficult doctrinal issues but they were united in support of church order.

On the other hand, Perpetua's picture had begun to be familiar; she was on the cusp of B list and A list celebrity; people were beginning to notice her clothes, gestures, hair style, speech patterns, eating habits, catch phrases and routines, even if they were not the least bit interested in what she said. There was a marginality, edginess, radicalism about her which attracted some of the more adventurous fashion house and lifestyle outfits. She was offered a perfume deal but said that cleanliness was more important than fragrance; she was offered a fashion deal on casuals but said that people were more important than what they wore; she was offered a topless model deal but said that showing your love was more important than showing your breasts.

The BBC offered her a daily chat show but she knew she would only be a front for researchers, producers and business promotion executives; so she turned the offer down. Trina was furious but the risks of being manipulated and of losing credibility were too great even with her miraculous powers. People enjoyed watching daytime television chat but that was quite separate from according respect. In some ways the shows were more easy to watch if the participants were not worthy of respect.

The greatest surprise of all, however, came when Smoother called on her mobile for a meeting. The previous day he had held a meeting with Varnish, the self-appointed head of the traditionalist faction, and Digger, who was spearheading "Fresh Expressions". New urgency had been injected by Archbishop Hawthorne's Ash Wednesday Homily which had flirted dangerously, though elliptically, with some of Perpetua's main ideas: Varnish wanted to keep the church orderly; Digger wanted to keep "Fresh Expressions" under (his) tight control; and Smoother wanted to head off this crisis in view of the much more important business of the Anglican Communion's Osborne Process for delaying schism over homosexuality; or was it women bishops?

Smoother had three proposals: first, that Perpetua be nominated as the external expert to the Liturgy Commission; secondly, that she be the Special Adviser on the "Fresh Expressions" Commission; and thirdly, that if she refused both he should be given a free hand.

They compromised on Tate Modern because neither of them would particularly stand out there and their discomfort levels with incoherent profanity were about equal. "We have been watching your progress with interest," said Smoother. "I know. Your counterpart, Trina, keeps me informed." "We have taken note of your refreshing views on a variety of subjects and would like you to help us." "I like to be constructive but I am not sure I can help. Or, put it this way, if the church was capable of reform from inside, God Our Parent would not have sent me to do what I am doing. Do you honestly believe that most people understand all that Old Testament cruelty and the Greek obscurities of the Creed? Do you think the people living in extreme degradation two miles from here care about the dispute over faith and good works in Romans? Do you suppose that communities where the only good that springs up comes from women are going to listen to an organisation that is institutionally misogynist? On behalf of Jesus My Brother I tell you and your people—and I have been very moderate so far—that love is more important than doctrine; if we feel the love of good shining through our neighbour then we will soon find our way to God. And, by the way, before you reply, I know about your special relationship with Sneer. What do you think you are doing?"

Smoother got away as quickly as he could. The meeting had been more painful than he had expected but at least he now had his free hand. He phoned a man in Nigeria who phoned contacts in North Dakota, Labrador and Rhode Island who put out inflammatory statements. Smoother wrote an urgent note pressing Archbishop Hawthorne to intervene directly to keep the Osborne process on track and to save the Lambeth Conference from collapsing. He told Sneer that Trina was on to their relationship so they might as well go all out.

Anonymous messages were followed by graffiti in the hallways and lifts; then faeces through the letterbox; then petrol through the letterbox with a message: "Next time it will come with a match". Perpetua wanted to run away. Clearly Dexter's downstairs rota wasn't adequate. Bill offered her his retirement home some miles away, but she would not go. O'Helly would rather cross the street than talk to her; he had lost most of his people and did not know what to do. His homosexuality, long suppressed, surfaced more and more often; and his drinking was getting out of control. Miles called round and told Perpetua she had better leave. What Grunge Park needed was a steady build up of discipline as a precursor to some self-discipline rather than her sort of fireworks and forgiveness. What these people did should be condemned, not condoned; and Perpetua was eroding middle class support for mission.

G4U IN GANG WAR

shrieked the TT.

DISORDER BREEDS DISORDER

said C&S.

BAD COMPANY BACKLASH

thundered the cannon from The Fortress.

Will and Annie were ashamed when they saw the TT headline but they were so happy together.

31

As soon as the TT campaign started it began to experience odd technological problems. First, and most worrying, advertising files seemed to get lost between the final sub-edit and the presses; valuable revenue was lost, particularly from Hypo. Smaller but significant revenue was lost from soft porn ads (which the TT only printed in defence of press freedom); and in the editorial sections pictures of drugged or topless girls and boys with guns and knives regularly went missing. Then there was the strange way in which final copy got altered which was funny at first but which soon made the TT into a laughing stock. For instance during one week in Lent its first headline was printed as edited:

PERPETUA VOWS TO SLUG IT OUT

But the next day's:

WE WILL STOP AT NOTHING G4U GANG VOW

mysteriously turned into:

WE WILL GO ON LOVING G4U VOW

between the editing and printing processes.
This was followed the next day by:

PERPETUA MOLE IN TT SCAM

but the day after, instead of the planned:

PERPETUA SLAMS PRESS FREEDOM

The headline came out as:

PERPETUA EXCLUSIVE IN TT

with 400 words on the leader page where the latest attack should have been.

Sneer could not explain this to management. There was a feverish internal security drive and the paper was produced in the "Exclusives pen" so that only a few people knew what would be on the first few pages; but the inconsistency went on.

The headline that most upset Smoother had been edited as:

HAWTHORNE DENOUNCES PERPETUA

but had appeared as:

which the poor, torn Archbishop was forced to deny.

After the mysterious copy switch on the leader page Sneer decided to cut his losses. The thought never crossed his mind that the accidents were directly linked to Perpetua's self-proclaimed and frequently reported powers yet his accusations of infiltration were only half-hearted. But he did not like coincidence. Things had continued to go wrong even when production went to the "pen" and that was unheard of.

Down at CEC, incidents were less spectacular but equally puzzling. g4u-TV kept cutting into CEC transmissions. After a relaxation of the adult material regulations as the result of a victory by porn king libertarians over religious minority control freaks, Will's late night Fang had been superseded by an American porn series called Bang! But there had never been a complete episode. Every time there was even a foreshadowing of violence or exploitative sex, G4U would cut in. It was usually Perpetua speaking quietly about love and respect.

At Hypo the technology was also playing up. The tills would not read bar codes of goods specified in the walk-out of Perpetua's people so that hot cross buns and Easter eggs piled up in the warehouse as the contractors went on delivering. Sometimes when they were brought out, they went through the tills at £00.00 and at other times they just jammed the tills altogether. In a scandalous breach of triopoly solidarity Jambo had gone back on its initial tough stance and had caved in to god4u demands. Its tills were working perfectly and it began to gain market share from its superior check out speed. People found that they could do without the hot cross buns and Easter eggs for a while. As Lent went by, its extra sales exceeded the forecast sales loss for Good Friday.

"When you are getting ready for God," said Perpetua, standing near the Hypo entrance, "it is important to put that first; what that means is delayed gratification. It is not 'me' and 'now!' It is 'You' and 'Later'."

Annie came out to protest. "You have taken things too far, preaching against people buying things at my very front door." "But I am not against people buying things; I am just against the obsession with instant gratification; with the headlong drive to make the future the present: Christmas in August; Easter in February; Spring fashions in January; beachwear in April; Autumn suits in July and Winter coats in September. Nobody can wait for anything; and then, when it is hot in Summer or cold in Winter there are no appropriate clothes." "Hypo can now turn round fashion items in two weeks," said Annie, defensively. "I know it can, with the help of sweat shops, but that does not invalidate my main point."

Perpetua started to talk to a small crowd: "We all want to be the first on and the first off airlines; but travelling towards God is not like that. Those who wait, who are patient, who find a moment to pray, will meet God. Meeting God is standing still.

"Sometimes consuming is necessary—we all need to eat—but so often it is display, or competition or, right at the root, trying to fill a spiritual gap with things. But there is a limit to the benefit from things. There will never be enough. When we have laboured for something precious we should hold on to that and value it instead of always wanting more of the same. Instead of filling up space with things we should leave it empty for God.

"The organised church has been deeply suspicious of mystics because they cannot be controlled. They sit and God comes to them when nobody can see what is happening. It is wonderful to rejoice with God on big occasions—it is part of what we are to worship God together on a regular basis—but in our frenetic world what is most needed is to look for God in a stolen, quiet moment, to stop and look at a picture, to see God in our neighbour's face, to listen to the words of a song, to recognise that the joy of love-making is God-given. Look around now, at the car park and the gaudy shop front; and let us see if we can see God. See God in the sky above, in the distant trees, in the gifts of creation on the Special Offers board, in the light and the colour and the sound; but, most of all, in each other. God is the simple answer to why there is something rather than nothing, but God is not a weird, distant, unknown force; God made all of us and wants a relationship with all of us, and in a relationship there have to be two parties; God looks for us and we look for God, and we find each other through the life of My Brother Jesus; and we find each other in moments of joy and in moments of quiet; in moments when we are making space for ourselves and for other people. We do not find God in the rush and tumble, in the headlong pursuit, in the selfish grasp, but in the standing back, in the smile. If we imagine all the good in the world that there has ever been, all the kindnesses we have ever known, all the love we have ever seen, these are just tiny fragments of what God is. It is as if we are standing in a drizzle but never see the sea, as if we have only ever seen a bunch of flowers but never see a meadow, as if we see a line drawing but never see the motor car, as if we see a recipe book but are not allowed to eat. This earth is so wonderful but it is still only a shadow; and because we are not perfect, because we are created to choose, whatever the vision we might have of God is obscured, made dark and dirty, by our wrong choices."

Perpetua said a little prayer and went away. Annie had almost forgiven her.

32

Bob was reluctant to say goodbye to the bus he had been driving for the past eight months but Perpetua said it would not be needed any more. He was consoled slightly by her request to find an open-topped bus for Palm Sunday. Perpetua had also given up her Grunge Park flat, saying that they would be staying in a friend's large flat in Bleak Villas until Easter. She had said goodbye to Grunge Park the night before in an act of worship at the youth club. It was the most enthusiastic reception she had ever received perhaps because, for the first time, she really emphasised the way ahead, the time to come: "We should look at ourselves, knowing that together we will all find our way to God Our Parent. I will be killed before very long." "No!" they all shouted. "You will not die; we will protect you". Dexter tried to grab the mike but he did not need to as his voice cut through the air: "I will protect you to the end, even with my life." She smiled and went on: "But in a way I can not explain, I will come back and I will always be with you, as will my Sister the Spirit who will look after all of us." They had all volunteered to come into London the next day. Miles, who had changed profoundly in the last few months, was enthusiastic.

Buses came from all over the country and thousands of Londoners, too, converged on Royal Park. Each set of house groups had its own banner and they were ranged in a circle round a central platform with the rest of the huge crowd spread out behind. Perpetua arrived in the open-topped bus like a rock star. She held up a massive palm branch and people cheered. Using her radio mike she led the chant: "Blessed be Jesus Our Brother"; but the Ten had worked out a different strategy. Brian cut off her mike and switched on those in the hands of her followers who began to chant: "Blessed be Perpetua, True Sister of Jesus and True God".

This was a bit of a mouthful and was soon reduced to: "Sister and God!"

Contrary to previous practice, she let it happen. A few of the crowd had come with misgivings but were carried away with emotion. To his acute embarrassment a group of Miles' former Toran friends took turns with a megaphone to shout insults, accusing Perpetua of blasphemy and of corrupting the people. O'Helly had lost the energy to do much himself but had found a strong Petran advocate who shouted such slogans as: "Church wrecker!" and "Gay lover!". Bill Midway was deeply involved with what Perpetua was saying but he was aware of some former colleagues on the fringe. The Church of England had chosen not to mount a public protest but he had spotted Varnish and he was almost certain he had seen Smoother talking to a knot of journalists.

The BBC had not asked Perpetua's permission to broadcast the event as this was classified as news not as a special programme. It was the first time it had scheduled live coverage of one of Perpetua's events. Annie, after a lot of thought, had also forgiven Perpetua and Corporate Centre had agreed that this would be a brilliant PR opportunity. There were special Hypo stands with hot cross buns, Easter eggs, crosses and crucifixes, chocolate rabbits, palm branches and palm crosses, Holy Week books and budget CD's of Bach Passions and various Lamentations.

"This is the day on which Jesus My Brother rode into Jerusalem on a donkey; the crowd cheered him, his own followers and all the people; and inside a week he was dead; the people had called for his crucifixion and his followers had run away.

"That is what is going to happen to me. You might shout 'Sister and God' now—and so I am—but within a week I will be dead; and most of you will not care and my followers will have run away. The only difference between my fate and that of Jesus My Brother is that He was killed by religious passion, I will be overwhelmed by the hopeless failure of Christianity to heal the broken who bind their wounds with booze, drugs and exploitation, taking revenge on the people and the society that have let them down.

"That, however, is not the main point. We are here today to celebrate two things: first, in the week before his death, the wonderful life of Jesus My Brother; secondly, the wonderful turning to Jesus that I have seen in the past few months with sisters and brothers from different sections of our torn society coming together. They have often had to leave behind their comfort zone in lovely, settled church communities and go into places they have previously been frightened to enter; and many of the clergy that have listened to this message of direct concern have bravely gone with them to witness to my Brother in sad and sometimes dangerous places. This has been very difficult for the established Christian Churches; but how they feel about me and the issues I have raised is far more important than how they feel about the sexuality and gender issues that currently divide them.

"When my life here comes to an end, try to remember that God Our Parent, Jesus My Brother, My Sister the Spirit and I will not abandon you; we will be with you until you join us at your death."

"Blasphemy!" chorused Miles' friends.

"Forget words like that," said Perpetua. "You are doing so well trying to help the poor and the unfortunate; stick to love and forget the theology!"

She asked Jim to lead the people into a song and, leaving the bus behind, she raised her wooden cross and started to walk Eastwards.

After a tumultuous day, when everything had been cleared away, her followers joined her in Bleak Villas, beneath the airport flight path.

"When I have gone," she said, "it will not be enough to remember me in England. Travel and communications are so easy now that my message should go all over the world."

"Remember, we asked you at the beginning," said Wayne, "about whether non-Christians should join us." "Yes," said Perpetua, "I remember. God Our Parent, who made the world, is the parent of all and, through Jesus My Brother, all people can enjoy direct two-way communication with God; and they are here to decide whether to do that. But people can only decide if they are given the choice and it is the responsibility of Christians to offer not to judge; offer the Word Made Human in my Brother to everyone; there is a world communications system. It is useless and unworthy to say to people who look for God in other ways that they are wrong or that they will be barred from uniting with God Our Parent; make them the offer, do your best but do not condemn; to say that people are wrong is either to say that we have not communicated effectively—which may be true—or, much worse, to say that God has not communicated effectively with them. Remember, you cannot say that God created everything and then say that Islam or Hinduism are an exception."

33

For once, Sneer was swept away by popular emotion. He had tried to buck the trend and diverge from his main competitors—always a high risk—and it had failed. The Perpetua campaign had been a flop and it was now time to cut his losses. He had not been carried away as part of the crowd—journalists were always at, yet not of, situations—but he had been impressed. He had actually wanted to interview Perpetua about the death threats but she had disappeared. He was collared by Smoother as he left the Park. Smoother had never seen him like this; instead of the calm which gave nothing away, he was agitated. "What did you think about that show?" asked Smoother. "A straight copy of Palm Sunday in the Gospels except it's a blasphemous woman hinting at death threats to drum up sympathy." Sneer said nothing, sensing that if he left Smoother for long enough he would say something useful. "It is bad enough having this disruption at a time when we thought church attendance was beginning to consolidate and even grow in some places but now Hawthorne is beginning to undercut our stance by hinting that Perpetua might have something. And all this is on top of the Osborne process which looks as if it is falling apart. Well, that is not quite true but," and here Sneer had his reward, "it is important to keep the fire stoked up in various parts of the Anglican Communion as it will give Hawthorne something to do while we try to sort out this attack on our structures. It is highly unusual for the ABC to be away from home base at Easter—highly unusual—but I think we can make this necessary."

Sneer, who had no time for the complexities of Church or any other kind of politics, saw "two birds" immediately, so clearly that he needed no additional guidance from Dowte. He could change his stance on Perpetua under the cover of maintaining his attack on Hawthorne:

WORLD EXCLUSIVE

HAWTHORNE DITCHED

AS PERPETUA DEATH THREAT LOOMS

In a World Exclusive the TT has learned that high Church of England officials are plotting to overthrow Archbishop Hawthorne of Canterbury for being "soft" over the Perpetua issue. As an interim measure the beleaguered and confused Primate is being shunted off to distant parts of the Anglican Communion to damp down dissent which is being deliberately stoked by senior Church House insiders.

In a related development Perpetua announced the startling news yesterday that she has received anonymous death threats to be carried out at Easter. Hawthorne is said to sympathise with some of Perpetua's views in spite of her attacks on traditional Christianity which have left officials fuming as congregations plunge.

Not surprisingly, given Perpetua's high profile threat to established churches, no Christian spokesman was prepared to condemn the death threats and one senior Toran who refused to be named said: "She has been trying to wreck the church and introduce her own blasphemous heresies; you know what they say about people who play with fire."

Perpetua's sensational news came in a triumphal rally yesterday at Royal Park when followers from all over the country came to celebrate the success of the *god4u* mission. Hundreds of people were in tears as she gave her message of darkness and hope: "I didn't know whether to laugh or cry," said a stalwart who had travelled all the way from Stumpy Knoll.

In general, media coverage was split between populist adulation and establishment cynicism. The news bulletins and the tabloids had a new hero who was exciting, glamorous and now under a death threat. The discussion programmes and Berliners thought the claim of anyone to be God was not serious. Most clever people did not believe in God but those who did knew that the big questions had been settled long ago. It was unthinkable to re-write the basic Christian doctrines; they were all settled. The kind of Christianity which was now practised was mercifully mute and had some social cohesion value but there was enough fundamentalism about without the Church of England being undermined. Naturally there were a few Toran extremists who wanted a Spartan church reminiscent of Oliver Cromwell's extremists and there were some Petrans who wanted to take the church on a return journey to Rome but the majority needed to stay firmly in the middle. The country was entitled to expect its established church to behave in proper English fashion, with a lack of emotion, a degree of understatement, a great deal of pragmatism and an appropriate level of hypocrisy. It would not be long before the nation would need a Coronation ceremony and the established church was the monopoly provider. The Archbishop of Canterbury and his fellow Bishops might, in this respect, be the ecclesiastical equivalent of the monkeys of Gibraltar; they were not very important but people would feel very uncomfortable if they became extinct.

Smoother was furious that he had let his guard drop. It almost wrecked his plans but Hawthorne had finally agreed to prolong his stay in North America in spite of his feeling that he was being manipulated and his sense that Perpetua's initiative could give new vigour to divided and exhausted Christianity. It did not matter what he did about the factions struggling over homosexuality while the core of the Church rotted. It was worse than the clichés about fiddling while Rome burned or re-arranging the deck chairs on the Titanic; this was a power struggle being waged by the clergy in direct and clear contradiction of the teaching of Jesus. They had become so power mad that they were blind; and there was nothing he could do. This made the decision about staying or coming home almost impossible.

Over and above the Hawthorne episode, Smoother's position was difficult. Sympathy for Perpetua had measurably increased in recent days and the Church had been implicitly linked to death threats against her. He needed her to be discredited by proxy. He could not trust the Torans because they were apt to sound off without checking with colleagues. He went back to the database and looked at reports of Perpetua's followers. Surely he could get something really serious from the Grunge Park ghetto. He called his daughter, Poppy.

Heather had been growing restless. In the world of drug dealing she had been a rising star, fuelling her own delusions with as much cocaine as she needed, still leaving enough money for whatever else she wanted. The Perpetua experience had been brilliant at first, offering new opportunities; and for a while she had enjoyed the return of clarity and order to her thoughts. As time went by, however, the lure of money and her kind of power became stronger. She had decided to give Perpetua one last chance at the Palm Sunday event but it had been a disaster; just a lot of talk by one person. Her followers were supposed to share the celebrity which Perpetua now enjoyed but she was not sharing it. As if it had never been different, Heather caught Jo's eye on the way out of Royal Park. They said nothing as they headed in the opposite direction to Perpetua and the rest of her followers, back to Grunge Park. Heather contacted Roy, Dexter's gang leader successor, enlisted with her old supplier and they both scored.

Next morning, sour and slightly disoriented after their first session in months, Heather and Jo talked about Perpetua. "She keeps talking about drugs," said Heather, "but she doesn't know anything about the joy and the danger, the ups and the downs." "Why not," said Jo, "give her a big dose of medicine and see how she reacts?" "That would show her; that would take the pious smile off her face and bring her right up against reality. We can always get her down here by saying that somebody desperately needs her and then we can do what we like; we will have plenty of help. A lot of the dealers and gang people have got fed up of her and want to go back to their old, familiar ways."

Poppy Smoother approached the girls cautiously. "Didn't I see you with Perpetua yesterday?" "No, not us," said Heather. "We don't have time for that pious weirdo. She was brought up here but thought she was better." "But surely I saw you yesterday?" "No you didn't," said Jo. "We were down here with some of the gang." "But if I go back into my folder for yesterday I am certain I will find your pictures." "Look; we've told you. Anyway, what do you want? If you don't watch yourself you will be in trouble. You might accidentally drop your phone down that grate and then where will your precious folders be?" "OK!" said Poppy, nervously. "I am making an investigative documentary on the drug scene in Grunge Park. Not the usual sort of stuff with experts and doctors and MPs; no, I want some real shots of real people doing real things." "Well, it's quite complicated," said Heather, "but we could do something—depending, of course, on the money. There is a drug scene in Grunge Park but it's not just locals. People come in from outside to enjoy the genuine gangland experience. We call them RIFs, 'rich fakes'. There's a group coming down this weekend so you can check out the genuine scene: locals, RIFs and—wow, yes—what about … No! … why not! Look, we need you to keep a secret for a few days if you want a really good programme."

She called on her mobile. A few minutes later a boy came round the corner on a motorbike. "Roy, this is Poppy; she wants to make a television programme about gang life. It would be good for us because loads more kids would learn about the way we live and that would mean bigger sales from richer kids; but we want a special feature and this will only work if we can plan and also if she knows what we're planning; but she has to swear to keep silent and not share the story." "But I never share stories," said Poppy. "But this is so big you might want to share it and take the money. All journalists are only in it for what they can get out of it." "Well, what's the big story then?" asked Poppy, petulantly but still nervously. "Well," said Heather, "Perpetua used to be a drug dealer." "What!" "Yeh-No, that's interesting but it's not the real story. If you come down on Friday night you can watch the pious Perpetua taking drugs!"

Poppy only just controlled her urge to dial her office. This was the biggest story she had ever had; and it was a massive break in her first week at CEC where she had replaced Will who had been fired at the same time that the Chief Accountant retired. "Well, I am going to have to tell my bosses as we want this to be real, actuality, live TV; no cuts; no fancy edits; just reality as it is out on the streets." "Suits us," said Heather. "But if it gets out," she looked at Roy, "you will be in serious trouble."

Poppy went straight to the top at CEC and got the resources she needed. This was a case of boom or bust. The station was in serious trouble but it had promised its audience and its bankers a spectacular Easter. The promise had been hollow when it was made but now it looked as if there would be a real story over the holiday weekend. Poppy also got permission for CEC to team up with the TT on the story; and she also told her father to prove that she was a real journalist, a chip off the old block. Smoother said it was best if he knew nothing in advance.

Sneer, who had quickly grown bored with and somewhat ashamed of his

Perpetua euphoria, had no trouble adjusting to the old, more familiar pattern after a rather breathless call from Poppy:

PERPETUA OUTED AS DRUG DEALER

In a shock development Perpetua has been outed as a former Grunge Park drug dealer. In a sensational programme this weekend CEC will reveal that the self-proclaimed saint used to deal in drugs before taking up her pious mantle.

Sources say that the shocking news was revealed by one of Perpetua's inner circle who is: "Sick and tired of her soppy face all over the media telling everybody what an angel she is. When she lived in Grunge Park she was as good and as bad as the rest of us. How do you suppose she got her glamorous *god4u* clothes? It wasn't by praying or even shelf stacking at Hypo. She thought she was too good for honest work so drugs was the easy thing to do."

A Church of England spokesman said: "We have to be careful how we deal with allegations of wrongdoing, particularly when the person involved claims a special closeness to God, but on the face of it this looks grim. We were always worried about her followers and now, it seems, one of them has told us what many have suspected for a long time."

The police, who would not normally bother about a trivial allegation of drug dealing, were quickly onto the case. As clear-up rates fell they were ever more aware of the need to give high profile people as much grief as possible. They had had a grand old time with the Prime Minster over Cash for Peerages; Perpetua was only a medium sized fish but it would fill an Easter weekend when competition was not so tough for front page stories.

Trina, horrified, immediately identified Heather and Jo as the culprits and wanted to have them disowned; but Perpetua said that they must have the opportunity to say sorry and start afresh; the life of people involved with drugs was complex and unhappy.

Whatever the outcome of that issue, however, Trina insisted that Perpetua should hold a news conference the next day.

34

"I am not in the habit of making formal statements," said Perpetua, "so this one will be very short. I have never been a drug dealer and I have never used any illegal drugs, nor have I ever drunk alcohol, other than the Sacrament."

"So are you saying that your own followers are liars?" "I have no idea as they have not told me what you say they told you; but, taking the worst case that they are the people who accused me and that they are therefore liars, the key issue is not what they said about me but that they should recognise their lie and we should forgive them so that we can all start again." "Isn't that just a bit cosy?" "No; admitting you are wrong is difficult; and forgiving people who hurt us is difficult. What you call 'cosy' is the toughest thing of all. The easiest course would be for us to do what most of us do; to avoid each other so that we never make a new start. Whoever accused me of drug dealing, whether a supposed informant or a fraudulent journalist, should say sorry to God and to me; and then we can start again."

Trina did not know whether this was a good or a bad move; it would certainly get the journalists off the drugs story; they were always much more interested in themselves than anything else. "Are you saying that a journalist on CEC or the TT would manufacture a story about you which involved a criminal offence?" "I certainly am. It may not be so, it probably is not so in this case, but that does not mean such a situation is not possible. The press is not, as it pompously calls itself 'The Fourth Estate' or the 'Guardian of Liberty'. The commercial sector is interested in profit and others, such as the BBC, are interested in power and ego. Still, I do not blame you all that much; there is so much temptation in money and power. Jesus My Brother said the rich would find it more difficult to be virtuous than the poor. The people I really blame are Christian churches which have tried to make a better world by controlling what journalists do (the supply side) instead of concentrating on changing the hearts and minds of people so that they voluntarily refrain from buying what journalists produce (the demand side). Torans and Petrans are obsessed with controlling supply but the essence of Christianity is growing demand." "Isn't this just the usual case of blaming the messenger instead of the message?" "No; I am not blaming the messenger. As I said, to describe what you do and to try to understand how tempted you are is not the same as blaming you. But that is not the issue here. Can you, any of you, honestly say that you never print or broadcast anything unless you are sure that it is accurate? And, even if it is accurate, can you honestly say that you think about the hurt it might cause?" "Are you prepared to give yourself up to the police?" "I will do precisely what the law of the land requires. Just because I love God Our Parent and Jesus My

Brother I am not obliged to pretend to do things I have not done; and I am not obliged to make it easier for anybody to convict me. I am at peace with God and that is what really matters; but the law must be observed. I doubt, however, that the police will find anything to interest them. When you began to trawl through the histories of my followers what you came up with was pretty pathetic and you found nothing about me. I have created enough grudges since I started fighting the drugs business and yet you have produced nothing until now. What does that say about your journalistic professionalism? Or perhaps, as I claim, I am totally innocent and an unchecked story was published." "What do you think of the church's attitude to your predicament?" "It is difficult to make a generalisation from a few anonymous comments but I get the impression that the Christian establishment is pretty pleased. It is much more interested in being the establishment than in being Christian. Since I began to lead people back to Jesus My Brother, the issue has not been what I have said, although some of this, I recognise, is quite difficult for traditional Christians; the real issue has been what I have done. If I had gone from church to church preaching my radical theology I would have been tolerated, even welcomed, by most except the most extreme Torans and Petrans; but what has made things tense is my insistence that the physical assets and hierarchy of the church are the chief barriers between God Our Parent and us. Even when people start by arguing about what they think are important issues, they end up arguing about one of these. Torans say that if the rest of the church does not agree with them they will stop contributing to any central fund and will just look after their own. Petrans, on the other hand, are most concerned, no matter how a discussion starts, with authority. The vast majority of Medians are frightened of losing any more money or authority; they want a bit of both and a monopoly of neither." "Are you saying that the church is corrupt?" "No, just misled. It happened when Jesus My Brother wanted the Chosen People to turn back to God; there was a terrible obsession with the minutiae of the Law. We have the same problem now and it is sad that we have not learned from the past. I am not, however, going to hurl accusations. It is so difficult for a church besieged by atheism and materialism, indifference and relativism, to imagine how it can survive without its Bishops and Cathedrals, priests and churches; or, alternatively, its Scriptures and rules, moral certainties and power to judge. Christians need to have faith in God Our Parent and Jesus My Brother and listen to My Sister the Spirit because faith is the most difficult thing of all; it is so much easier to cling to buildings and traditions, to lovely old churches and lovely old rituals, to safety and power. No doubt the Jews at the time of Jesus thought that their lovely old building and lovely old rituals were essential to their spiritual life; but it is so easy to persuade ourselves that what we like is what is good for us."

"What do you think the church should do, then, just walk away from its buildings and sack its clergy?" "No; that would be such a wrench that it would do much more harm than good, like a forty-a-day smoker suddenly giving up altogether. The Petrans need, over time, to feel less need to be in charge and everybody, over time, needs to feel less need for buildings. As their faith builds, their need for these physical supports should reduce. At the same time, Torans need time to modify their obsession with Scripture and judgment.

"Let me put it like this: an old man who was a millionaire built a school. He wanted the children to learn through thinking and creating, through discussion and experiment, through collaborative rather than individual effort; in other words, it was to be a place of mutual love and respect where everybody accorded everybody mutual concern and respect. There was no rigid curriculum because you could never forecast what would happen with a pool of creative young minds working together in numberless combinations; and you could not control outcomes. At the beginning, the children were as thoughtful and creative as the old man could have wished but after he died the school gradually became more and more like other schools. Children began to spend more time on standard tasks set by teachers and because they ended up doing the same things they began to make comparisons with each other and became competitive. Then, because they became competitive, abandoning the self discipline of collaboration, teachers had to impose discipline and set boundaries; and in the end they had to punish children for being aggressive. That is what happened to the world after God Our Parent created it. That is what happened to the Church after Jesus My Brother visited it. I was sent to reinstate that old man's dream, God's wish, the wish of Jesus My Brother."

"Well, that's very nice," said Sneer, "but why should we listen to all this cant from a hypocrite?" "I am prepared to be judged on how well I represent and live by the standards of God Our Parent and Jesus My Brother. Your question implies that only totally pure people can ever give an opinion about the behaviour of others; this goes back to Jesus saying that he who is without sin should cast the first stone but casting a stone in individual judgment of a fellow human being is quite different from expressing a view of how people individually and collectively should try to behave towards themselves, each other and God. If journalists are saying that only the pure should pontificate, then he who is without sin should write the first story."

Trina knew by now that no matter how well the news conference had gone it would make no difference to the coverage which would be disastrous for Perpetua. It was. She had made the mistake of denying an accusation and refusing to say sorry but, much worse, she had attacked the media. They would have no mercy.

35

Perpetua set up a stand within reach of the Orthodox Petran, Anglican and Toran headquarters, right in the heart of Government. She was surrounded by followers but Heather and Jo were missing.

"I have brought the message of God Our Parent and Jesus My Brother to poor and desolate people; but I would be failing if I did not bring it to the rich and powerful.

"It is easy to make predictions like a canny fortune teller: everybody knows that our economic system of injustice is unsustainable; everybody knows that liberal democracy has lost the will to fight for liberalism; everybody knows that we have the dreadful combination of free market capitalism and sneering elitism; everybody knows what the solutions are to our problems but we will not face the truth or meet the cost.

"My mission, then, is not to tell people in this centre of power what they already know. My message is one of affirmation. There is no point hankering after a church filled with people who do not want to be there, filled with serfs and servants, the backbone of the conforming church; we will not see it in our lifetime. We are called upon, as a minority, to be the affirming church; not to cower in corners of vast, empty, expensive heritage sites, but to walk out into the light, as small tokens of the love of Jesus. Just as the Church which My Brother founded was first for the poor, then taken over by the powerful and the rich and then made into an instrument of social control, now we are back at the beginning. I am re-founding the Church as My Brother founded it, as a reservoir of affirmation, as the vibrant meeting place of My Sister the Spirit. I know why people hanker after the past, looking for security and comfort; and we must always be respectful and sympathetic to those who have such needs; but the church which I have come to re-constitute is a place of outwardness and adventure, of resource and risk.

"There are many that say that the Church is dead. It is not, it is just facing the wrong way; it is facing inwards towards those who, no matter how imperfectly, have glimpsed the vision of oneness with God Our Parent. They have become trapped in the spell of the mirror, of seeing themselves instead of seeing God. They are good people but have lost the capacity to be good to anybody else; they are, only in a static sense, good. We have to look outwards to where we fear to go. Fear is the consequence of weakening faith. If we trust in God we will walk out into the world without fear.

"This whole superstructure of conforming will disintegrate. As God gave human beings, as their quintessential quality, the power to choose to love; and as God also gave free will and freedom of conscience, organising a Church through social control is doomed.

"There is only affirmation, there is nothing else."

"But," asked Dexter, "what are we to do about all the dead wood, about the massive financial and human investment in churches and hierarchies?"

"What I showed in leading people out was only a demonstration of what is needed. I do not mean to trigger a massive exodus, making people disoriented and powerless. My aim is to make people powerful. Leading out only took place when we were there to provide the right support.

"The superstructure of Western Christendom will collapse because it is in fundamental conflict with the purposes of God Our Parent as articulated by Jesus My Brother. He brought good news for the poor; it brings comfortable news for the rich. He placed love above the law; it places law above love. He warned against judgment; it is mired in judgment.

"Every day people leave the Church because of their personal disagreement with hymns, vestments, incense, bells, textual translation, candles, the attitude of the Vicar, financial pressures, peer unkindness, standing and kneeling, orders of service and the variety of communion wine. They are saying that all these trivial things are more important than God; and so they are saying there is no God. If God is inferior in importance to ritual and rubric then whatever phenomenon they seek to worship it is not God.

"The Church, in fellowship with those who bear the burdens of state, needs courage and simplicity: without them the world will plunge into ever worse crises of man's making; with them there will still be crises but people will face them better if there is genuine, uncontaminated hope.

"When I have gone this will all be made even more plain to you. My Sister the Spirit will find a way, after you have abandoned me, into your injured hearts. The Spirit has always been in the church of Christ My Brother but this will create a new level of hope. You are frightened now of hostility but what will make you really afraid will be indifference. When you talk about God you will not be attacked, you will not be laughing stocks, you will not be threatened or injured; you will be marginalised, made unimportant and obscure. People will want to make you the subject of mild humour and vague nostalgia. You will be the sacred equivalent of town criers; dressed up, ornate, lovable, figures of pageant but of another time and place.

"There will be no measurable triumph; there will be no victory; there will be no conversion of thousands; there will be no grand gestures; there will be no sudden gifts; there will be no imposing churches; there will be no letters from Bishops; there will be no thanks. There will only be the Word Made Flesh in quiet people, of Jesus living in humble hearts, of the Spirit protecting the distant and dispersed, the pioneers and the persistent.

"When you go out and see the churches empty do not rejoice; this is the sadness of the bygone age, of the failed dictatorship of piety. Learn from the grim doors and grimy windows. Do not resent those who love our heritage but do not mistake heritage for hope. Do not be nostalgic for the age of Paul, or the age of Augustine, or Luther, or Wesley, or Newman, or any other figure of the Church. Search instead for God in children whose lives lean forward; search for Christ in his sisters and brothers whose energy is pent up and contaminated by parental materialism. Set them free from the harm done to them.

"You are witnesses of God living in all of us, not in the Church, not in the articulate, not in the listed building, not in the charity fête; but God living in the discontented and the disconnected, in the fragment of prayerful anger, in the word hardly said, in the flicker between nothingness and nothingness when a faint spark leaps."

36

Perpetua texted Heather and Jo and said that they should come to the evening worship. She had heard rumours that they were the source of the bad press coverage but that made no difference.

Heather and Jo hung back but, even though Perpetua greeted them as warmly as the rest, they received some very hostile looks and some of the others began to whisper. "Let us look at ourselves," said Perpetua. "We are all capable of making mistakes, of being proud or thoughtless. We all have moments of weakness. Heather and Jo may have said things they should not have said but before the Easter Vigil you will all have let me down." "Not me," said Dexter. "You more than anyone," said Perpetua. They all went quiet.

As each of The Ten arrived, she told them to take off their shoes. She lined them up and started cleaning them. "You can't do that," said Dexter; but she said: "You have to see that I can only lead if I am your servant." Dexter replied: "Well, if that is how it must be you can wash my underpants." "There is no need to go over the top; the shoes will be enough. The important thing is that you must all behave like servants not like masters. Just as I have been your servant, you must serve the world. When things go badly you will be safe but when things go well you will be tempted by power. Then, when things go badly again, you will be tempted to blame other people and want even more power to ensure that things go well. But the power of God works in people when they choose to love; and remember what I have always said to you: love is creating space for others because everyone is a child of God Our Parent; and, in creating space for others, you are creating space for God within you."

When she had finished cleaning the shoes she made each sit on a stool. She put the shoes on their feet and carefully tied the laces, each according to the individual fashion, remembering the different configurations. "This is our farewell party," she said. "Concentrate, remember how it feels so you can carry the memory with you." "Why are we talking about farewells?" asked Wayne. "Are you going somewhere else without us? We've stuck together in spite of difficulties." "Is that why you sold the bus?" asked Bob. "I am travelling into the unimaginable but you cannot ever reach there unless I go first and send back more strength for your journey. If I stay now we will not move on. You will have to learn to do without the physical me; but I will always be with you."

As it began to grow dark they gathered round the table. "I have ordered a takeaway but it is a bit special. I have ordered dishes from many lands to remind us that we must go out into the world. We must try to eat things outside our comfort zone. So if you usually stick to pizza you must try something different."

All the food was put in the middle of the table on a revolving stand and they helped each other. For the time that they were eating they almost forgot their sadness but they kept wondering what Perpetua meant when she said this was a farewell party. "Just as Jesus My Brother came into the world for a while and then went back to join God Our Parent, so I must leave. He was betrayed and I will be betrayed; He was killed and I will be killed; but He came back from the dead and I will come back."

When the meal was over, Heather and Jo got ready to leave but Perpetua said: "Not yet; just one more thing before you go.

"Ever since Jesus offered the bread and wine on what we call Maundy Thursday, Christians have celebrated the sacred mystery of His true body and blood in these simple things. The Church has remembered the steadiness of the bread but has forgotten the risk of the wine, remembered the solidity of flesh but forgotten the trickling away of the blood. It has kept the body and blood in silver and gold. I will offer the sacrifice of the body and blood of Jesus but the bread and wine will be in glass so that all may see it in its fragile containers. The glass represents me; I am the Sacred Vessel which contains the body and blood of Jesus My Brother, I am the special vessel of His inheritance. I am not Him but I am of Him as I am of God Our Parent. Never again hide My Brother in silver and gold; never again dress Him in jewels; never again make His presence a secret. Jesus here with us is a mystery not a secret. God has given us My Sister the Spirit so that we may approach the mystery in faith.

"I call upon My Sister the Spirit to bless these gifts and to unite us with the whole world in the offering of this sacrifice."

Taking the bread she said: "This is my body given for the whole world so that all of God's children, filled with this immortal food, may learn to love." And taking the wine, she said: "This is my blood, renewed in the Third Covenant for the Third Millennium, shed for all the world, to be shown to all the world, to be carried into every street and every home. Whenever you sacrifice this bread and wine remember Jesus My Brother and, in the light and clarity of the glass which bears Him, remember me." When they had finished passing the bread and wine round the table, Heather and Jo slipped out. They sang a hymn and half of them left but Perpetua asked Dexter, Trina, Andy and Kylie to stay behind. She wanted them to pray with her but their minds kept wandering, sometimes thinking about the stories in the press, sometimes trying to blot them out by inventing bright futures for them all. In the end, Perpetua said they should leave her alone. The sadness she felt after all the time they had spent together was unbearable; even now they could not focus on what mattered, their minds so easily wandered back to their own concerns.

Perpetua shut the door gently and began to cry.

37

Bill Midway's congregation came home on Good Friday, bringing new friends from the house groups who had never been in a church before. They had processed through Grunge Park, alternating hymns and silence, led by Bill and Perpetua who took turns to carry the cross. They had gone on steadily through the taunts and the traffic, through the noise and the nastiness; they had a sense of purpose and momentum which they had never felt before.

In the whole of Bill's time there had never been so many people in church on Good Friday. Bill led the two hours by the Cross, with Perpetua sitting quietly at the back with all of the Ten except Heather and Jo.

Just after two o'clock, as Bill was standing at the West door about to walk through the church with the cross, all the lights went out, the organ pump stopped and there was complete silence. More candles were lit; there was obviously a power cut as neighbouring buildings had lost their lights which would now have been visible as the sky grew ever darker. There was thunder in the air.

When Bill steadied himself, Perpetua became agitated. And when he raised the cross and walked down the aisle intoning "This is the wood of the cross" she threw herself to the floor and put her face in her hands. Bill invited the congregation to venerate the Cross, either by coming to kiss the wood, kneeling in front of it, or "Venerating it in your heart from where you are in your own way". Perpetua struggled to her feet and began to stagger down the aisle; Trina and Dexter tried to stop her but she had a desperate, jerking force that carried her forward. They did not want to be embarrassed so they edged away. On she went, half walking, half kneeling, as if in a crazy dance; and when she reached the chancel steps she stood up, shakily, and turned to the congregation.

"Follow me!" she said urgently. "How can you sit there at the hour of My Brother's death? He walked with a cross to His death; the least you can do is walk the few steps to touch the wood. You can not sit there after two hours of Bill's reflections, thinking that this is just an intellectual event, an exercise in salvation accountancy. Feel the thorns, feel the nails, feel the lance; feel the blood ebbing away; feel the sorrow; feel like His mother; feel like His sisters and brothers which is what you ought most to feel. Follow me!"

Given new impetus, Dexter and Trina came forward, followed by the others and then by braver members of the congregation, mostly the new house group people who did not understand the niceties of Anglican liturgical understatement. They followed the example of Perpetua and knelt before the cross and kissed it; then others, with a mixture of embarrassment and determination, came forward.

Perpetua went to the back of the church and stayed there until Bill had finished. She said she would stay a while. Bob, Andy, Wayne and Brian had already disappeared. Kylie made a slight gesture of farewell and walked slowly out. Trina and Dexter hovered, muttered something about the Sunday worship and slipped away. Then she saw Jim coming from behind a pillar: "It is all right Jim. It is not a day for music. Stick close to Father Bill, he is expecting you to stay until after Easter. He needs company and he likes music." With utter faith, without a question, Jim went.

Meanwhile, the outside world was in chaos. There had been a nationwide power cut since two o'clock and there were fears of flooding as the rain poured down. A tornado sliced laterally through central London, tearing the great doors from London Minster, cutting a channel right through the Toran Fortress, blasting out all the windows at the Toxic Times and smashing all its production machinery. The few who knew what day it was said this was a judgment on the others who did not. On millions of tiny, crackling portable radios, the disaster news, the weather reports, the traffic grid-locks, were interspersed with doom-laden messages as if the BBC had been getting them ready, the sociological equivalent of obituaries.

Perpetua lay on the cold marble of the chancel at the foot of the cross which she had put there after Bill had finished. This was the strange time between the burial of Jesus Her Brother and His rising again 30 hours later, preceded by flower ladies and a last minute choir practice.

She felt the cold of the floor and the cold of Her Brother's body. "Do I really have to die like You?" she asked. "Is there no other way through which these people will recognise the depth of God's love and the depth of their rejection of it? Your death seemed to put everything right for a time but the Church you made has become part of the problem, not the solution. What else can I do now but die? There is no other way. Nothing I can say will make any difference now; but if I die like You, the memory will be more powerful than the reality. Or will it?" She shook violently and then began to cry again.

"It was so wonderful at the beginning, when people wanted to believe in justice and love, when the sun shone, when there was growth and hope. Even the debates and disagreements, the doubts and the divisions, were symptoms of growth but everything has become bleak and hostile. You know that, My Parent, of course You know. I wish I knew now what You plan for me, how You want me to die; but I know it will be painful and degrading; I know I will have to die that way to be worthy of the Brotherhood of Jesus. At times I have wondered what kind of life I am leading, whether I am really a special messenger of God or whether this is an illusion I have built up for myself to protect me from my own mediocrity. I wish I could know."

She took up the cross and began to dance with it as her partner.

Then the training from countless hours of praying kicked in. She forced herself to lie perfectly still and to listen.

"Now I only know two things clearly: that You want me to die a painful death for Your sake and the sake of the whole world, worthy of Jesus My Brother; and that I will do what You say, no matter how much I hesitate on the way."

Hours later her mobile phone signalled a text message, as she knew it would. It was from Heather.

38

There was an unusual level of activity at the Hollow. There was a police cordon around it at a distance but the police had made it clear to Poppy and her crew and to those who ran affairs in that part of Grunge Park that they would not be able to intervene if things got out of hand. The Commissioner of the Respect and Order Directorate had seen the CEC broadcasting proposal and thought that it would do no harm for the public to see the nastiest the community could provide without any decent people being involved. It was in the public interest for broadcasters to make realistic portrayals of social ills such as drug taking and violence. The Directorate of Independent Media agreed. Once shooting began the priority would be to keep respectable people out of the way.

The local gang leaders had sorted out all the arrangements for the evening but they were only facilitators. If the RIFs had a really good time, the gang could spread its influence outside this low margin area and start to operate in Excelsior Gardens and other much more lucrative patches. Poppy had a slight worry because she was almost certain she would know some of the RIFs who were coming. The original idea had been to shoot gang locals dealing and addicts taking stuff and then behaving outrageously; but the RIF complication had been accepted on the grounds that it would be even better to see middle class kids degrading themselves.

The visitors were led by Rory Varnish and Oliver O'Helly who had met just before they dropped out of theological college. They now ran a highly exclusive internet porn operation (nothing less than platinum cards) and, in spite of their age, were the central figures in the Excelsior youth scene on account of their outrageous behaviour. "Theology," said Roy. "That's handy because one of your playmates for the evening is Perpetua who's a bit theological; you could have some fun there."

Heather and Jo hovered nervously at the edge of the Hollow's territory, frightened that Perpetua would not come. They should have known better. She walked towards them steadily, not altering her pace, not looking to the right nor to the left, not smiling, until she saw them. Then without speaking, she followed them down a slope towards a piece of scruffy waste ground at the centre of the Hollow. They glanced at Roy and the rest of the reception party and at her and then turned away as if to get past her but Perpetua put out her hand and patted each of them on the head.

Rory and his pals were standing on the edge of the waste ground drinking export lager. They did not know it but they were looking straight at Poppy's central camera which was hidden in the boarded up shell of what had been a community centre. The locals would keep their hoods down and their guests well fuelled and they would nudge them round into camera if they showed signs of straying. Poppy had told her producer that there could be no fixed rules of engagement; he would have to put the feed on a delayer and cut to commercials if there were bits where the public interest was outweighed by the offensiveness of the material. The police had said that this was just a normal journalistic sting so they had no public interest problems.

"Don't move," said Rory. "There's a knife at the back of your neck and if you move it will be the last time. We wondered how you might justify all the mess you've been making lately, attacking the church, people like my dad and Olly's uncle." "I think the church is doing its best but failing; not failing people like you with intelligence and means who ought to know better but people like those I grew up with. There is more gunfire in Grunge Park than lawn mowing; more rap than singing; more drunkenness than dancing; more fear than friendship..." Oliver hit her on the face. "Are you blaming respectable people for the problem because little slum rats like you can't behave properly?" "The other thing," said Rory, working himself up to a pitch of anger, "is that you are so pious. Well, you keep talking about drugs as if they were the end of the world but you say you've never tried any. This is your night babe, we're going to enjoy watching you get out of your holy head." "There is a better way to be happy," she said just before she was pulled down from behind so that she sprawled on her back in the mud. "We were thinking of helping you to get out of your skull immediately," said Rory, "but you wouldn't enjoy us so much if we did that."

Oliver pulled off her jeans and they stood in a circle chanting: "Dirty bitch! Slut!" and obscene expletives as each boy took his turn to rape her. It was cruel and clinical, almost military.

When they had finished, Rory took a syringe and injected Perpetua just above her bikini line while Oliver and others held her down. Then they all took their own fixes and went on drinking beer as they waited.

Two of the boys started fighting over Perpetua's *god4u* top which they wanted as a souvenir for their girlfriends. "Don't be stupid," said Roy, "toss for it."

Nearby, Jo and Heather were in a top floor flat drinking vodka. They got into a terrible row over what had happened to Perpetua and whose fault it was. They began to hit each other and somehow they reeled onto the balcony. Whether Heather was pushed or took her own life, Jo did not know. She sent a shaky text to Dexter, finished the vodka and jumped.

Dexter texted Trina. He reached the police cordon in minutes. "What's going on?" he asked. "Just a bit of filming. Haven't I seen you before?" "No." "Yes I have; I saw you in Royal Park with that Perpetua preacher." "No you didn't; I'm an atheist."

He pushed past the cordon without any more bother and was confronted by Poppy's roving interviewer. "Who are you? No, don't tell me, even in this bad light I know I've seen you before somewhere. Yes, I saw you outside Hypo with Perpetua." "No you didn't, you can't see properly in this light and, anyway, I shop at Lakshmo." "No, you weren't shopping, you were one of her gang." "No I wasn't; stop pestering me or I'll ram that mike down your rotten throat."

He almost knocked the microphone out of the interviewer's hand and went headlong towards the middle of the Hollow before he was stopped by a loud scream. He crept forward until he could see a group clearly outlined; strange, as it was usually pitch dark. As he focused, he saw Perpetua's face writhing in pain; but she struggled to regain control. She saw him just as he had decided to run for it, and held his gaze for just a moment with what felt like a blessing. And then, in blind panic, he ran; he did not know where, he just had to get away. He could not live with his cowardice but he would not live without it. He knew his love had failed.

When Trina got the message she assembled the pieces rapidly. Desperate to get to Perpetua, she felt no remorse when she found the bodies. Heather's mobile was smashed but Jo's was working. She checked the history and went screaming towards the Hollow. She had almost reached the waste ground when Roy blocked her progress. "If you move a step further I'll kill you." "What about Perpetua?" "What about Perpetua?" "She's there; I know she's there." "She's enjoying herself with a few friends; leave her alone." "They are not her friends." "They are now." "I need to see Poppy." "No you don't. You need to leave before I lose my cool and kill you."

He took a step towards her and she saw the gun. Her resolve broke and she turned and walked slowly, very slowly, away. As soon as she felt safe she bombarded Poppy's phone with voice mails and texts; but there was no answer.

The drugs, alcohol and anger had made the whole group mad. Somebody stamped on Perpetua's hand so that the wrist broke; Oliver threw up over her; Rory pissed on her; and as they degraded her they swore at her, telling her that her dose had been adulterated so that she would be no better than she ought. There was a price for piety, for purity, for being po-faced; there was a price for all that she claimed for the world. She was paying that price, Oliver said, in a strange echo of his theological training, because somebody had to pay for all the world's wickedness.

"I know," she replied, just about audibly. "I am paying willingly for my Father and my Brother because I love the world God made; and I love you."

Thus was all the degradation and wickedness poured upon and into Perpetua as God's Sacred Vessel set aside to receive it. They kicked her, ground broken glass into her face, burnt her with cigarette ends, broke all her bones with their heavy boots, turned her onto her face and left her in the mud for dead.

39

Varnish looked in fascinated horror as the group wheeled round the girl. He thought he recognised her and then, in a moment of horror, he thought he saw the figure of his hooded son. It was impossible. Surely what he had heard from Smoother could not go wrong. He had had a terrible day, the usual Good Friday rigours augmented by the disaster at London Minster. He poured himself another glass of claret, and then another, and finally dozed off before he finished the bottle.

O'Helly, exhausted with disappointment, snored and, twitching in his sleep, knocked the empty whiskey bottle off the table.

Sneer watched with professional detachment—"two birds"—Perpetua was done for and Poppy would become a celebrity. He hoped this story would bring them closer. The camera settled greedily on the battered figure in the mud; along the bottom ran a loop of text: "Perpetua, Daughter of God Our Parent, Sister of Jesus, God's Sacred vessel."

The image was faded out, replaced by a Hypo commercial apologising for the disruption of service at Grunge Park and promising extra bumper Easter bargains at all its neighbouring stores.

During the break Poppy reluctantly consulted her producer. "That was brilliant," he said. "There will be some argument about whether what we have shown is in the public interest but we can't lose. Things look as if they are about to go dead but don't stop shooting because you never know; and while you're shooting the police will stay out. I don't know what we will do with the recorded footage; it depends on official and public reaction; but once we have had the complaints and a bit of a tussle with the Directorate for Independent Media we will have the basis for some good documentaries and tidy overseas sales."

Hypo was pulling out all the stops to recoup its store loss by bombarding local radio as well as television with emergency advertising. People stopped in flat screen departments and looked at the pictures of boxing, shoot-outs, Perpetua being kicked, domestic violence, almost naked singers, terrorism in Jerusalem and Renaissance pictures of the Crucifixion without sorting out the fact from the fiction, the now from the history.

Two broken figures crept towards her supine figure. The first said: "She's got nothing, damn it!" The other said: "Poor girl, she doesn't deserve it the way we do. I wish even we could help a bit." "Damn it!" "Be quiet, be gentle." "You hardly know how you will be rewarded for what you have said," Perpetua whispered. "God has seen your love.

"I am thirsty," she said, and the compassionate addict found a half-drunk can of lager and gave it to her. She took a sip, coughed violently and dropped it. "But thank you for trying. It is the best thing you have ever done."

As the numbing effect of the drugs wore off, the pain became greater as the effects of the adulteration and the violence done to her were increasingly unmasked. "Jesus, look down on Your Sister and forgive the world." "Even us?" "Particularly the poor and weak; those who do not know what they are doing."

Poppy stopped filming. It was best to get out while the girl was still alive and could be reported as such to the police.

Jim and Father Bill emerged on to the open ground, leaving behind some of the new house group members, and knelt down next to Perpetua. "No," she said, "I will never move from here alive; it is almost over. I do not want to die in a church or a hospital. Just here. Bill, I am sorry if I have been harsh; I know you are a good man. Love Jim for me; and Jim, Father Bill needs love as well as someone to love."

Bill had to put his ear very close to her mouth as she signalled with her eyes for him to come closer: "I am going to God Our Parent and to be reunited with Jesus My Brother. Do not cry. I am going home but you will never be alone".

With a last effort she raised her head slightly, looked at Jim and said: "I believe in the God of love."

And then she died.

Jim and Bill took up her body and, passing Roy and the remnants of the gang, Bill said: "Best for all concerned if we move the body. You can let the police back in a few minutes."

They were already moving in, after Poppy's report as she left, but Bill and Jim, with their helpers, hurried down a cut between two tower blocks and put the body into the back of Bill's car.

At the church they cleaned up Perpetua in the vestry and Bill wrapped her in some old, dark red choir robes and locked the door. He would have to be back in the morning with the police before the flower ladies arrived.

As the TT had an exclusive tie-up with CEC, Poppy told Sneer as quickly as she could what had happened. The deadline was close and there was a lot of messy detail and some things she would have to hide, even from her father. As usual, Sneer wanted two birds for his stone. With the power cuts and the freak storms to report and the paper reduced in size so that it could be produced on hired presses, this story would have to fight for its life if it were not to end up near the bottom of page 5:

PERPETUA IN MYSTERY GANG OUTRAGE

> In a sensational development late last night, gangland fig-
> ures in Grunge Park reported that the episode involving Perpetua
> shown on CEC was a staged event for rich outsiders.
>
> A CEC film crew source said that rich thrill seekers paid up
> to £1,000 a night for a genuine gangland booze, drugs, sex and
> violence experience. The customers, known as rifs (rich fakes),
> were said to include Rory Varnish the son of the Archdeacon of
> Patchminster.

And then, in a piece of unethical spite which he could not help, in spite of his designs on the girl, the story went on:

> The controversial and often gratuitously brutal coverage of
> gang activities on CEC was masterminded by Poppy Smoother,
> daughter of the Church of England's chief media spokesman.
>
> Sources within the Church warn that the Varnish and
> Smoother connections with the distasteful events at Grunge Park
> may do damage to their careers and the Church.

Two-and-a-half birds!

When the police arrived at the Hollow there was nobody to be seen. Perpetua must have been taken away. Local hospitals were checked without success but on Friday nights the Grunge Park A&E was more interested in handling violence and its results than keeping up-to-the-minute statistics. She might have been taken to a friend's house. Whatever the situation, all that the police could say was that there had been a TV gang sting and although the scenes were said to be unpleasant, no crime had been reported.

Very early on Saturday morning, that curiously empty day before the Res- urrection, Bill came to St. Simple's. To his surprise, the main door was open. The vestry door was open and the body of Perpetua had disappeared. He was frightened and did not know what to do. He sat on a tombstone and said a prayer. Then he remembered what she had said: "I will die very soon but I will return. You will not even have to wait three days." Still, he did not want to fall foul of the authorities so he reported her missing.

Somehow he got through the day, the flowers, the Easter egg buying; somehow he got through the Vigil and First Mass of Easter without breaking down. Every time he read the word Jesus he kept seeing her name in its place. He had risen again; but she was dead; dead but disappeared; on the very day His Resurrection was being celebrated.

He went to bed exhausted.

40

There had never been such a chaotic Sunday in the history of the media. First, an enraged and bewildered Sneer went on breakfast television to say that the TT news operation had been sabotaged in its temporary production facilities, by *god4u* infiltrators. Sneer had written a front page lead saying:

PERPETUA DEAD
BODY SOUGHT

It is widely reported that Perpetua died as the result of a drugs overdose on Friday night in a Grunge Park gang orgy of sex, drugs and violence. It is not known whether she was part of the main activity or was accidentally involved but CEC coverage clearly showed her in a highly deranged state. After filming stopped police moved in but Perpetua had disappeared and has not been seen since.

During a day of frantic activity the reports of Perpetua's death multiplied but there is still no clue as to where she finally met her end. *god4u* leaders have all gone to ground and the g4u-TV network is temporarily out of action.

In a related development, Church of England spokesman Chris Smoother defended his daughter's CEC coverage: "Poppy was standing up for the freedom of the media and she was exposing the horrors of our inner cities. I don't know what Perpetua was doing there but I watched the coverage carefully and it looked to me as if Perpetua was a more than willing partner in what was going on. We have to be so careful when people claim special virtue as she did."

"As for reports that Archdeacon Varnish's son was involved, this is pure speculation. There are thousands of others who would look like him wearing a hood. In any case, he might well have been part of the investigating team."

Sneer brandished the TT so that the cameras could pick up the banner headline:

PERPETUA RISEN FROM DEAD
BODY SOUGHT

The camera then moved down to the first paragraph:

It is widely reported that Perpetua, reported dead, has come back to life. She was raped, forcibly drugged and violently assault-

ed by rich thrill seekers before being left for dead but there are
widespread reports that she will make herself known later today.

I would never have written that rubbish!" shouted Sneer. "It's pure speculation, it's without foundation. It's an insult to honest journalists like me."

Early in the morning Jim completed the reunion of the remaining core
group. Trina had got there first, and over Saturday Perpetua's followers had
gradually assembled at Bleak Villas where they had eaten their last meal with
Perpetua. Trina, Dexter, Andy, Wayne and Bob had met up and agreed it was
safest if they stuck together. Nobody knew about this house; they would all be
looking in Grunge Park. Once they felt safe, they contacted Brian and Kylie.
Dexter went to see what had happened to Heather and Jo; their deaths had
been too routine to command any news coverage. They had missed Jim and
were relived and pleased when he came in, followed by Bill who had, unprec-
edentedly, left his Easter Family Eucharist to the Curate.

They were sitting around listlessly, not even reading the newspapers. Jim
said: "Perpetua is alive again; it says so in the TT." They just laughed, sadly, thinking of all the damage it had done.

Brian was sitting at the computer. He clicked on the g4u-TV website and
saw the logo and a picture of Perpetua.

Her eyes moved.

The rather solemn face broke into a smile.

Perpetua said:

"I promised that I would never leave you. God Our Parent and Jesus My
Brother want you to know that everything they have done has been re-confirmed in me as their Sacred Vessel.

"You do not need to do anything drastic. Remember what we learned
together. You must now go out and practice what you have learned. It says in
the Gospel that there were fifty days between the Resurrection of Jesus My
Brother, His return to God Our Parent and the sending of My Sister the Spirit;
but the world does not work like that any more. Be ready at noon today to
receive further help for what you have to do."

Without thinking, Dexter asked: "Where are you now? It looks like the
top of a tall building."

"I am alive but not in the way I was when we were together. I am taking
this earthly shape so that we can talk. If you think back to all the things that I
have told you, it will become clear."

Then Perpetua reminded her followers what she had said about her death
and return to life, and their mission to be God's witnesses.

They could not understand what had happened or how. Only when Perpetua had gone did they realise that they had been talking to her and she had

been hearing what they said. Brian fiddled with the computer but the *g4u* site showed only the logo and the picture.

They were still talking and arguing when the screen sprang into life again. This was the point at which all television channels, radio stations and internet broadcasters lost control of their output.

"I have taken the highly unusual step of speaking to you all on every media channel on planet earth in your own language because I want you to know that God Our Parent loves all of you. That love was shown when Jesus My Brother was sent to demonstrate God's love on earth; and it was shown again when I was sent as a witness, as the Sacred Vessel of God's fullness. I was killed but I have returned to proclaim God's love afresh to all the world.

"In matters concerning God, forget complexity, hierarchy, tidiness, cleverness and calculation; these are simply human attributes for human situations."

Sneer, breaking off from a somewhat acrimonious wipe-up session with Poppy said: "Jesus!" "No," she said, "Perpetua."

"When you think of the divine love of God for everyone, think only of returning God's faith in you, expressed in creation, with faith in God; God's hope in you, expressed in the Resurrection, with your hope in God; and return God's love for you, expressed in my space, through your love of God; and in all three, recognise the constancy of My Sister the Spirit."

The screen reverted to the station logo. Will and Annie, looking out over the bay, wondered how they had heard these words in English on a Spanish television station. There was a knock at the door and a maid came in. She opened the Champagne and uncovered a bowl of nuts. She made the sign of the cross (as Spanish people will) and only then did they recognise Perpetua.

I do not know how this story got into my computer but I have checked all the information that is checkable and confirm that it is correct.

JACK

CLAIRE

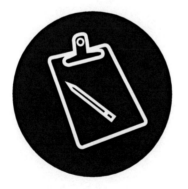

1.

"This is Bad Morning with Craig Knocker and with me, Owen Grumpy, at the end of the worst week in the Prime Minister's long career: Teachers leaders have rejected a set of Government proposals before they are announced; police morale is at rock bottom; nurses say the Health Service is falling apart; doctors say the only way to put the patient first is to give them a pay rise; business leaders are calling for lower taxes; and a senior Labour back bencher says the Prime Minister should resign in case he wins another election. Norma Sniff, our Political Correspondent, is at Westminster. Norma, can it get any worse?" "Of course it can, Owen. This is the worst of many worst weeks for the Prime Minister but it would be even worse if the Conservatives could cash in." "And are there any other troubles on the horizon?" "Yes, there are always troubles on the horizon but, worse still, there are always troubles over the horizon where you can't see them, Owen." "So what can the Government do about all this?" "Nothing, of course; if it does anything right, it's taken for granted and it gets none of the credit but if anything goes wrong, for whatever reason, or no reason at all, it gets all the blame." "Thank you Norma. Now for some more bad news..."

The precise circumstances of the birth of Perpetua (her refusal to take a proper surname caused considerable administrative complexity) are unknown but it is widely accepted that she was born in early June 1987. Grunge Park residents who were questioned by SAD (Social Action Directorate) officials once Perpetua was brought to its particular attention, say that she was born on the Estate and that the neighbours "rallied round"; and some say that there were "unusual events" associated with her arrival.

The confidential SAD Report (and the reason for its confidentiality will become clear) says that Perpetua came to immediate prominence because of a breakdown of communication. Thinking that their party leader had called for a much more interventionist approach in areas of urban deprivation, a delegation of senior Councillors and officials arranged a visit to Grunge Park. Wishing to achieve the appropriate 'spin' (a phenomenon which pre-dates 1997; cf Philip Larkin on sex), they made a reciprocal deal with the regional television news: the coverage would be positive and the station's application for a (rather ugly and unpopular) building extension would be granted.

SAD's access to private medical records indicates that Perpetua was born in an unoccupied, severely vandalised, one bedroom flat overlooking The Hollow. Her mother, Concepcion, was a promiscuous substance abuser of Afro-Caribbean origin with Latino connections, and with no official papers, although there is evidence from the records that she had been in the neighbourhood for three months. There is no record of the child's father.

The Council, through its CANT (Community Action for Nurturing Transition) programme, arranged temporary accommodation for Perpetua and her mother in a refurbished flat awaiting new tenants, the HIT (Health Inter-sectoral Task force) arranged round-the-clock support for the mother and child, and the CRASH (Community Rehabilitation and Action for Self Help) agency hired furniture, white goods and house plants. Local traders were approached and, through a combination of regulatory imposition and relaxation, were persuaded to provide baby clothes, soft toys, toiletries, canned and frozen food, bed linen, towels and even a pair of garish prints. Consequently, when SLOT (South LOndon Television) arrived, Councillors would be able to show that the various strands of special provision to support urban regeneration were fully integrated; but they were unable to avail themselves of that opportunity. When the Conservative Head of Media read the draft SLOT evening news schedule she immediately saw the possibility of gaining some easy air time for Cabinet Ministers promoted in the post Election re-shuffle rather than mere Councillors. These were small but easy pickings for a slack June Friday. SLOT coverage was confined to the Ministers. They entered, simpered, made wooden statements about the Government's commitment to urban renewal and presented the child with a Baby Bond, a toiletries voucher and free funeral insurance. There were later unofficial reports that the Councillors had complained to Central Office; and further rumours that they were compensated with comfortable positions on Statutory Boards.

This unusual combination of circumstances explains the persistent urban myth prevalent in Grunge Park that Perpetua was a peculiarly important baby, commanding the benevolence of local traders and the visit of three Cabinet Ministers. So persistent is the myth that SAD officials found a considerable number of people who claimed to have been intimately involved with the events shortly after Perpetua's birth who could not possibly have been so by virtue of their age or residence profile.

The conclusion is difficult to avoid that the opportunistic political intervention had no collateral benefit. Notwithstanding the (unusually combined) protests of SMEAR (Special MEasures Against Racism), DAMN (the Diversity, Alienation, Malnutrition and Neglect agency), and DEATH (the Division for Encouraging the Achievement of Targets in Health), Concepcion and Perpetua were forcibly evicted from their temporary accommodation within hours of the departure of the SLOT team and, because they were deemed to have taken up premium public sector housing and to have abandoned it without giving due notice, they were placed at the bottom of the housing waiting list. Without any recorded protest or assistance from their neighbours, they were left in the street with nothing.

The record of Perpetua's Baptism at St. Simple the Lesser presents some curious circumstances. A brief article in the parish magazine (preserved under the auspices of CHART (Community History Archive Technology initiative), says that the baby cried so vehemently while the Godparents (none of whom, it turns out, were churchgoers) were trying to say their vows that the Rev. Comfort was forced to move directly to the font at which point he apparently experienced some kind of hallucinatory episode. He had, he said, for the first time in his life, directly experienced the Lord's presence. He was pouring the water and blessing the child when there was a loud thunder clap (although meteorological records show that the weather was calm) and a voice told him that Perpetua was God's Sacred Vessel. It was not this supposedly remarkable event which had prompted the article but the trivial circumstance that, at the end of the service, Perpetua had been observed crossing herself. Such, concluded the Vicar, are the ways of God.

In spite of extensive efforts using the SAD NESS (National Electronic Surveillance System) there is only one record of Perpetua's pre-school existence and this is contained in the Stumpy Knoll CRASH Register which shows that Concepcion received a loan to purchase a push chair. There is no record of repayment.

Perpetua was enrolled at Grunge Park Primary where she stayed for six years without any special needs either for under-achievement or over-achievement. Records of the INEPT (Integrated Education Through Participatory Targeting) Bureau shows that her first choice secondary school was the Excelsior Gardens Grammar School for which she had achieved the minimum entrance grades but for reasons which are not stated on her INEPT record, she was assigned to Grunge Park Comprehensive where, again, she achieved average grades in all subjects except Religious Education where her performance was spectacularly erratic. She also obtained a special credit for a voluntary social action module.

Perpetua was, however, an almost immediate cause for concern because of her refusal to accept the authority of teachers in matters of pastoral care and discipline. She insisted on hugging distressed children and when there were disputes she intervened to make peace, telling teachers that their disciplinary rules were not only unnecessary but harmful. She led a campaign against physical punishment and, when that succeeded, she campaigned against what she called "verbal humiliation". When she met with resistance she established a so-called Pupil Circle for Social Responsibility which sent a Declaration to the Head Teacher, Mr. Laydon, saying that if pupils needed mediation over and above that which the Circle provided, they would ask him for it but until that time discipline should be self-imposed. Incidents of violent and disruptive behaviour fell steadily during this period but teachers and parents were so angry that the matter was raised in Parliament.

"Norma, we heard from the Minister yesterday that he is minded to intervene in

the affairs of Grunge Park Comprehensive in spite of the fact that pupil discipline is improving there." "Yes, Craig, it isn't the outcome that matters, it's the principle. Ministers are worried that there has been a breakdown of authority in the school, depriving teachers and parents of their right to discipline pupils." "Yes, such a breakdown is very bad news. We also gather that somebody at the Inland Revenue has mislaid a tax return…"

She was so argumentative in Religious Education classes that they were frequently brought to a standstill and lesson plans were left incomplete. This was a matter of great concern to Mr. Laydon and Governors because it threatened the School's already low place in the league tables which, in turn, affected the budget.

After a particularly disruptive episode the Rev. Comfort, as a School Governor, was invited to sit in at a series of RE classes involving Perpetua. His report says that there was a rather bewildering discussion in which the teacher, Miss Dawkins, explained the development of the Christian doctrine of the Holy Trinity as formulated by early Church Councils. Perpetua said that all Christian doctrine, being metaphorical, was necessarily inadequate and provisional; and that a Trinitarian doctrine was a derivative of Greek logic and was a closed theorem using the methodology of geometry; and that God, being infinite, should always be treated in human language as an open-ended phenomenon. There might be new Members of the Trinity at any time according to the will of God to intervene in human affairs.

Miss Dawkins said that she could not speak on behalf of the early Councils of the Church nor even the present Councils such as they were. It was not the intention of the curriculum to pass any kind of judgment on the formulations of the religious authorities but simply to explain what they had said and, to the best of our knowledge, to explain why they had reached their conclusions. Perpetua then asked why, if teachers and pupils were allowed to express controversial views on Dickens and Picasso, they were not allowed to comment on Nicaea and Chalcedon. Miss Dawkins replied that religion was so important to the different faith communities that it was best not to say anything about it in case people were offended. At this point there was considerable disruption because Perpetua called for a poll of Muslims in the class to see how many of them were offended. Asked to intervene, the Rev. Comfort said that religion was like fire, it was very beneficial but it could also be terribly dangerous if it was not handled carefully. Too much information was as dangerous as too little.

Following the submission of the Rev. Comfort's Report, Mr. Laydon called Perpetua in for an informal discussion (which was taped but the tape was found to be blank). Perpetua was told that it was the purpose of the school to deliver the curriculum and that individual disruptive behaviour would damage the prospects of other children and the school. In reply to a (non-transcribed) intervention, Laydon said that the school was not the least bit interested in what Perpetua thought about Christian doctrine but only in ensuring that she and her peers knew what the church thought about it.

There are no further records of Perpetua's education and at this point there is a gap in her life profile except for references which possibly connect her with menial work at Grunge Park Infirmary and a care job at Paradise Lodge home for the elderly.

2.

"This is Bad Morning with Craig Knocker and Rod Stirrer on the day that the Government is set to announce its long overdue proposals for tackling global warming. Norma Sniff, our Political Correspondent, is standing by; Norma, I gather you have not been able to read the proposals but what do they say?" "Well, Craig, the Government is facing a serious problem because many people think it is too late to do anything; and that if it does anything, for instance trying to cut the consumption of energy, raw materials and so on, that there will be a political catastrophe. There are, of course, many critics who think that whatever the Government does it will either be too little too late or too much too soon. So whatever it does there will be a crisis." "How much do we know about the real situation?" "From all the scientific data it is clear that there is a possibility that there might be a complete Himalayan meltdown more disastrous than anything we have ever seen before." "Well, Norma, we will await developments with extreme cynicism, or do I mean scepticism? Rod." "There are reports from the major supermarkets that they face financial meltdown unless the Government lifts all procurement regulation. Mr. Lakshmo, tell us what is about to go wrong…"

Perpetua first came to the attention of SAD when she came to speak on behalf of Beth, a teenager with a record of shoplifting. Beth had been apprehended by the Head of Security at the Grunge Park Hypo for attempting to leave the store with goods she had not paid for. Beth said that when she reached the check-out there had been some confusion because some of her goods (baked beans, she said) did not register on the till's bar code reader (an unlikely story) and that the Store Manager, Annie Price, had waived the payment. Because of an (unrelated) technical problem, the Manager could not be questioned at the time but the Head of Security had apprehended the girl in the car park. When he told her he was reporting her to the police, Perpetua, who was mounting some kind of (ridiculous) protest against excess consumption, latched on to the couple and waited with them until the police arrived. At the Station Beth said that the Head of Security had promised that he would not press charges if she gave him "a good time". Perpetua sided with the girl and said that while she was standing with her placard she had seen the man aggressively attempting to engage a number of young women instead of attending to his duties during a crisis in the store. She said that if the girl did not already have a criminal record the police should not be interested. She knew why the till had malfunctioned (an unlikely story) but, as Hypo would not bring a charge, it hardly mattered. Beth had been grudgingly released with an informal caution and left with Perpetua. The Head of Security was dismissed a month later and joined the police.

A few days later, Perpetua began to recruit followers from Hypo, supplemented by some unemployed teenagers.

- Andy, a school drop-out who had twice been charged with theft but discharged for lack of evidence. His parents had barred him from their house and he was a rough sleeper until he registered with the Big Issue.
- Bob, who had been in care since birth and who had been found guilty of joy-riding and been committed to a YOC (Youth Offending Centre.
- Brian, a school drop-out with a record of repeated classroom disruption; some reports said that he had special educational needs but others said that he was lazy.
- Dexter (Afro-Caribbean), a local gangster with a criminal record for repeated threatening behaviour and an assault, widely recognised as a gang leader in The Hollow. No known father. When he was abandoned by his mother (for a new partner) he had five fostering placements before dropping out of the system.
- Heather, a 'known' drug dealer found guilty of possession with intent to supply. Her parents had been forced to move to Grunge Park from Excelsior Gardens after her father had been made redundant in a corporate takeover.
- Jim, a Down's Syndrome sufferer with moderate special needs. His parents had taken care of him until their marriage broke up as a result of stress.
- Jo, cautioned for possession of a small amount of cannabis. Both unemployed parents had problems with alcohol abuse.
- Kylie, brought up by a bewilderingly complex combination of partners, suffered from low self-esteem; medical record of extreme obesity.
- Trina, a university graduate, with high-powered parents, had turned down job matches to work for Hypo.
- Wayne, standard normative in all records (except gay).

Almost as soon as she had established her core group, Perpetua began to conform to the pattern established at school. She was hostile to professional community leaders, notably SAD officials, and established a network of community cells for social responsibility. This immediately attracted opposition not only from SAD officials but also from established community mechanisms on the Estate such as churches and social groups. The two major opponents from the faith sector were Father Joseph O'Helly, the local Roman Catholic Priest, and Miles Wycliffe, a community youth leader. In a joint statement they said that whatever their doctrinal differences, they were united in their view that socially vulnerable people required firm moral guidance from well trained pastors who should not be usurped by a self-proclaimed community leader. They would welcome Perpetua as a social care volunteer undertaking such tasks as SAD was unable to perform because of its recent (savage) budget cuts; and there was always the opportunity to undertake those little extras for the house bound such as shopping and cleaning. They gathered that Perpetua had denigrated their wholehearted efforts by saying that their solutions did not seem to work and that there was need for an examination of root causes such as poverty and the lack of love and self-esteem in the community—if, she said, it was accurate to use the word community—but O'Helly and Wycliffe said that they had dedicated themselves to instilling responsibility and respect into the community. "The problem with Perpetua's so-called solution," said O'Helly to a SAD official, "is that this talk of love is just sentimental nonsense. We all know that there are many people suffering from deprivation who still go to church and observe the common decencies." "And what is more," Wycliffe added, "in an age of selfishness and relativism it is important for people like us to set standards and see that they are honoured. There is far too much soft talk about love and not enough regard paid to God's judgment".

Perpetua's initiatives were also denounced by the Muslim community because of her gender (in this more honest than the Christians); and community leaders who maintained contact with problem elements said that female leadership was culturally inappropriate.

Perpetua said she did not wish to be drawn into a dispute with hard working, committed community leaders who were doing their best in difficult circumstances and they were welcome to become members of her social responsibility cells. At one of these (taped by an undercover official) she said that those who were making money out of drug dealing would never be happy. "If you think about it, you know that you were hooked to make money for somebody else and you will hook other people to make money for you, forming a chain of wreckage. If you look at yourself in the mirror, how can you want to make other people the way you are? You thought that dealing would bring you untold wealth because of the enormous profits in the business; but you do not get the profits. As time goes by, whatever you make will go on your own consumption; and in feeding your habit you are dragging other people down after you." "But what about rich people who don't work at all?" asked Dexter. "One of our problems is that there is no longer any real contact between rich and poor people so that we do not understand each other. We will put that right by bringing some prosperous people from places like Excelsior Gardens into our small groups so that we can learn about each other."

"Well, Rod, there are unofficial reports that there has been an improvement in the crime statistics in Grunge Park but everybody is pretty confident that it is only a blip and that things will soon return to their former poor state. One official has said that

the good news was leaked by a junior Minister in an attempt to weaken SAD's case for a rise in its budget in the forthcoming SPAR." "Thank you Norma; and now we turn to the extraordinary case of a young woman called Perpetua who says we are all consuming too much. Now, Mr. Jambo, as the head of one of our most successful supermarket chains, what do you think about this remarkably audacious claim..."

At this time SAD recorded a measurable decline in reported crime and antisocial behaviour. As a matter of course, statistics were only published when there was a measurable improvement but on this occasion SAD officials put pressure on DID (the Directorate of Impartial Data) to withhold the statistics in case Perpetua received credit for the improvement on the one hand or in case this was taken to mean SAD needed fewer personnel; either way this would make the current SPAR (SPending and Acquisition Review) even more difficult. The Government was determined to privatise social services by engaging (gullible) charities in 'burden sharing' so there was enough of a problem without Perpetua.

Matters grew worse as SAD caseloads began to decline. A typical example is Ruby who was well known around The Hollow as a petty criminal and all-round nuisance. Perpetua asked her if she could hold a group meeting at her house. Ruby said it did not matter. The group discussed responsibility. Perpetua said that responsibility was more important than respect because respect involved altering behaviour and this could be achieved through self control, incentives and penalties; but responsibility involved a genuine change inside. Because of extremely difficult conditions, people lost their sense of collective and, most important, individual responsibility but they could reclaim it. "What Father O'Helly and Miles are saying is that they can get our sense of responsibility back for us but what they really want to get back is respect. It is not like getting a parcel out of lost property; God does not run a parcel office or hand out presents. Only we can look into ourselves, deep down where My Sister the Spirit has her true home." (Fanciful.)

Ruby says that she cannot understand why she ended up crying in front of this young girl, pouring out her messy life story. "Perpetua didn't say anything, she just held my hand and listened, and when I had finished she asked me to remember the stories I had heard about Jesus Her Brother. I shouldn't get worried about all the grief from SAD and other so-called leaders but should find a few minutes every day to sit quietly and try to work out how I had got where I was. If I worked out where I wanted to go, she promised to help. I didn't actually need very much help. I recognised that I had just let things happen to me from the time I wasted my talent at school because I just wanted fun. Look what kind of fun I've got in a dump, in The Hollow; three kids by three different fathers and all of them gone, and the kids running riot. The only help I needed from Perpetua was to gain the self confidence to lead instead of being led.

"She never said a word against me." (Even privately.)

3.

"The time is ten past eight, and you are listening to Bad Morning with Rod Stirrer and with me, Janet Burns. After a set of rogue and possibly fraudulent statistics from the Government suggesting that violent crime is falling in London, including notorious trouble spots like Grunge Park, a recent spate of stabbings has restored a sense of reality. Now, Minister, what is the Government going to do about all this stabbing?" "Well, Janet, as you know, we take this kind of thing immensely seriously. We will listen to what people say; so, for example, if people want five years' imprisonment for possession of an offensive weapon, we will double it." "But so far your punitive policies have not been effective." "It depends what you mean by effective. I mean we can't exactly take all fifteen-year-old boys off the street and lock them up without some kind of evidence that they might be a danger to the community. Last time we tried to institute a law to lock people up in case they were harmful, the House of Lords threw it out, ranking a notional civil liberty higher than the liberty of all citizens not to be assaulted." "Does that mean you are considering new legislation of this kind?" "Of course we are; decent, respectable people are crying out for more protection." "But is it not true that most criminals are also victims, that crime is a symptom of poverty and alienation?" "I thought I would never hear that discredited Old Labour rubbish ever again.""Thank you Minister. Now here is the sport with Barry." "England have finally won a game but one spectator said he had never seen such a poor display..."

While Barry was talking, the Minister said to Janet: "The real problem is that we can't talk about this frankly any more. The fact of the matter is that most of the criminal activity is the result of immigration; at one time it was Afro-Caribbean youth without proper male role models but now there are hordes of criminals from Eastern Europe and a new cohort of Islamic malcontents. As long as they are knifing each other nobody bothers much except for the occasional high profile child murder; but we really have no leverage."

There was a feud between Roy and Kish to succeed Dexter as the leader of the Grunge Park territory. Brokers had tried to make a Granita-type deal with one of the two leading for a fixed period to be followed by the other but the stakes were too high: there was no substitute for power and profit now, and for any gang to be effective the boss needed real power; and with real power all deals would be off and he would eliminate his rivals. Kish and Roy both knew that.

Where Kish was charismatic, Roy was outwardly careful. Kish went around with his close followers in a show of strength. Roy checked his supply lines with dealers. They wanted a steady operation. They were not against violence by any means but it needed to be effective. Roy thought that Kish might be useful, if he could be brought under control; he had the kind of personality that would be very effective with middle class kids in Excelsior Gardens, all gadgets and games. Kish was the expander, Roy was the consolidator; but below the surface, Roy had a terrible temper, particularly when he felt belittled.

When they met to see if something could be sorted, things got out of hand and somebody stabbed Kish in the chest and everybody, including his own people, ran away, leaving him to bleed to death. Perpetua was with Kish's mother Miriam when the bleeding body of her son was dumped on the front doorstep. It was not the first time that he had been attacked. This time it looked fatal but Miriam worked with the hard-lipped determination that the will to live induces. Perpetua, who was also familiar with such scenes, knew that her job was only to do exactly what she was told. The wound was deep but they did not know how deep. He was bleeding heavily but still breathing. He was in a state of shock which made handling him much easier. They managed a clumsy bundling operation to check the bleeding but Miriam said it was hopeless. An ambulance would take too long even if it was allowed (by the controllers) to answer the call. There was no doctor nearby; not even special incentives had made that a reality.

Perpetua suddenly changed her attitude. She gently but firmly put Miriam to one side and said: "I will take care of this." She (is supposed to have) prayed to (somebody called) "God Our Parent" and asked that she be given the power of healing. She laid her hands on the boy's chest and the bleeding stopped. Within a few minutes he was sleeping.

The story does not add up. Although there were strong rumours of the stabbing no witness has ever come forward, and there is no indication in Kish's medical records (he was comprehensively examined when he signed on with Excelsior United) that he ever suffered any assault.

Perpetua sat with Miriam as Kish slept. "And what good will it do that I have put this right for now?" she asked. "I can cure people physically as a sign that God Our Parent is never absent; that all the children of creation are valuable. I can cure people physically so that they can see the power of God working on earth. I can cure people because, like now, it is just too painful not to. After all, you looked after me when my mother was unable to, and Kish and I have known each other all our lives. And although the physical comfort that I bring is valuable to you and to me, what does it really do to change anything? Kish will get better and learn from what has happened. But somebody else will bleed to death tomorrow night and the next night.

"I am always talking about love but it does not come out of nowhere. Because we are creatures made to live in a community we can only learn love from a community; not our own narrow, geographical community, but the wider community that has made *how* we are *what* we are. God knows how difficult it is to grow love in a wilderness which is why the forlorn are so readily forgiven; but we are here now in this shattered place because the rich have turned their backs. All they want to do is to punish us all; Kish, Roy and all the others. If love ought to come from anywhere it is from those who have the resources. But they, too, are in a wilderness, a wilderness of goods and services, a wilderness of packaging and denial. In many ways they are as desperately lost as we are here but it is so difficult for us to sympathise with their loss.

"But there are those who are not quite lost, who know what needs to be done; but they have grown cautious as the grip of selfishness tightens. This is why I am here. This is why I have come. God Our Parent sees that the wilderness needs to be watered. The churches are bleeding themselves dry; they have so little strength to give to others.

"I do not think anybody will want to admit to seeing Kish when he was being stabbed or afterwards. Say nothing. It is not yet time for the community to know my power."

Perpetua went back to her house and spent the night praying. She thought: "With this kind of power I could become a celebrity. I could sweep the world. It would be for the good, of course, but I could do so much." Then she remembered and said: "Lead me not into temptation. I have no power except through You, My Parent." But when her concentration lapsed she thought: "It would be better if I was in power, stopping all this wickedness." But then she flexed her tired spirit and said: "No. I am only a channel. True love will not come, as many Christians think today, through making rules and urging discipline. The only solution is to be a channel into the souls of my brothers and sisters so that the love can flow through." And then she grew frightened: "If I go on like this I will get into trouble either with the authorities who want to keep things as they are, no matter what they say, or with the criminals who want to keep things as they are.

"I must remember Jesus My Brother and have courage."

In the morning she went to Roy's headquarters and walked straight in. "You are safe," she said. Roy, looking at her carefully said: "I don't know what you are talking about. Get out or I will make sure you never come here again, interfering with us. We are only doing what they are doing. They use lawyers, we use knives; they use slave labour, we use drugs. They use many words, we use few." "What they do does not excuse us." "We don't need an excuse. We are where we are. What else can we do?" "You can be their slave, as you call it, and stand alongside other oppressed people. You behave as badly as them; you have admitted as much. That is a good start."

"If you do not get out I will make sure you are finished off. There is no nice, soft, easy solution, there is no magic wand." "I was not thinking of magic, I was urging you to remember where you came from, from God Our Parent." "I remember that; I remember my father who beat me and I remember God the Father in Sunday School on behalf of whom they beat me." "I know; they did God an injustice." "And me, too." "And you, too. I know it is hard but I will always be with you."

He looked as if he was going to grab her by the throat but, without any sudden movement which might have provoked him, she turned slowly and walked out, fixing a *god4u* sticker on the inside of the door before she opened it steadily, closed it gently, and walked out. Once she left he began to shake.

4.

"Now for a light hearted item before Barry brings you the sport. We have received a press release from a character by the the name of Perpetua who is going to launch a mission to the poor from a golf club. We asked her to come on the programme but she said that the BBC was too establishment; but how can you get more establishment than a golf club? Professor Trend is a leading sociologist. Is it likely that any reform movement launched from a golf club will succeed?" "Well, Rod, there have been cases of reform emanating from the middle classes but there have also been cases of it emanating from grass roots movements. It can come from anywhere." "Yes but what about this particular launch, where does it fit into the pattern?" "We don't have any data on social reform movements being launched from golf clubs, indeed I can find no link between sporting establishments and social change. It is frequently asserted that, for example, rugby union supporters are more conservative than rugby league supporters; but there's no evidence." "So it's going to fail, then, is it?" "I could not commit myself." "Thank you Professor; very enlightening. Janet." "Thank you Rod. I should think it will be a miracle if anything comes of it. Now for the latest news of England's gloomy prospects, here is the sport with Barry."

The SAD MASS (Media Assessment and Screening Service) reacted nervously to Perpetua's launch at the Excelsior Golf Club. During the previous week there had been various alerts from local press cuttings analysis that she was up to something. She had made unauthorised visits to a number of medical, social and educational facilities and strange stories began to emerge, alleging that she had calmed hyperactive children, cured the sick and persuaded delinquents to undertake volunteer community action. The objective was clearly to garner publicity material and when the video was played at the launch the results were ambiguous. Very cleverly it was implied that Perpetua had special powers but there was no evidence. It is easy to splice together a clip of a man claiming to have been cured and a shot of Perpetua leaving the hospital. It is the kind of technique that politicians use all the time, notably when they arrange photo calls with successful sports teams as if they had played in the game (which perhaps explains in part why our politicians are so unpopular at the moment!)

In fairness, if you believe in God then what Perpetua said made a lot of sense. If you believe in God then that implies absolute dependence. MASS was not particularly concerned with the faith aspects of her speech. There is, after all, some potential in the naïvite of faith communities which say, at least, that they are doing what they are doing out of commitment, wanting nothing in return. The Number 10 PACS (PArtnerships with Civil Society) is in rare agreement with Number 11 that faith groups can be 'milked'.

What concerned MASS was the socio-economic radicalism into which Perpetua strayed. 1960s radicals now at the top of the political parties and the civil service are comfortable with the relatively stable political consensus following the departure of Mrs. Thatcher and Michael Foot. It may be necessary to implement apparently radical policies like the minimum wage but this is all part of a settled policy of containment. The crime rate is a price worth paying for majoritarian prosperity. All the polling evidence shows that fear of crime is much less than the fear of the falling standard of living which would result from any substantial redistribution of income and wealth. Although governments lose some credibility because they cannot eliminate crime, the public hysteria which is inevitable in a democracy is much better directed at a minority, intractable problem than it is at an issue which might de-stabilise the democratic consensus. Everybody in SAD recognises at least that poverty is a root cause of crime but the risks of doing anything about it are so great (not least to professionals who earn their living from working in deprived communities) that containment is the only realistic option.

In spite of the radicalism of the message, it went down remarkably well with most of the middle class audience which applauded politely at various points throughout the speech and showed a degree of enthusiasm at the end, confirmed in the size of the collection that was taken. A careful analysis of the coverage, however, indicates that there was a small knot of men in their early 20s who were making obscene signs and seemed intent on disrupting the occasion; two of them were known troublemakers and university drop-outs. Dexter kept a close eye on them and there seemed to be mutual recognition. Without any fuss, Dexter edged steadily towards the group and it edged steadily away. There were some muffled shouts off camera before Dexter came back into shot.

It was reported later that Perpetua gave Dexter a severe ticking off, telling him that he must forget his old rough ways and learn to listen to himself instead of taking any notice of the taunts of others.

SAD decided to put Perpetua under low level surveillance (through a regular but informal arrangement sanctioned by the police; left wing newspapers characterise this as "illegal snooping") through offering Grunge Park contacts minor regulatory concessions in exchange for information. New miniature technology is cheap. There was also a proposal to watch the core group but this was rejected on the basis that it would be easier to persuade a vulnerable member of the group to make regular reports. It was, however, agreed that the nascent *god4u* organisation's finances should be investigated as it had benefited from an unauthorised collection.

Miles Wycliffe agreed to be the SAD liaison point which was useful because he could move in and out of the community easily and did not want anything in return for his services (another instance of faith community altruism).

As July drew to a close, Perpetua showed signs of preparing to leave. Bob (improbably) passed a standard and then a special passenger transport driving test arranged by Heather, the SAD opposite number in the regulatory minefield. Before she went, she was visited by Miles. He was shown in by Trina who was working on a post-Excelsior event analysis.

It was a strange meeting. Miles, naturally hostile to Perpetua because of her gender, her religious outlook and her encroachment on his patch, nonetheless had to be emollient because of his new role. She gave him no time to settle. "Look, Miles, I know you have agreed to organise surveillance for SAD and I am very grateful. I do not intend to say anything private and there is just a chance that some of your contacts who hear what I have to say will be moved by it in some beneficial way." "How do you know?" "You are basically a good man, Miles which means that you are a terrible liar. Your pretext for coming here was flimsy. I know you resent me for all kinds of reasons and I know that you have been in contact with SAD because the number is at the top of the contacts list in your mobile. Let me show you." She took out her mobile phone and went down a menu until she reached his name and then she showed him the complete contacts book from his phone. "I will sue you!" he shouted. "Calm down, Miles, what will you sue me for?" "For stealing private information." "But all the numbers in your book are public. You seem not to have any private numbers such as friends. I would like to help you. You are so lonely."

He wanted to get up and leave but instead he sat in silence, trying not to shake. "It would be good for you to have something better to organise than the youth club where you are so brave; and the SAD operation is no better. It gives you nothing. You are so full of pent up love and there is such a shortage of love in Grunge Park. You need to find some way of letting it out. You are so worried about losing control but love is all about not having any control; it is about leaving yourself open." "What I do not understand is what you want." "That is such a strange question because in the way you understand it, I do not want anything. Apart from my general message that I want everybody to want less, I want everybody to stop using the word 'want'." "But don't you want people to live better lives?" "Yes but I am not going to try to make them do that. Miles, you are confusing what you want with their need to want it. You also mistake codes for ethics. You are trying to get people to live by a code but I am trying to persuade them to accept an ethic for themselves, a tool which will allow them to assess the validity of different kinds of codes. In spite of all the desperation and brokenness around here I profoundly believe that, with the help of God Our Parent, by looking into themselves to find My Sister the Spirit, they can attain a degree of self esteem and, from there, take responsibility, so much responsibility that they can distinguish between different kinds of codes. For example, many of us have a code that we will not give others away to SAD or the police, or anybody else; but there is an ethic of confidentiality which helps us to distinguish between when we tell and when we do not tell; and, behind that, it tells us when we should promise not to tell and when we should promise nothing."

"But the Bible sets out God's code." "Yes, there are codes in the Bible but Jesus My Brother, who is the crowning point of the whole Bible, gave us an ethic of love over judgment through which to interpret the codes. He gave us a way of working out which code to accept when." "I can't grasp that." "I know," said Perpetua. "Not yet. But you will. By then I will no longer be here; but I know that you will."

Trina followed Miles outside. "It hurts me to do this but Perpetua says we must jump to no conclusions. So, were you the 'highly respected Christian youth organiser' in the TT story who was 'worried'—nice weasel word—that Perpetua might be recruiting gays and selling drugs? And before you reply, I can promise you that if I find out that you are lying I will get Dexter to come and exert some pressure; not much point being accused of being thugs by your media friends and then being as nice as pie to nasty little liars like you."

Miles had little choice; there was hardly a wide range of Christian youth leaders to choose from in Grunge Park. "They misquoted me; they took what I said out of context." "Of course they did. I wouldn't expect anything else but what did you give them to go on?" "I was worried about that time Perpetua and the *god4u* gang came to our club and took everything over; and when she got into the papers I thought I would warn people that she is not Biblical." "Not Biblical! What does that mean? Are you Biblical, then?" "Well, you see, a lot of people think that Wayne is gay and that this presents a danger to youth." "I wish I knew what all the fuss is about men who are interested in each other. At a practical level you don't go round recruiting gay people the way you recruit nurses or even soldiers. People are gay or they are not; gays don't go round trying to turn heterosexuals into gays."

"But the Bible." "But the Bible nothing. Well, not quite nothing. The whole central point of the Bible, its purpose for existing, although Jews and Moslems would disagree with this, is the incarnation of Jesus. I'm not very theologically trained like you, Miles, but my rule of thumb is to try to see things from the Jesus point of view, not to guess what he would have done in that silly 'What would Jesus Do?' phrase which simply makes him validate whatever we think he would have done, because he was wonderfully left field; and from our human brokenness it's foolish to speculate; but if there is a choice between the ethics-based non-judgmental approach of Jesus and the codified particularity of the Books of Moses, I know which I would take. No wonder people call you Torans rather than Christians!"

Perpetua came out. "Trina, you are too harsh. Miles, all I have to say is that we all hope that no harm comes to Wayne because of what you are supposed to have said."

5.

"The time is ten past eight. The shooting last night in Stumpy Knoll brings the total of fatal gun crimes during the last week to three. The opposition says that the Government has overseen the most rapid rise in violent crime and murder since records began. Minister, when are you finally going to admit responsibility for the rise in crime?" "Well, Owen, I will probably get sacked for this, but it hardly matters, since ministers in charge of this area don't usually last long, but that is possibly the stupidest question you have ever asked, and there have been an awful lot of stupid questions." "I am here to represent the public and I don't expect Government ministers to insult me or the public on behalf of whom I ask the questions. I suppose you think that reply will get you off the hook; are you going to answer the question?" "Yes, when you let me finish a sentence and stop talking. First of all, you might claim to represent the public but I was actually elected by it. Secondly, the Government is not, in the very nature of the meaning of the word, 'responsible' for crime; criminals are responsible for crime; they can choose to commit crime or not." "What an extraordinary statement. Are you therefore admitting that you can do nothing about gun crime and we should all sit about waiting to be shot?" "Of course not. There is growing pressure on us to increase sentences for the possession and use of guns—and knives, for that matter—and that might make people feel better but it won't reduce the crime rate. We know—and here's another nail in my Ministerial red box—that being caught and found guilty is a more powerful deterrent than the actual sentence but our conviction rates are very low." "And what are you going to do about that?" "Well, we have floated various proposals to 're-balance' the system in favour of the community and against criminals in the court system but the media and the House of Lords always kick up a terrible fuss about civil liberties. The fact of the matter is…" "Briefly if you will, Minister, there's the sport coming up…" "The fact of the matter is that we need much smarter policing which isn't helped by incessant bleating about 'bobbies on the beat' as if organised crime syndicates walk about our streets dodging Constables." "Thank you minister. Follow that, Barry."

Off-air Owen said: "Superb interview, well done Minister. I hope you don't get sacked; we could do with a few more of those. As far as I'm concerned you can't get rude enough but we have to play the game, don't we?" The opposition was so pleased with the series of Ministerial gaffes that it said nothing; the Prime Minister hated sacking Ministers; and so, surprisingly, he lived to gaffe another day.

During their retreat, Perpetua led the group in an exercise to define ten commandments. "I will give you as a starter the two governing principles of the Jewish Ten Commandments as set out by Jesus My Brother: love God and love your neighbour; or, just to expand slightly, love God; and treat your neighbour as you would want to be treated."

"Taking the first one," said Heather, "What do we get out of it? We have given up our freedom and our lifestyles to follow you, so will we get into heaven and when we are there, will we be the bosses, just one level down from God?" "First of all," said Perpetua, "there will not be a hierarchy in heaven with God Our Parent at the top and everybody else in layers. We will all be equally enfolded back into God's unlimited love. But the more we come to learn about the love of God, the more responsible we are to live in the knowledge of it and to spread that to other people; so in a strange kind of way it is more difficult for Christians to reach God than it is for others, particularly if they refuse the help they are offered by My Sister the Spirit. We need all the help we can get; and now you are in, there is no getting out. You cannot pretend you have not heard what I have told you."

"But," said Jo, "it isn't possible to do anything unconditionally, there is always a deal to be done." "There is no deal with God. In the Old Testament there are some fascinating stories about deals that the Jewish people made with God Our Parent but the deal making broke down which is why Jesus My Brother came to earth from God Our Parent and confirmed God's unconditional commitment to us; so there are no conditions we can put on an unconditional commitment. We cannot say to God: 'Now that you have made an unconditional offer we want to slap on some conditions'."

"What about people praying for stuff, then?" asked Jim. "At its best, prayer is establishing a terminal in ourselves so that God's love, what we call Grace, can be sent between God's terminal and ours like electricity. When we pray for somebody who is sick we are not making a deal or asking God to alter the course of history or medicine, we are simply bringing our distress to God and saying that what we want lies entirely in the hands of an all-loving parent. In a way the Bible makes these ideas rather difficult to come to terms with; as God is so different from humans, the Creator and the Created, there is a profound sense in which the two kinds of 'person' are so different that no deal can be made. Imagine a single, poorly paid worker trying to make a solo deal with the boss of a multinational. The distance between humanity and God is infinitely wider than the difference between the two people. And even if you combine the power of every human creature that has ever lived it is puny in the face of God's power. There is no deal to be made. So, Dexter, all deals are off."

"Yes, Perpetua. I know. I really know. At moments when I have that terminal feeling inside me I can feel what you are saying; but it isn't always there. The more I listen to you the more I feel in touch because of your special mission from God Our Parent. Let's agree, then, that our love of God should be unconditional."

"As this is a quite abstract idea at first it is, paradoxically, easier to handle at a superficial level than the idea that we must love each other unconditionally."

"That isn't possible," said Heather. "How can you love somebody like a sneak from SAD?" "We do not necessarily have to like everybody and we must particularly try to love the people we do not like. Because we are all so much more mobile than we used to be, we can avoid people we do not like. We put old people into homes and expect social workers to take care of what we call 'problem' or 'dysfunctional' families. We dump many people with learning and mental health problems in prison. We are exchanging what we must love for what we like.

"Love can be defined in many ways but one way is that it is our attempt to imitate the life of Jesus My Brother; another way of saying this is that love is seeing Jesus in everyone. Conversely, the way for us to think about sin is to see it as deliberately putting distance between ourselves and God, through what we do and say and think and what we do not do and say and think."

"So does that mean that all crimes or sins are equal?" asked Brian. "Superficially, we can rank actions but this is usually done in connection with human justice rather than our ethic of love. You will hear some wise people say that you must hate the crime but love the criminal. That is a good start. We never will know how people got to be where they are; only God Our Parent knows why we do things. Think about a woman who is almost driven mad by a cruel husband so that she kills him; then think about a rich person who methodically exploits his workers for his personal profit so that they can hardly feed their families and die prematurely, leaving mothers and children destitute. Superficially, most people will always rank murder above every other crime and I have only put a very approximate case. We always have to remember that these are matters for God."

"Does that mean that poor people are less guilty of the same crime than rich people?" asked Heather. "There was a man whose father left his mother before he was born; and his mother tried very hard but he was lazy at school and got no qualifications; and he turned to drug dealing for a quick profit; and he became a gang leader; and in a turf war he stabbed his rival. There were things he could not help, like the father's behaviour, but there were so many things that he could help, such as commitment to study, choice of lifestyle and whether to carry and use a knife. As soon as people say that their conduct is the result of deprivation, they could be making an excuse but they could be thinking seriously. If they can think seriously about root causes, they can think seriously about their own behaviour. Seriously deprived people are much more likely than well-off people to commit crime because of the pressures under which they live; but Jesus My Brother had a special love of the poor and promised that God Our Parent would be merciful to them; He was less optimistic about the rich. Because we must be subject to human justice, the poor get the worst of it but that does not reflect the position of God Our Parent."

"Well," said Heather, "it's not very practical." "We always have to ask ourselves questions as followers of Jesus My Brother before we get to grips with secular justice. For example, we need to determine our ethical attitude to imprisonment before we engage in a political debate about it. As I have said, we must never make up our own minds and then attribute our conclusion to Jesus My Brother. It is not realistic to try to have one set of Christian ethics and a separate set of secular ethics. I think what you mean, Heather, is that if we based our criminal justice system on Christian love it would not work. Of course it would not; but we need to work to establish the primacy and universality of the love of God Our Parent on the earth; love cannot wait until there is a right time."

They finally agreed the following at the end of their retreat:

1. Love God and all humanity unconditionally
2. Worship God and not people or things
3. Reserve a special time for God every day
4. Never call on God irreverently
5. Act justly and fight injustice
6. Protect the vulnerable
7. Do no violence without justification
8. Thank God and be content with what you have
9. Respect and preserve God's creation
10. Never be indifferent.

"Remember," said Perpetua, signing off the work and telling everybody how well they had done, "Remember, no deals!"

6.

"There are still tensions inside the Government as Junior Ministers compete for funding. Norma, I suppose there is a lot of in-fighting?" "Yes Janet; officials are fighting for the last penny, so to speak, going through budgets line by line; but they also want to get away for their holidays, so the atmosphere is very bitter." "Tell us the place where it is worst." "There is no doubt that the Social Action Directorate is under pressure because of its rivalries with other parts of Government." "So what will happen?" "If there is no final settlement before the Summer break this will cause severe disruption; but if there is a settlement it will unravel in the Autumn." "Thank you Norma. Now we turn to the vexed issue of faith schools".

The SAD operation to keep tabs on Perpetua lapsed for a few weeks. It was late July, Parliament had risen, Ministers were either making last minute arrangements or leaving for holidays and it was usually the time when there was no pressure but, after the completion of the SPAR, SAD was still trying to get its final budget settlement out of the Minister. Some of its enemies in the Cabinet had said it needed less money because it was doing well and could do its job with fewer resources while another hostile faction said that it was wasting money and should be down-sized and merged with the CICU (Citizen Information and Consultation Unit—ostensibly for obtaining information about grass roots opinion but actually yet another intelligence gathering operation loosely controlled by the police) and these arguments were now raging at a lower level. The problem was that contesting one view tended to reinforce the other: it was not politic to admit to failure; but there was also a budget penalty for being efficient. The natural course of action would be to argue that there was a rapidly expanding work load but it was Government policy to say that everything was getting better. As long as SAD could be distanced from the crime debate it was likely that there would be a reasonable settlement but there were many in the (Left wing) press who insisted that there was a link between social policy and crime.

"The recent controversy over wearing the Muslim hijab and the Christian crucifix have caused complete chaos in our education and employment sectors. Our Social Policy Correspondent has seen a leaked memo that says there are only a handful of cases but we have found a man in Bradford…"

SAD was requested by Hypo to send a representative to its (generally ineffective and infrequently convened) Community Forum. It contained a cross section of religious leaders although, curiously, there were no Christian representatives. On this occasion Hypo had allowed two self-appointed (shelf stacker) Christians to attend and store Manager Annie Price had made a last minute decision to invite Perpetua as a "Special Adviser".

As the lead agency (the local council did not have a clue) SAD kicked off by supporting the Hypo policy which broadly states that Christians do not mind other religions having festivals but their adherents do mind Christian festivals. One of the community representatives (rudely and irrelevantly) interrupted by saying that if they disliked Christianity they could go home. "Where to?" shouted the Mullah. "You won't get rid of us sending us down the road to where we were born." Annie cut in: "That isn't the issue, let's get back to business." SAD went on to say that all its survey work had shown that Christians were extremely tolerant; some people said this was because of the foundations of their faith, others said it was because they were now too weak and lacking in social confidence to be anything else. Still, the data showed that they would put up with more or less anything, including extended drinking hours, super casinos and even hard porn. Their hierarchy called for heavy regulation of the supply side but Christians "in the pew" (polite chuckles) were not in the least bit interested in curbing the demand side. They wanted somebody else to do all the work, regulating social and economic affairs, while they just lived their own (presumably virtuous) lives. On this basis, SAD concluded, Hypo could do anything it liked and there would be no comeback; Christians would have to buy their turkeys, carols or no carols. "But why should they have to?" asked the Rabbi. "This is a Christian country, after all, so people are entitled to expect Christmas music; I don't mean the reindeer and Santa type but the occasional carol." (He must have been some sort of progressive.) He had hardly finished when the Mullah said: "That's right. We people from the Abramic tradition" (whatever that is) "must stick together. Particularly after 9/11 we don't have the leverage to push through official recognition of the Hijab but we can make an alliance with those who want the Christian Cross." "True," said the Sikh, "we were founded to bring peace between Islam and Hinduism and we would be delighted to do the same between Islam and Christianity, even Judaism".

This was unlikely enough and a complete contradiction of what the media say about religious tension but, to cap it all, Annie Price made the meeting more or less superfluous: "You are all right. If Christians are so tolerant they will shop here no matter what we do or don't do; but Hypo has steadily been taking sales away from high street chemists, greengrocers, music shops and tobacconists, so why not niche faith shops, too? The Hypo Manual clearly needs re-writing."

"I wonder whether I might be permitted to say a few words?" said Perpetua. "I am sorry that SAD did not say this" (cheeky bitch) "but we should not follow the line that we can do anything to people simply on the basis of relative superiority of force, because we are strong and they are weak. It is socially stupid to punish altruism. The Government says that it wants to work with faith communities to deliver social care and other public benefits and so it is very strange that it simultaneously wants to weaken faith communities. People turn to religion because it is collective, because it provides superstructure, a degree of predictability, mutual support and outreach, geography, shape, comfort. Why does a supposedly 'moral' Government allow people to be exposed to pornography while it wants to protect them from the Sermon on the Mount?

"If you devalue Christmas that is just another element—in addition to the general materialism of our society—which will help to weaken religion. It is very strange for a society to damage itself by throwing away its social capital at a time when it has never been more precious. In a very real sense the fewer Christmas carols we hear the more violence there will be in our deprived communities, not because 'Carols stop crime'..." "You can just see that headline," said Trina, who had somehow slipped into the meeting, "...but," continued Perpetua, "there is a link between carols and Christianity, between Christianity and social capital, and between social capital and crime reduction."

"Count us in, too," said the Sikh. "We have social capital to contribute but we are worried at this perverse social trend which attacks Christianity on the basis that it offends us, always supposing, of course, that policy makers know who we are. Most people in this country with its grand imperial tradition don't know the difference between Muslims, Sikhs and Hindus."

"We remember the thin end of the wedge which led to Hitler," said the Rabbi. "There's no difference in principle between banning carols and burning books".

SAD maintained that its policy of sensitivity towards minority faith communities was even-handed but one of the Councillors muttered something about "incumbent blight".

Annie Price seemed very pleased with herself and thanked the two self-appointed shelf stackers for coming. She mentioned the prospect of constructing a crib outside the store but SAS (the Security and Safety Directorate) pointed out that Hypo would need permission under the STAR (Self-standing Temporary Artefacts Regulations) in order to proceed. Annie said that what she did in her own car park was her own business but if the SAS wanted to sue it was welcome; it would look very silly making rules about cribs. The SAS said it didn't mind looking silly as long as everybody kept the rules and was kept safe.

Annie asked Perpetua if she was still running her campaign against conspicuous consumption because, she said, almost laughing: "it is quite difficult to isolate factors but it looks as if your intervention in July gave us a slight profits uplift." "It was not a campaign," Perpetua replied, also smiling, "I just wanted to get a message across at a time when there were stories about the melting Himalayan glaciers, but you have to change your angle all the time. It only goes to show that theologians are not necessarily good economists nor even good at public relations. Still, we cannot go on just consuming and not caring about the consequences." "But we have all these green initiatives." "Yes, but that is a response to an economic and not a moral crisis. If you knew nothing about ecology you would go on selling regardless of the damage that does to individuals and society. The problem with the green movement as a whole is that it is purely pragmatic, utilitarian, there is nothing moral about it. The moral position is that we must protect the poor of the world from the downstream results of our selfishness; and then we must curb consumption for our own moral well being. If we were morally well we would not have to wait for some scientific evidence to force us to be pragmatic about resource management, we would be doing that anyway."

"We will have to agree to disagree," said Annie. "No hard feelings, I hope?" "No," said Perpetua, "but the time for hard feelings is approaching fast." "Talking of which, how can you complain about consumption when your followers have just insisted on Hypo bringing in all these extra Christmas items?" "There is a balance between social capital and physical resources depletion. Unless we build social capital there will be nothing left, neither physical nor spiritual. God Our Parent only rarely and sporadically speaks to hermits; Jesus My Brother created a church so that God's Spirit, My Sister, has a point for constant communication. You are doing your bit for Christmas. Learn to sing some of the Carols you have not sung since you left school."

7.

"Norma, what is the reaction in Westminster to the Minister's claim that crime is *falling in the inner cities?*" "Most Government back benchers think the move has back-*fired. They acknowledge that there might have been some improvement but to talk about it is simply to make the Government a laughing-stock. If Ministers go around claiming that things have improved they simply leave themselves open to ridicule. When they say that problems are difficult to solve they meet with cynicism; when they say things are worse they meet with contempt; on balance, they prefer cynicism or contempt to ridicule. So they are left with the problem that when they issue a set of statistics everybody believes in the rises but nobody believes in the falls."* "Thank you Norma. Now we turn to *the claim that people are leaving hospital totally cured...*"

It was a relief when Perpetua started her September tour. She had made Grunge Park decidedly edgy. The pirate radios had been replaced by a *god4u* community channel, drug dealing seemed to have disappeared and there were weeks when there was no recorded gang violence; but far from creating a sense of well-being the effect was surreal; people did not know how to handle a situation they all thought they wanted. This lull could not have come at a worse time for SAD which was (again) grappling with a budget crisis. As had been forecast, the hurried mid-Summer settlement was unravelling. It was easy enough to persuade journalists not to disseminate good news but it was more difficult to manage the steady stream of hostile briefing from inside the Cabinet. Fortunately, when a Minister quoted the favourable Grunge Park statistics on Colosseum, the BBC's flagship political discussion forum, he was overwhelmed by a hostile and incredulous response from the audience. One of the problems which the Government now faces is that even when it succeeds nobody believes what it says and no journalist will report it; but, then, although people enjoy journalism as the cheer-leader against 'spin', nobody believes journalists. It was a relief, too, when the spotlight temporarily moved to other places and other Directorates.

On her tour Perpetua left a trail of administrative chaos behind her which took weeks to sort out. First, she visited a school in Grimestack which had just been handed over to SMEAR because of poor performance. Without clearance, she and her *god4u* followers ran after-school activities for a week and, (incredibly) it was reported (confidentially for obvious reasons) that there had been a complete turn-around in the attitude of the most difficult children. Officials were almost immediately aware that they would have to report SMEAR's success after the next round of assessments and that this would present a credibility problem. The *god4u* local channel showed pictures of teenagers of different races singing together, playing together and even holding hands. There was an impromptu concert at the end of the week organised by Jim which, one teacher reported, was of a higher standard than anything the school had ever produced before. Nobody would have believed this if it had not been broadcast on *god4u*. In an accompanying interview Perpetua was asked to reveal her secret. "There is no secret," she said, "we just asked the pupils to imagine themselves into the position of other pupils. We asked the white children to imagine themselves into the position of black children and vice versa. We asked the really macho guys to imagine what it would be like to have a special need and we asked the special needs children to imagine how they might help the macho guys. Then we talked about how everybody is a child of God Our Parent with different gifts and how they are all loved all the time when they try to see Jesus My Brother in each other. When we had got a degree of understanding between the children it then became possible to get them to collaborate constructively. It is not very difficult to see that what really unites children in our culture is not drama or novels but music. White children really like black music so that seemed a good place to start; but we also got black children to understand something of European culture by teaching them one of the easier Chorales of Bach."

Secondly, and more difficult to sort out, was Perpetua's impact on an old people's home in Siltup-on-Sea. Again, the group preyed upon a hard pressed Matron by offering a week's relief services. They stopped day-time television in the main lounge, gave people a choice of meals and, much more serious, a choice of eating times. Each member of the group facilitated a different activity and residents were helped to fill in an activity timetable. Competitions were organised and little prizes were presented at a party on Friday evening. The owners asked Perpetua to leave on Saturday morning because, they said, she was raising unsustainable expectations. She said that some of the residents were perfectly capable of organising themselves and, given a constructive approach, it would not be difficult to get volunteers. She also said (which the owners found most offensive) that the objective of running a home was to make the residents happy while gaining a modest living for the owners. If they could not afford to feed people properly and help them to live fulfilling lives they should not be running a home at all. After Perpetua's enforced departure the residents became aggressive and said they wanted to keep things going in the new way. They elected a committee and insisted on a high degree of self-governance. The problem was then to work out whether they would be better left where they were or re-distributed throughout the system. SAD (mistakenly, as it turned out) decided on the latter course of action and the word spread.

Thirdly, and most damaging of all, Perpetua wreaked havoc in Eastmorland Royal by emptying its long stay wards. Fortunately *god4u*'s (primitive) PR operation decided to keep this confidential but SAD was seriously worried that cured patients would talk even though Perpetua told them to go home and say nothing. As usual, the danger was over-delivery. Fortunately, the computer records seemed simply to show a high degree of coincidence in the discharges but there was a red alert for some weeks. There were some personal stories in the free newspapers but it all died down most satisfactorily. If word had got out there would have been problems in areas with a poorer performance and accusations of a 'post code lottery'.

Perhaps even more disturbing was the general level of contentment brought about by Perpetua's worship events. The first murmurings came from the established Christian churches. Perpetua agreed not to hold any of her meetings during the weekend but she still drew huge crowds. The churches said that they would not be able to collaborate with SAD if it could not somehow keep Perpetua under control. The SAS were brought in to assess safety but a three-way meeting between its officials, SAD and Heather ended in stalemate. There were complaints from pubs, off-licenses, tobacconists and even fashion outlets that people were buying fewer 'comfort items'.

For the record here is an extract from the speech which Perpetua made at the major events on her tour:

"How many of us know what it feels like when we lose something we really care for? Let us imagine that our cat goes astray. We spend the whole evening searching, we knock on the doors of neighbours, we put a notice in the newsagent's window, we never really settle. And then imagine our joy when we find it, thin and straggly but still our beloved cat. We feed it, we take it to the vet to have its ear fixed and to give it precautionary jabs. For a while we think that cat is the most important creature in the world. That is what God Our Parent thinks of us; not just for a few days, but all the time. It does not matter how often we go astray, we are still precious and our return is celebrated by Jesus My Brother.

"Or imagine that we have been working on a really important project on the computer and, suddenly, the file just disappears. We spend the whole day trying to find out where it has gone and in the end we call upon an expert to use special utilities to get the file back. How relieved we are. Well, in our case we do not need an expert to bring us back, we need My Sister the Spirit to be with us. Whenever things become difficult we can always turn to God, of whose being I am a part.

"Or imagine that we are trying to make our house beautiful and we know that there is one exquisite object that will complete our work; we can see it in our head even though we have never seen exactly what we want. We go around shops rejecting objects that are almost what we want because 'almost' is not good enough; and, at last, in a really obscure, dingy old shop, we find what we want. It is covered in dust but we somehow know immediately that we have found what we have been looking for, that with a little time and care it will shine, making our design complete. That is how we should look for God Our Parent because without the presence of God we are not complete.

"But instead of only looking for God in obvious places we have to remember that God is also to be found in the darkest of places, in the most physically unprepossessing places and people; and sometimes it is difficult for us to see the God that shines when there is so much earthly dust.

"For a start, we must all see God in each other. After all, we only have each other to go on. Some people say that we can reach God through doctrine and theology but we can only find them through what human beings have done. As most of us can only think of God in terms of human language we are always seeking after a great mystery; but the search is so important, it is the only search that counts.

"So just as God always rejoices when we return after going astray, so we are in the process of devoting our lives to the search for God. This only works if we see our lives as a series of searches where we hope that each time we set out we will get nearer to God. This is what happens when we read a good book. We start out on a journey, knowing quite soon how we would like it to finish. And then the author takes us away from the conclusion we want and we cannot see how she will get back. Then we are drawn towards the conclusion we want and it is just about to happen when there is a disaster and we think that the conclusion we want can never happen. Then, right at the end, the author reaches the conclusion we wanted from the beginning.

"Look at the person next to you. There is more God in what you are looking at than there is in the library of a theological college. However tired we are, we must keep on looking."

At the end of one of her meetings, a man who had been looking on from a distance, walking up and down restlessly, suddenly rushed through the crowd towards Perpetua. Immediately Dexter sprang in front of her and blocked the man's way. "Let him come," she said. "Everybody must be allowed to come. Look at him, he is not dangerous, he is shaking. What do you want?" "I know you are The Daughter of God Our Parent, you can heal me. I am" (he paused) "A paedophile." At this point the crowd pressed in waving their fists and threatening to push him to the ground and stamp on him but Perpetua shouted: "Stop! This man has bravely come to seek forgiveness; and you think you are so much better than him that you can commit an act of violence against him? We are so fortunate that God Our Parent never gives up on us. Stand back!" Reluctantly, the crowd shuffled backwards a few paces. "It must have been so frightening for you to say what you have said in front of all these people. You are cured and your sins are forgiven; your humility and courage have saved you. Dexter, call a taxi and see that he gets safely into it."

Then a journalist and photographer pushed forward: "You're not a minister of religion, what makes you think you can forgive sins? And what's all this bogus nonsense about a cure? You're just a fraud; but you won't get away with it because we've got pictures of the man who has admitted to being a child molester."

"I am not surprised as you clearly know nothing whatsoever about God Our Parent which is very sad; but now would be a good time to learn. What do you know about the power to forgive sin and to cure people? What, for that matter, do you know about the dynamics of paedophilia? But to show you just a little of the power that God Our Parent has especially vested in me as a Sacred Vessel, I hereby wipe all the pictures you have taken since you arrived here tonight in an attempt to ridicule what God is doing through me." The photographer reviewed the pictures and saw that everything was there up until 18:43. He stepped forward threateningly. "If you want to keep the rest of today's pictures I would be very restrained, if I were you," said Perpetua. "It is more than the matter of what is in your camera. To show the great love God Our Parent has for all of us, your sins, too, are forgiven; but you will have to learn humility if you are not to fall back into the trap that your job sets for you."

8.

"The time is ten past seven. The Government says that the obesity rate is rising alarmingly, particularly among children and teenagers but the Bureau for Active Teenagers has just published a report saying that there is a sharp rise in eating disorders. Professor Dabbler, are we too fat or too thin?"

On the last leg of her tour Perpetua, at Brian's insistence, visited Silicon Ridge. She set up a portable stand outside the Eye of the Needle dress shop and Jezebel's beauty salon and engaged the bored-looking women going in and out. "I can see why you might look a bit worried going in," she said to a young woman, "in case they do not have the kind of things you want in your size; but there you are with two big Delilah bags and a pretty package from Esther's and you are still not smiling; what is it all for?"

After half an hour she had a small crowd of listeners, mainly prosperous-looking women. "Follow me," she said, leading them to the top of the hill which gave a view for miles around. "Look over there at Brickton; and over there at Slatethorpe. It is such a lovely Autumn day that we can see such long distances. To the North and to the West we can just see ugly factories and cramped houses. I know some of us came from places like that and never want to go back but how can we ignore people who are within a few miles of us who need our help. We send chickens to Africa and goats to Asia and seeds to Latin America but should we not also get in our cars and listen to children reading in that deprived primary school over there? How many of you have ever been in Slatethorpe?" The women looked embarrassed. "Let us go and get a bit of lunch and meet in the car park and we can go down and look." As they walked down into town a few women slipped away but the majority stayed.

Instead of dispersing, they seemed anxious to gather round Perpetua. "I suppose," said one, "you are against unhealthy food." "We do not have to be religious to support principles like moderation and proportionality; but often we hear about 'comfort food' which leads me to believe that we should find less unhealthy ways to achieve the same end, like learning to love ourselves as a way of loving others."

After they came out of the school Perpetua said: "I think you have found today more interesting than another tour of the fashion shops; and I am glad that you have agreed to set up a support group for Slatethorpe Primary. Remember how lucky you are to live on Silicon Ridge."

Perpetua stood in the car park of GLINT (The GLobal INstitute of Technology) waiting for the workers to leave when she was approached by a band of people in their early twenties who asked to look at the materials on display, mostly made by Wayne and Brian. "Some of this stuff is fine but some of it is a bit strange. Perpetua, are you saved?" "In a manner of speaking but I doubt I mean it the way you mean it." "Well, have you been born again?" "Actually no. I was a Sister to Jesus My Brother forever and from the time I was born; I was spared being born again." "But how can you claim to be a Christian if you have not been saved and born again?" "The problem with these expressions is that they are anthropocentric, they are centred round human experience. The core of Christianity is the mystery of incarnation and resurrection, of how Jesus was, in a way, saved and born again; Christianity is not about our emotional or intellectual response to Jesus but about God's response to us as children in sending Jesus Our Brother. Please let me look at your brochures.

"I see you are teaching a course called LIFT, about the way in which God will raise us on high as long as we praise 'Him'." "Yes, Life In the Father Today. What's wrong with that?" "It is essentially correct but I think that many people, particularly vulnerable women and abused people, may find the male metaphor rather discouraging." "But God is our Father, it says so in the Bible and the Christian churches, in the Trinity, have always used that language." "That does not make it helpful. The Jewish people occasionally had women leaders like Judith but they could not imagine a female idea of God. Neither could the male-dominated early and Medieval church but we should know better now. We know that God is in a different 'class' from human expression and so if we are going to use a metaphor would not 'Parent' be much better?" "But there is the idea of 'male headship' in the Church." "Yes, it is a problem particularly experienced by men lacking in self-confidence who impose it on women." "Saying that, you can't be a Christian." "This is so simple: Christianity is focused in Jesus My Brother and how we must try to live like Him; and how we must try to understand the mystery of His birth, death and rising again; and there is the mystery of the Church which He established; but we must use the material of the Bible given to us by God not to use as ammunition against each other but to try to explore the mysteries of God. Different people will be in tune with different metaphors for God; theologians call it 'different hermeneutical horizons'. As we are all different, we might find it necessary in secular society to impose rigid laws for the purposes of criminal and civil justice but it is pointless to try to impose our personal metaphors on others as if we possessed some kind of truth." "We thought it would be nice if you joined us in our act of worship at GLINT but it seems that you are in denial of God's word." "Which would be difficult as I am God's Sacred Vessel sent to earth to repeat the work of Jesus My Brother for a new millennium."

The group were so appalled by this heresy that they disappeared inside and left Perpetua to talk to the majority who left the building, weary and worried, as the sun set. As she had with the women, she gathered a group together. "You have been there all day and, apart from the money, what have you got for it? Earlier today I saw some of your partners almost throwing money away in the shops and getting no pleasure from it, and so it is not sensible for you to insist that you only work such damaging hours in order to earn the money you need. If you spent slightly less time here and earned slightly less and you and your partners spent slightly less on things you do not want in the futile attempt to stave off misery, your bank balances would be the same but you and your partners would be happier." A GLINT senior executive intervened: "I am sorry but we do not want any sedition preached on our own premises." "This is not sedition. You have a big research department; ask it to see where the optimum point is between productivity and hours worked.

"Much more important, even than your partners, is your self worth. I know so many of you came with high hopes of contributing, working together to produce amazing new technologies and all the enthusiasm has been squeezed out of you by corporate politics and egotistical agendas. The important thing is to make ourselves real to ourselves and to others. We can only do that by communicating from our hearts and with our brains; otherwise we are like robots working to formulae. There is no point in grumbling to ourselves or to those who can do nothing about our concerns. And there is no virtue in obedience which causes harm.

"Look at it like this. One of your colleagues is rather secretive. He is polite to people but nobody knows anything about him. He says very little at meetings and people resent him because he does not share his ideas. Then, one day, he looks very nervous and somebody hears that he has somehow got an appointment to see the Managing Director. Colleagues smile encouragingly as he leaves silently; but within half an hour he is back, shaking. 'I am so ashamed and angry,' he says, 'He just took no notice of me. First he said that the Department is not performing and then he said my idea was totally impractical. See what you think.' Still shaking, he forces himself to calm down as he gives some instructions to his computer. Suddenly there are wonderful, gleaming 3-D objects that appear to be floating in space but which, he says, can be manipulated so that they can be seen from different angles in different combinations; it looks like an enlarged child's kaleidoscope. 'This is early work on a computer methodology for assembling materials for a major project using colour, shape and volume', he says. Everybody thinks it is wonderful but nobody knows whether to try again with the MD or whether to form a small company to sell the idea elsewhere.

"You may not be as inventive as the man in the story but you have to value what you are doing and have the courage to speak up for it even if bosses reject it. There is no point in self-censoring and grumbling. God Our Parent has given us brains and if we pray to My Sister the Spirit we will receive courage. We are never given any task in life without the resources to undertake it."

The LIFT people came out with their followers and tried to dash past

Perpetua. "It is not worth the effort," she said. "Just because you do not respect my Christian metaphor it does not mean that I do not respect yours. I disagree with the way you are seeing things but we must always listen to each other. Next time LIFT comes to visit GLINT, go along and give it a try. Only through spending some time with Christian people will you be able to make a start in your relationship with God Our Parent."

One of the LIFT leaders stayed back while the others put things into their cars. "I thought you disagreed with us; and we certainly disagree with you." "Yes but we are disagreeing over perspective and metaphor. You see that people are saved and re-born I see that Jesus died and was re-born; you are anthropocentric, I am theocentric; I look at Jesus, you look at what Jesus has done for people; I believe that what Jesus has done is a mystery, you believe that it is obvious. But what Jesus is and has done he is and has done regardless of our differences. You are doing wonderful work here bringing God Our Parent to the rich and the sad."

Next morning Perpetua made her usual visit to the local Hypo to discuss the *god4u* project along with its sponsoring leader, in this case Brian. Then she went with the women's group to Slatethorpe Primary and listened to the children reading. Perpetua told them a story about her Auntie Mary and how they would all see her at Christmas. When she referred to Jesus as her Brother but his mother as her Auntie Mary, one child asked how this could be. She said it was a mystery.

9.

"This is Bad Morning with Rod Stirrer and with me, Craig Knocker. And the main story today is that Parliament has passed its twelfth Criminal Justice Bill in as many years. Norma, will this be the last in the series?" "I don't think so, Craig. Most MPs now wearily admit that legislation—even tougher prison sentences—will not solve the crime problem; there are even some who say that the Government only introduces bills to try to convince the public that it is doing something." "How cynical; thank you Norma. The other major story is the rise in the number of families living in poverty..."

While Perpetua was on tour, Roy was getting a grip on Grunge Park. After the initial buzz, most people looked back to the reign of Dexter as a golden age. Where Dexter had managed to rule by threat, Roy felt that because he was physically slight (and lacking in self-esteem, according to a rather 'soft' report) he had to act rather than talk. Power made him careless.

His major target was the youth club from which he intended to dislodge Miles. Coming in early one evening he found Miles and a girl setting up tables. He told Miles that if he did not leave immediately he would regret it. Miles, who was scared beyond anything he could have imagined, held his ground. Roy, who was not quite sure what to do, hid his indecisiveness by grabbing the girl and saying: "If you don't get out this moment I will spoil the face of this pretty little thing." Miles was rigid with fear, he could neither speak nor run. Roy felt that he had lost control, downgrading his threat from Miles to the girl. This was when he was most dangerous, when he lost control and just needed to assert; that is what had happened with Kish. He had gone to sort things out but because Kish was 'talking clever' he had just lost control. The girl, who had been temporarily startled, was now working out whether to scream or stay quiet, to try to allure, to do nothing or make a run for it. Roy had a knife in his right hand and was pinning the girl against a table with his left but she could tell he was not very strong. In a sudden rush of bravery Miles lunged at Roy who lunged at the girl. They both missed but this made Roy dangerously angry. He managed to kick Miles in the face while he was trying to get up without losing control of the girl who was half sprawled on the table. His temper rose to a terrible pitch and he was about to stab her in the chest when: "Stop!" shouted Perpetua. Dexter gripped his upper arm and shouted: "Drop it!" He then went to the door and asked Trina to bring in some coffee from the bus and Perpetua told the other three to sit down.

Roy had crumpled. The girl was curious and Miles was just coming down from his unaccustomed bravery, seeing now how close he had been to real danger.

Perpetua said: "First of all, we need to listen, without interruption or judgment, to what Roy has to say." "There isn't much to say. I'm the boss round here and Miles is in my way. I came to give him a quiet warning but the girl got tangled up in it." Silence. "Is that all, Roy?" Silence. "All right, you have had first turn. Now, setting aside whether you are boss, why do you want to be the boss?" "I had a difficult childhood; my dad was violent and my mum was a user. I never got a fair deal at school." Silence. "So that makes you entitled to threaten people with knives?" "How else can we get control of our own lives?" Silence. "But you have control of your life; the problem is that you want to control the lives of other people. Have you finished?" Silence. "All right, if that is all you have to say. First, your dad was not violent. He was a gentle, hard working man who was desperately unhappy because of you. Secondly, your mother was a virtuous woman who was also terribly upset by the way you treated her. Thirdly, the reason why they were both so upset was that you were very bright but chose to be lazy at school; that was your choice." (all confirmed by INEPT). "Liar!" "Do not start again. I know all about you. None of us can do anything until we have faced up to ourselves."

Dexter was becoming impatient. "Calm down Dexter, you are not a gang leader any more. Sit down." The girl asked to leave. "I would prefer you not to go," said Perpetua, "because the healing process has to involve everybody who was part of the injury, including the injured people. So far we have heard Roy tell some lies. Do you have anything to say about adding lies to your threatening behaviour?" No. "He was threatening you with a knife, what do you have to say?" "Not much. It was a bit frightening but nothing happened. We don't want to involve anybody else." "So do you forgive him?" "I am not sure what that means, really. I mean it would have been better if he hadn't been so nasty but nothing happened really." "Miles, what about you?" "I can't forgive him. He's a thug. He threatened me and then he threatened a girl." "But if the girl can forgive him, or at least come as close to it as she knows, why are you not prepared to?" "People who are sinners need to be punished." "Oh Miles, what about the Prodigal Son?" "Who's he?" asked the girl.

"There were identical twin boys, James and John, so identical that not even their parents could tell them apart at first. But as they began to walk and then talk, James was jolly and active but John was grumpy and inert. As they grew up, James worked hard at school and gave his parents great joy but John did nothing, which made his parents very sad: 'But,' he thought, 'they love me, so they will not punish me. They will see that I am all right whatever I do.'

"When they were sixteen, James, through very hard work, qualified for a car mechanics course and used his savings to make a down payment but John, who was much more talented, did not turn up for his exams and asked his father whether he could have some money to take driving lessons. Relieved that he wanted to do something, his father gave him the money and he passed his test. 'Look,' said his father, 'that proves that you are capable of doing things when you want to.' The boy only growled and went away; but later, he thought: 'I can use this situation to my advantage. I will ask him to give me the money for a car as a reward for my hard work.' His father offered him all the spare cash that he had to put a deposit on a car but John was dissatisfied. He accepted the money but one evening when his parents were out he gathered up all the valuables he could carry. He took his father's credit cards and diary where he found all his PINs and in the next few days he took as much money as he could until the cards were stopped. His father knew what had happened but did not report his son saying: 'I know I should but he will get into trouble; one day, with God's help, all will be well.'

"John joined a gang of tearaways who stole cars for joy-riding, got drunk and used drugs but when his money began to run out they dropped him. At last he began to steal to buy drink, drugs and food. He thought it would be easier to steal in a familiar place but there was a greater risk of being identified. His father picked up rumours that John had been seen in the neighbourhood. Without telling his family, he steeled himself to go into parts of the town he had only heard about. He found John, skinny, dirty and insensible in a squat. He was so limp and light that, with a great effort, he could lift him. He took him to a doctor friend who said there was no danger; John just needed looking after. The father took John to a farmhouse where they had spent happy holidays. He told his wife he would be away for a couple of nights. She did not ask why or where; she trusted him.

"Next day, his father sat by John's bed until he woke up. 'Father', he said, 'I feel like killing myself.' 'You must think no such thing. You are very run down and need help.' 'But I have stolen so that I can live. How can you, who are so honest, bear to look at me?' 'The first thing we must do is put together a list of those you have stolen from so they can be quietly paid back.' 'But you do not have the money.' 'The Lord will see that we are all right.' 'I feel so ashamed. I have let you down so badly.' 'No, my son, you have let yourself down.'

"The father quietly told his wife what had happened. They were very worried about the reaction of James. They wanted to hold a family party but when they told him the story he was very angry. 'I struggled to get through my car mechanics course while he stole your money and spent it all. You have never let me bring my friends round for a party and now you want to throw a party for him.' 'Yes,' said his father, 'but we need to celebrate as he was lost to us and now he has come back. You have been here all the time and so we have enjoyed a warm family relationship but he is coming back to join that relationship.' 'But look at what he has done.' 'None of us will ever forget what he has done; he will remember most of all; but we must all love John as he has remembered how to love us.'

"James would not come to the party and this pained his mother and fa-ther but, as the weeks passed by, the family worked hard to knit itself back together."

"Sentimental crap!" said Roy. "You might think so," said Perpetua, "but without that kind of forgiveness at the private end of the spectrum there would be no mercy at the public end of the spectrum. "Why should I care?" "Because it is only a matter of time before you are asking a court for mercy. However, the main point of the story is that the father's forgiveness is wonderful but it is incalculably small compared with the forgiveness of God Our Parent. I want you to know, Roy, that no matter what you do, you will always be forgiven if you turn to God." The girl said: "I forgot to thank you for getting me out of this situation." Miles said: "As a private person, the father can do what he likes but in the public arena punishment must go hand-in-hand with forgiveness."

"We need to go now," said Perpetua. "We were only dropping in to see that everything was all right; but Trina says she wants to stay, if that's all right with you; and, Miles, you are doing such a good job."

10.

"The Government is becoming increasingly concerned with the number of foreign women who are illegally entering the country to work as prostitutes. Minister, I presume that the latest crackdown on these women has failed." "No.We are using a three-pronged approach: tightening up on immigration, increasing the sentences for prostitution and taxing immoral earnings." "But what about the men who run the whole business, the people traffickers and pimps?" "Well, Janet, that is a much more difficult problem but we are tackling that too." "And what about the customers?" "Well, there really is nothing you can do about that; boys will be boys, you know, Janet." "Thank you Minister. Now we turn to the news that the Directorate of Independent Media has lost its court case to keep hard core porn off television. The Coalition for Adult Self and Health has said that it brought the case to defend freedom of speech..."

It was relatively easy to keep tabs on Perpetua and her *god4u* followers during their month-long visit to Stumpy Knoll. They all stayed together and all the set pieces were captured but it was more difficult to keep track of her less formal activities. Before her arrival there had been some racial tension and she spent the first week shuttling between the two disgruntled groups but they were gradually brought together. The first signs were the usual kind of thing, football matches, talent contests, dances, but it was not long before there was a mixed race community choir and a park restoration project. There were the usual stories that filtered out from schools, nursing homes and hospitals about the unusual consequences of Perpetua's visits but their frequency meant that SAD simply logged them. The DISC (Democracy Interchange for Senior Citizens) was causing some concern but SAD was only interested in statistics and locations; personal stories were no use.

There was, however, the curious incident of an open air music event at which Perpetua handed out free soft drinks and burgers to more than a thousand people. None of the local traders took credit (though Perpetua had been in Hypo, Lakshmo and Jambo) and no other supply was sourced. There was a report that they had deposited 50 jumbo black plastic bags at the tip on their way out of town. One eye witness (suffering from some kind of religious delusion) later reported that Perpetua had somehow conjured all the food and drink out of nothing, saying that she had divine powers as the "Sacred Vessel" (curious word; a dish or a ship) of God. He tried to get the local paper interested but the story was so clearly a 'wind-up' that it went no further. Nonetheless, the file on the Party for 1000 is still open.

Father O'Helly was never comfortable when he came out of his local paper shop; but even before he could look carefully up and down the street he bumped into Perpetua. "Good morning, Father. I am glad I have bumped into you as I wanted to ask you to join the media literacy task force which we are setting up to educate people about the dangers of pornography." "Ah yes, pornography", said Father O'Helly. "You know what I mean Father, the kind of material that people carry away in brown paper bags ... like that one you are holding." Father O'Helly blushed. "It's all right, Father. I will not say anything but you really should not be buying *man4man* and *Onan*. Perhaps you are not exactly the right person to help with the task force; I will have to rely on Miles, Father Midway and my own people."

At this moment Miles came out of the shop clutching a brown paper bag. "I am not sure I like what is in there," said Perpetua. "I would almost prefer you to have pictures of girls than guns. You hardly seem right for a media literacy task force." As if they had contracted Perpetua's infection, O'Helly and Miles started looking at what people were carrying out of the paper shop or, rather, what they were hiding. They had (of course) imagined a stereotype person but, as they were themselves brown bag carriers, the stereotype no longer worked.

"One of the problems with Christianity," Perpetua said, "is that it is so code based rather than ethic based that the ethical sense becomes atrophied. We are so used to giving orders that we no longer have to analyse our own behaviour. This happens in the positive as well as the negative sense. The Commandments say "Thou shalt not..." but we have added to these a whole list of "thou shalts...". There is so much work to be done in the vineyard but we have all become self-appointed supervisors expecting somebody else to do all the digging and pruning. Nowhere is this worse than with the media. We are forever complaining about the prurience, the violence, the sexualisation of teenagers but all that we do is call on other people to regulate supply. We sign petitions about people trafficking but there would not be any if people did not buy slaves and prostitutes. Girls would not be exploited if people did not buy pornography. There are those poor souls who might want to make a crude pornographic movie for their own consumption and pleasure but most of the industry is driven by demand from people who consider themselves to be 'respectable'.

"It is, however, too easy to put labels on people. All of us know, the suppliers, the buyers and the standers-bye, that damage is being done to people in their doomed effort to mend what is broken in them. Anybody who buys anything that needs to be put into a brown paper bag to save them from shame must ask why they are buying, who suffers and whether there is a better way of finding ourselves.

"Christianity has become a formula competing with its arch rivals, cynicism and materialism, but it will only live if it becomes a lively, muscular ethic which grows out of the Spirit of God and the life of Jesus My Brother." "I wish you would not keep on using that clumsy title," said O'Helly, recovering his aggression a little. "We are all brothers and sisters of Jesus." "True, but I am a Sister of Jesus in a very special way because I am the Daughter of God Our Parent in a very special way. You will see when you get home. Our problem is that a rigid ethic, no matter how well intentioned, springs from the same blinkered view of creation as the cynical and consumerist syndromes. The cynics say that only extreme caution, mistrust and monitoring, can keep order in a society where everybody is only motivated by material gain. The icon of cynicism is incentive. The consumerists say that all ills can be cured by acquiring something or using a service. The icon of consumerism is therapy. The Christians who are obsessed with codes—Petrans like You, Father; Torans like you, Miles—think that there is some clear cut way of saving people if they follow a rigid code. The icon of Christianity is control.

"But, to paraphrase St. Paul, I know a better way which we should talk about when I get back in time for Advent."

Perpetua walked down a grimy street full of houses with highly unusual levels of security. As she went by, bars were snapped, windows were broken and locks were sprung. Women and men in all states of undress, poured out into the streets. Their owners came afterwards shouting and brandishing weapons. "Stop!" shouted Perpetua, and all the weapons clattered to the ground. Wayne and Bob began to collect the weapons, Dexter rounded up all the men and Kylie and Jo worked with the women. As each house was emptied, they went back in for their few possessions. Perpetua took a long look at the men. Apart from the owners there were the usual categories: one of Bill Midway's Churchwardens, a TT leader writer who berated the country for its immorality, a senior magistrate, a dancing tutor, a policeman, the owner of a bridal shop, a city councillor, two nurses and two teachers, but there were also the empty shells of men who were incapable of adult relationships with women (or other men) for whom prostitution was the only form of control they could exercise; and Miles. "You do not need to worry," she said, looking at him and those who thought they could be identified, "I have nobody to tell; but you must tell yourselves what you have done and resolve never to do it again. All of us, in different ways, feel that we are inadequate in our relationships but we must never try to mend ourselves by breaking other people. The only true healer is God Our Parent through the Grace of My Sister the Spirit and the highest relationship we can have while on earth is with Jesus My Brother. We must all look into our hearts; and if we need help to confront ourselves we must seek it in those who love Jesus.

"As for you exploiters, I will say nothing this time but you must look into yourselves and ask whether the money you make is worth ruining the lives of so many people, treating them like sex machines that have to be fuelled with drugs to keep them going until they disintegrate. As for you 'clients', it is bad enough that you exploit vulnerable people but it is even worse that you are public moralists, hypocrites, condemning others for doing what you do yourselves. You know this; you hurl the word 'Hypocrite' around often enough in your talk and your writing, your rules and your judgments."

As usual when Perpetua pulled one of her stunts, there were problems with finding homes for the people she had 'liberated'. Even before the SAD contact had reported, Perpetua had phoned the RED (Regional Executive Director) and asked her (conversation taped) for an emergency team. This was highly irregular as, technically, it needed SAD clearance. Those who could be placed were given cash by Andy, and Perpetua and her other followers took the rest back to their rented flats. This was also highly irregular but Perpetua could never understand the importance of rules. There was also the question of the weapons that *god4u* had seized; a large number were deposited at the Police Station but nobody knows how many were held back.

When Father O'Helly got home, he was almost wild with guilty desire. He tore the brown bag open and stared at the plain cover of *mary4me* and the equally prosaic *Theotokos*. When he recovered, he wondered what Miles had found in his brown bag.

11.

"Professor, why have you chosen to make this ferocious attack on the concept of God?" "Because it's unscientific." "So what is so wonderful about concepts that are scientific? I mean, is enjoying a sunset or crying when you hear a favourite piece of music scientific?" "Of course it is, these emotions are triggered by concrete phenomena." "But the same phenomena don't always trigger the same emotions." "Of course not, because we are all different." "So what is wrong with the difference which means that some people are disposed to believe in God?" "It's unscientific."

In mid-November plans for Christmas were discussed at a quiet day attended by the *god4u* core group and delegations from all over the country. Perpetua said that they would be leading a movement to encourage people to communicate with God through house groups rather than conventional church services. This (not surprisingly) did not go down well. Although her followers had moved on since they were first recruited, they were still emotionally and intellectually tied to received tradition. They expected Perpetua to support struggling churches and saw house groups as additional activity but Perpetua said that most conventional churches were an obstacle to communication with God: "There is no point theorising," she said. "How many of you who are defending conventional church go there other than at Christmas and Easter?" Two hands went up. "Precisely. That tells us how effective almost all of you think it is. Our objective, then, will be to establish cell churches and gradually build them with cross-sections of people. I do not want cell churches for the poor and cell churches for the rich, not just because I want the poor to benefit from the experience and wealth of the rich but also because the rich are operating under a terrible handicap in their pursuit of a relationship with God.

"Before we set out on Christmas morning to start these new cell churches I am going to preside at an unconventional celebration of the Eucharist of Jesus My Brother to show how it can be opened up." "But," objected Wayne, "you are not ordained." "The point is that nobody can perform the Eucharistic right without the direct intervention of My Sister the Spirit; it is She, not the minister presiding, that makes Jesus My Brother truly present in the sacred elements, conventionally but not necessarily bread and wine. What we need to preside at the Eucharist is the will of the people that we should be their link to the Spirit and the Spirit's confirmation that we are a suitable link. The problem is that in the Christian tradition, the first part of this process has been almost forgotten and the second part has become like an interview for a job with assessment centres, profiling and, worst of all, the power of the process to tell people they do not have a calling from the Spirit; not just individual people but whole blocks of people such as women, people who are gay, people who do not conform with the paradigm psychological profile. To listen to most people in the churches, My Sister the Spirit only seems to like mild-mannered, indecisive loners. St. Paul would not pass a Selection Conference today; nor would I."

"Why are the Christian churches so rigid?" asked Brian. "The problem with the theologians who drive the churches," said Perpetua, "is that they forget that theology is a metaphor; and then they, and their more militant adherents, start trying to impose their metaphors on other people. It is hard enough to impose a code on other people, even harder to impose an ethic, but most difficult to impose a metaphor. Having said that, they have all been very set on the metaphor of the Church as the 'Bride of Christ' which means, as the Church is the creation of Christ and, therefore, in a 'lower' category (it is inconceivable that the created should be equal to the Creator), so women, styled as brides, must be 'lower' than men. The metaphor for the communication of God is the Trinity which also manages two males and the Spirit.

"When all our inner resources are turned towards the mystery of the relationship between creatures and the Creator, between the 'saved' and the Redeemer, between sinners and the Sanctifier, we all have individual experiences of it. Churches are not belief systems they are collections of individual believers who come together for mutual support and celebration. In churches people naturally hold onto formulae which they think bind them together but actually they do not. What binds people is the search, not what they think is the answer. Churches are questions not answers and it is their forgetfulness of this, of their anthropocentric transference from questions into answers, that has stultified them.

"We are going to go out and energise the world so that it can better apprehend the mystery of the relationship between Creator and Created and between all of us and Jesus My Brother; and we will help people to leave themselves open to My Sister the Spirit.

"It is important that, at least for the time being, you are not to say anything about my true nature. The Spirit will tell you when it is time, after I have been murdered." "But," said Dexter, (getting very angry), "if you are part of the Godhead you can use your divine powers to stop yourself being murdered." "As could have Jesus My Brother but he chose to hold such power in abeyance. But that is not the point. He died and I am to die because there is no other way in which humanity, the Creatures of God, can both understand the depth of their wickedness and the depth of the love of God for all of them. I could stop myself being killed but I must not, no matter how frightened I am. Only when I am dead will people realise how the love of God lived in me in a special way and therefore lives in all who recognise God in themselves and others; only then will they see that the death of Jesus My Brother was not only an event in history, it is an event in the story of humanity that must happen over and over again. Already there are those, notably in the established Christian churches, who are very angry at what I am doing and would like to stop me. They think that the story of Christianity is over, that it has reached a kind of 'end of history'; but as God Our Parent's Sacred Vessel I am the living proof that the history of God on earth has not ended."

"You keep talking about being a Vessel," said Wayne, "but what does that mean?" "I know that we are all children of God our Parent and brothers and sisters of Jesus and of the Spirit in a mysterious way," said Perpetua, "but I am a daughter of God and Sister of Jesus in a special way: I am the Daughter of God in the way that Jesus was the Son of God; I am an incarnated form of God." "Does that mean," asked Wayne, "that you claim to be part of the Godhead?" (Incredible! No wonder the Torans and Petrans were hostile!)

"I am as much a part of the Godhead as Jesus. I am the Sacred Vessel into which God Our Parent has poured the whole of Divinity without losing any but I am also the Vessel sent to carry all the wickedness of the world as My Brother Jesus carried it before me." "But," asked Wayne (who, according to INEPT, had a high grade in RE) "even if you are the Sister of Jesus, how can you be equally the Sister of the Spirit when the Spirit was not the Sister of Jesus but 'proceeded' from Jesus and God Our Parent?" "Because these relationships are not biological but divine," (cleverly) said Perpetua.

"I will give you the energy of life. Anyone who does not have this energy cannot live forever. I have brought this energy directly to you from God Our Parent." "But Christians say," said Wayne, "that Jesus was the last word; He made the final sacrifice." "His sacrifice of Himself upon the cross was full, sufficient, to save the world from its wickedness; but it was not final. How can human beings instruct God Our Parent that Jesus must be the last incarnated manifestation of Godhead? How do you know how many manifestations of the Godhead there have been in other planetary systems? You only know that, so far, Jesus is the only incarnate existence of God on Planet Earth."

"Nobody will believe what you say," said Trina (PR to the fore as usual) "unless you perform some sort of miracles to prove that you are who you say you are. Don't get me wrong, I believe you are who you say you are. Quite obviously you are the Sacred Vessel of God Our Parent in the way that none of us is but you can't just assert that to people in the twenty-first Century. They are so cynical or, at best, sceptical." "I only perform special acts in tribute to God Our Parent who has given me special powers. I will not perform special acts to buy people. I have already performed some special acts but these have been to help people to think about their relationship, through me, with God."

"Does this mean that we will be able to perform special acts?" "Not until you are past needing me to perform special acts to convince you of who I am. Once you have faith in me and my special relationship with God Our Parent you will, when you go out to spread the word, be able to perform special acts if My Sister the Spirit enables them with Her blessing.

"In the meantime, we need to work on the way we pray and we need to think about how we can build firm cell churches. We also need to understand our approach to Presiding at the Eucharist. Those whom the Spirit calls have special duties to perform; with my special relationship as the Daughter of God Our Parent I know from My Sister the Spirit that all of you have been called to follow me and to bear witness to God in your lives and in your mission. Each of you who leads a cell church will need the special strength to preside at the Eucharist."

She set up a table and placed upon it a simple glass jug of water and a plate of fresh apples. She followed the usual course of the Eucharist until the end of a Gospel reading and then called the leadership group to stand at the table. She said she must ask each of them three questions: Do you affirm that you have been called by the Spirit? Do you affirm that you will try to bear witness to God with every word, action and silence of your life? Do you affirm that you will try to see God in all humanity and to love regardless of personal prefer- ence? When they had each had answered positively, she put her hands gently upon their heads and said: "Receive the power of the Spirit"; she blessed them and gave them each a Bible and a notebook, saying: "Teach and learn, speak and listen."

She then blessed the water and the apples, called on the Spirit and used the words of Consecration, substituting "apples" for bread and "water" for wine.

At the end she said: Go out and tell the world that all is not lost; that life is worth living because it is a gift of God. Pick up materials from Wayne and a media pack from Trina."

Some people had already gone before the end. They had found Perpetua's description of herself too difficult to take. SAD picked up some of these in case their resentment might prove useful.

Perpetua then disappeared for a while. Trina would only say that she had gone away to pray (but this was clearly spin.)

12.

"Chief Constable, are there areas on your watch which are in a state of civil war?" "It depends on what you mean by 'civil war'; it's not a term we use." "I would have thought it's obvious." "Not to me.We measure criminal activity and our ability to keep on top of it." "Which, OF COURSE, you are not. But what people want to know..." "Which people?" "The public we represent; they want to know whether our inner cities are in a state of civil war." "Do they?You might be interested in the headline proclaiming a civil war but I think they are more interested in what is actually going on than an argument about the label you slap on it." "Thank you Chief Constable. Janet." "Well, Owen, the latest development in the cash for honours scandal is a shift from what happened to how it happened.We have moved from whether it happened to what people did wrong even if it didn't happen..."

In spite of a series of reckless forays, Roy did not feel that he had complete control of Grunge Park. The *god4u* movement still had a grip on local media with its own channel complementing the Community Channel. The pirates were not functioning because of technical difficulties they could not solve.The drugs revenue was at a disastrously low level and showed no signs of picking up and the neighbourhood in general seemed to be less threatening.As already noted, SAD was ambivalent about this phenomenon.

Then, without warning, the place erupted. It was as if all the selfishness that had been pent up inside people had to find its way out, as if inner devils needed room to move. The evening had started quietly enough. In spite of (counter-productive) SAS rules on the use of fireworks there were (inevitably) numerous unsupervised parties. One of these took place on the waste ground in The Hollow and it was unusual because Roy had invited some associates from Excelsior Gardens, notably Rory Varnish and Oliver O'Helly. There had been informal links for some time with Roy tentatively extending his sphere of influence into the Gardens through Rory and Oliver who were forming a RIF (RIch Fakes) group. (RIFs are well off people who take part in gang activity as a form of recreation.) When they were all, except Roy, high or drunk, he suggested that they should throw a few fireworks into a tower block undergoing refurbishment and, once that had excited everybody, he decided that it was time to put his main plan into operation. His target was the *god4u* Channel where Perpetua's followers put out a looped diet of her speeches and interviews, reflections and prayers and reports from nascent cells, supported by Jim's music. Roy's problem was that everybody got too excitable and began to set cars on fire and lob fireworks into windows at random. Things were getting out of control and so the only way he could appear to stay in control was to appear to be directing the mayhem. Frightened residents phoned the police who (as a matter of routine) decided to classify Grunge Park Estate as a 'Containment Area', hoping to keep any unrest strictly inside agreed limits. When people said they wanted "Bobbies on the beat" this did not mean a high profile police presence in run-down housing estates, it meant the ability of the fashionable watch-wearing middle class to ask the time of a reassuring young constable.

Trina, who was on duty at the *god4u* Channel, called Perpetua. She was not optimistic as her phone had been switched off for more than a week but this time she replied. "There is a disturbance in Grunge Park," said Trina "and there is a rumour that we are the target." "I know," said Perpetua. "So what should we do?" asked Trina. "Keep on broadcasting; stay where you are; I am coming right down; I am only a couple of miles away." "How did that happen?" "I have been praying for a few days. My Sister The Spirit said that you needed some special help; she knows how evil works."

The problem for Roy was that although he was not as focused as he need-ed to be, he did have the definite object of stamping his authority on Grunge Park in general and over *god4u* in particular but the RIFs lacked any sense of strategy, they were there to have a bit of fun. They were naturally particularly attracted to combustible items like cars and wooden structures and they loved the sound of breaking glass. Nonetheless, through the frenetic use of his mo-bile, Roy managed to tempt all the stragglers to get back together by promising a spectacular. In spite of the security risk *god4u* had based itself in a ground floor office to ensure easy access from the street. When Trina heard the sound of breaking glass coming towards her down the street and when she saw a firework explode under a nearby car, she was about to evacuate when Perpetua walked unhurriedly towards her. "Did you not believe me?" Trina blushed. "Go back in and broadcast what you can. Brian has come from his assignment and will be taking footage; but be careful how you use it; only general background until we know how things are. No close-ups of faces."

She walked unflinchingly towards the core of the violence, through threat-ening fires, flying fireworks and broken glass. There was a pall of smoke thick-ening overhead and there were sparks everywhere. She reached the youth club cross roads where Roy's nucleus of about twenty young men was milling: Ol-iver O'Helly was was supervising car overturning; Rory Varnish was priming a petrol bomb to throw at the tempting wood and glass club; and Roy was trying to keep them moving in the right direction. Miles was standing in the doorway, frozen between protest and flight, overwhelmed by the general sense of evil but oblivious to the particular threat from Rory. "Stop!" shouted Perpetua, whose amplified voice cut through the general noise. She stood (courageously) right in front of Miles. "Oliver, home, or I will tell your uncle; likewise, Rory I do not think your father the Archdeacon would enjoy a picture of you throwing a petrol bomb. Roy, get your people to come here." He bridled. "Now!" she said.

"Before we go any further," she said to Brian, "get those pictures to Trina and tell her to edit and release them to any other channel, starting with Cutting Edge. I will now phone the police.

"Officer, I know who you are and where you are. Get your people in here. … Nonsense … If you do not come in to help these people I will.…

"Roy, get your people to clean up and work out who has been damaged by your stupidity. This is not blackmail; I am not the police; there will be no attempt to identify faces; if the police will not come and collect evidence I am not going to do that for them. I just need you to put this right."

She went back to the *god4u* Channel office. "It is so sad," she said in an interview with Trina, "that there are so many self-inflicted wounds. It is significant that these people do not create mayhem outside their home ground; it shows that they are not really concerned with money. They want power in small places because they are sick. They are sick of how they live but they have so few routes out." "Is it, then, a question of resources?" "Not really, we could put unlimited money into urban renewal and it would not alter some of the underlying problems. What unhappy people need—and this kind of behaviour is the result of unhappiness—is love. They need to know that God Our Parent loves them; and they need to know that there are many people who love them because they see God in them. Social Services work so hard," (true) "but the ethic of non-involvement, borrowed from medicine, is entirely wrong. There is a difference between being objective, which is necessary, and being cold, which is counter-productive. Naturally, we cannot expect people in social services to like everybody but they must generate genuine regard and something as near to love as they can manage." (So interesting.)

"We must get all the material—minus shots that identify people—as background to my interview, to as many channels as possible, starting with CEC.

"We can work with most of these people. As for Roy, I can control what he does but there will come a time when he destroys me because that is how it must be." "Of course not," said Trina, (appalled) "Yes. There is no avoiding it. I am inevitably moving towards a terrible death."

The next day Perpetua called the almost defunct Ecumenical Partnership. Miles was grateful for what Perpetua had done but could not stop talking about punishment and judgment. He was angry that Perpetua had wiped what he called incriminating pictures. O'Helly was inclined to side with him but Perpetua asked him whether he would be quite so draconian if his own family were involved. "Be careful," said Perpetua and, sensing the warning, he was.

The police were understanding. They did not want complex cases to be brought against Roy and his people; they wanted to keep things as they were. The Council was grateful that things had not been worse and accepted the damage as part of the 'containment' policy. SAD had a routine for dealing with emergency need. Perpetua said that Kylie and Heather would be brought from their assignments to help with organising special help and she promised to see that the worst off got help before Christmas with a (really innovative) proposal to raise promises from the people of Excelsior Gardens.

Back at the Channel Perpetua was still thinking about the disturbance. "I think this foreshadows my own death. This is not important, really; what matters is that there is so much evil. I can use my special powers to stop things happening but that is not a long-term fix.." Miles came in to ask Trina if he could make a statement. "Not," said Perpetua intervening "if you are going to call for retribution. You are so brave and good Miles, you just need to learn about love." It was a rather rough attempt by Miles but as it was pre-recorded they made a good piece. "O'Helly next," said Trina.

From that time there was a (perfectly reasonable) attempt to downgrade SAD's interest in Perpetua. What she did was apparently irrelevant; much more important was her anomalous profile which made her look more like a person with special gifts than a makeshift radical.

13.

"Thank you Barry, it's good to see that England have lost again. Now we turn to the vexed question of overcrowding in prisons. Mr Leftside from Prison Is Terrible *joins me on the line. Your latest pamphlet—what you call research—says that putting people into prison is counter productive." "Yes, it does absolutely no good whatsoever in the case of most prisoners. If we had a population of the 10,000 most serious offenders in prison and let all the others out it would have a negligible effect on the crime rate. Most of these people need a job to keep them out of prison in the first place." "So taking people who have offended against society and not putting them in prison is good for them and society?" "Yes, with some qualifications that is correct." "But that is nonsense." "No, it is simply counter intuitive." "But there is no such thing as 'counter intuitive'; everybody knows that if you put somebody in prison they can't go on committing crimes. Anyway, there is another place where you call for more effective policing and judicial procedures to increase the rate of arrest and conviction. What's the point of going through all of that if you don't put them in prisons? The two things don't hang together." "It is vital that we use detection and due conviction as deterrents and that we use the period between detection and release back into society for problem solving; but prisons are a bad place for problem solving." "Well I am sure we will receive hundreds of emails ridiculing this rather contradictory thinking. Rod." "Thank you Craig. Now the case of a boy who has been cautioned for throwing a snowball at a police car..."*

Needless to say, Parkwood Prison had neither a park nor a wood. In fact, because it was so crammed in amongst urban developments, it had nothing much at all; only the high security prisons out in the real countryside had gyms. Never was forbidding stone so makeshift. Some prisons had workshops but because of the overcrowding these had been converted into makeshift offices so that an office block could be turned into makeshift cells. In spite of numerous attempts (genuine and fake) to reform the system, the basic statistics about Parkwood were stark: 80% of its inmates were forced to share cells whether they liked it or not; 75% had a substance abuse problem; 70% had never had a job; 65% were re-offenders and would offend again; 60% had literacy or learning problems; 30% were suffering from severe mental illness; 25% were black; 10% were ex-servicemen; 0% were receiving the kind of regime set out in a series of judicial, independent and internal reports on the purposes of prison.

One morning, shortly after the disturbances, Perpetua, Heather and Jo turned up at the gate and asked to be let in. They were told that this was highly irregular and that they would have to make an appointment to see an officer or come at the appropriate time to see inmates. "Oh dear!" said Perpetua, "I wonder how that gate got open. Calm down and it will close nicely behind me; there. I could have slipped through that next gate, officer, but I thought we better follow procedure." The gate officer could not work out how the gate had opened without proper authorisation and without triggering an alarm. He pressed a hidden button and four colleagues appeared. "I think we better put these young women into a holding cell until we can find a suitable person to question them." They were about to take hold of Perpetua when she said: "There is no need for that, we will gladly walk in front of you." So the four men escorted Perpetua and her companions to a tiny cell in the main court just inside the gate lodge. They locked the door and returned to file their rather puzzling paperwork but they had hardly started when there was a tap on the door. "As nobody came I thought we might dispense with any more procedure," said Perpetua. "I would be most grateful if you could introduce us to the residents." "This is highly irregular," said one of the officers. "So many things are," said Perpetua. "It is so sad that it is the bad irregular things that seem to be sanctioned and the good irregular things that are vetoed. We can say that I am a chaplain Emeritus; officials are always impressed by Latin—it is a man thing—that, anyway, is what I have entered in your records although this was a challenge because your IT system is so erratic.

The senior officer left the room and returned a few minutes later with the Governor. "It is so nice to meet you, Governor Bentky," said Perpetua. "I am sorry that our visit is so sudden." "That is nothing to worry about," said the Governor, "as long as we can have a picture of you with the caption 'Chaplain Emeritus', such a charming designation; you are quite a celebrity. I can hardly turn on CEC without seeing you discussing one serious issue or another." "You are very kind. I would be most grateful if we could talk with the two young men brought in after the disturbances and remanded in custody. There will be nothing private," said Perpetua, "so I do not mind how many accompany us but perhaps it would be appropriate for the regular Chaplain to be in attendance." "I am afraid we have a serious problem," said the Governor, "we have every variety of Chaplain except a Christian; I don't know why. I will accompany you myself."

As they went through the main court Jo said to Perpetua, "do that thing with the gates again; it was great. It really frightened them." "No," said Perpetua, "I do not perform tricks for entertainment, I simply witness to God Our Parent in unusual and special acts when this is strictly necessary to fulfill a purpose."

The two prisoners were brought to the visitors' area. "Well, Kelvin, I can guess how you got here but Thomas, how did you get here?" "I have now been officially listed," said Thomas, "as one of the 'Usual Suspects'." "Well I am sorry to hear that but at least it proves that not all alleged hooligans on deprived housing estates are black," said Perpetua (wryly). "What happened?" "Nothing, really," said Thomas. "We were hanging about, on the edges of the trouble, wondering whether there was anything we could get out of it but I don't see the sense in burning cars that are good to drive or breaking windows if you don't nip inside and take a look. Then you came and shouted at Roy and he disappeared and a few minutes later the police came and we ran for it, right into some other police. They seemed a bit worried that they had stayed out so long and needed to get their quota." "Kelvin, I have told you before and I am sure that Father O'Helly has told you, Thomas, to stay away from trouble." "But we didn't do anything." "That has nothing to do with it. People like Roy always make sure that people like you always get caught. What happened in the court?" "There were these three women," said Thomas, "and they were ever so nice. They called us 'Mr.' and after the police had spoken we had all the time we wanted but it was no good. The police described what had happened but it was a complete muddle because they didn't know the street layout at all; they kept making mistakes; but the women had never been round our way so they couldn't see the difficulty. Anyway, they said they had no choice because the police told them we had been flinging fireworks through windows." "Did you call for maps?" "Yes, but the ladies had problems with them. They said even if the details were a bit muddled, flinging fireworks was 'very serious' and so they remanded us."

"Let them out with that gate trick, if they're innocent," whispered Heather. "No. They will be all right. O'Helly and Miles will see everything is fixed. Now, Kelvin and Thomas, we will go and find help for you so that you are properly represented but, in the meantime, you must use your time in prison to reflect on your lives. You might not have been involved in the latest incidents but I dare say you have caused distress before whether you have been caught or not." (They were on numerous agency files, including CICU, as highly suspect). "But what are we supposed to do?" asked Kelvin. "We keep going on these schemes where they tell us how to fill out a CV, whatever that means." "Oh, Latin," said Perpetua, "it is a man thing! Speaking of which I will talk to our people. You do not want jobs with CVs, I know. Thomas, I know you like working with cars so I will ask Bob if you can help him. What about you, Kelvin, you never seem to have been interested in anything?" "I am; but everyone makes fun of me at school because I am so interested in tropical birds. They say I am behaving like a girl. Funny, years ago they say you got beaten up by the teachers if you didn't work hard and now the teachers let the other kids beat you up if you do. It is interest in my Caribbean heritage; not pirates and all that rubbish, something wonderful and liberating." "O God!" said Perpetua (almost crying) "You had nobody to tell, not even a teacher. I promise you can spend the rest of your life studying and writing about tropical birds. Such a small, small thing. Just look forward to that through these difficult few weeks. You can trust me. So can you, Thomas."

The room was was emptying as men moved towards lunch. "Excuse me," said Perpetua, "I have a little job to do. Could I possibly visit the kitchens?" "I am not sure," said the Governor but then his pager alerted him to an emergency call so he hurriedly detailed two officers to accompany Perpetua. Somehow on the way (a lengthy and muddled enquiry never found out why but I am beginning to form my own suspicions) Perpetua ended up on the wrong side of a security gate from her escort and they could not free it to follow her. They were still dithering when the kitchen staff rushed towards them saying that Perpetua had turned them out. There was about to be a breakdown of order when Perpetua appeared and said: "Everything is ready to carry in." The Governor appeared saying that there had been a false alarm. It was all rather confusing.

Gathered together in the association area, Perpetua said grace: "For the gifts we are about to receive may we thank God Our Parent." Most of the prisoners grimaced, knowing what lay ahead; but when the covers were taken off the dishes they were presented with the most wonderful meal that any prison had ever seen. The Governor did not know what to do but Perpetua said: "I will make this all right in a moment."

When the men had finished eating she said: "We must thank God Our Parent for the many gifts of creation. I know you do not enjoy many of these gifts while you are in here but I thought it was important for you to be reminded of the world outside so that you can aspire to be there and aspire to stay there. It is difficult in such crowded conditions but you must try not to repeat in here the mistakes you made out there. You were in pecking orders out there and you are in pecking orders in here; but God Our Parent looks upon you all as equal to the Governor himself."

"What am I to make of that?" asked the Governor. "How can I account for what has happened?" "It was, as I said, a gift from God; so it will certainly not appear in any official records" (as it did not) "as there is no such box designated to be ticked. God, you know, the being who makes all those Chaplains necessary. If the story gets out nobody will believe it. Just go on saying the same thing and people will dismiss the explanation; it can be a gift from anybody else but not God. Mind you, there may come a time when you have to choose between owning up to God and your next promotion."

14.

On the Third Sunday in Advent Perpetua and the *god4u* group went to church at St. Simple the Lesser. "I always like Advent," said Perpetua, "waiting for the commemoration of the birth of Jesus My Brother. I like getting ready. I like John the Baptist because he is the kind of person who would not be allowed into a church today; he would be stopped at the door and told to go away, half-dressed and hairy and telling everyone to repent. Clergy have a monopoly of telling people to repent."

At the end of the service Bill Midway supervised the lighting of the third candle in the Advent wreath. "Why is he lighting a pink one? Why are they different colours?" asked Kylie. "Oh, it is a man thing," said Perpetua. "Most people think that women are fussy about little things but it is clerical men. Purple for three Advent Sundays, pink for the third, not quite so penitential, and white for Christmas day. If you look in the back of that book you will see that the rules for what we pray, what texts we listen to and what they wear, are almost impenetrable." "Why?" "Oh, it is a man thing!"

At the Sunday School Perpetua sat on the floor and talked to the children and their teachers. As usual for that time of year, the subject was the materialism of Christmas. "People have always hoarded and feasted", said Perpetua. "There is nothing wrong with that. The problem arises when people condemn hoarding and feasting and then do it themselves. I hear lots of complaints but do not see that much action." "But it's so difficult to resist the demands of the children." "The demands arise in a context; they arise because we have made the world where they arise. I am only sorry that we are excited about the birth of Jesus My Brother but less concerned about the Triumph of His Resurrection. Hands up all those who will be coming to the Crib Service." All hands went up. "And the Easter Garden Service." Blank expressions. "This is a Christian Sunday School?" More blank expressions. "Of course it is," said one teacher, failing to hide her irritation. "So why is the Easter Garden Service not so well attended as the Crib Service?" "Parents aren't so interested." "That is terribly sad because we are not the children of the Nativity we are the children of the Resurrection. Let me show you how.

"Once upon a time in a bitter and bewildered land full of strict priests, extortionate tax collectors and occupying soldiers, My Brother Jesus was born. The stories are rather muddled as stories will be that are written down a long time after the events but we will do our best to put the pieces together. My Auntie Mary and her partner Joseph both believed that the baby she was going to bear was very special but everybody else shunned them because they were not married when Mary was known to be pregnant. Mary praised God for the baby and promised that this would be good news for the poor, that the rich and powerful would be made low and that the humble and meek would be lifted up. Jesus was born in a smelly cave on the outskirts of Bethlehem and was visited by outcast shepherds who had received the good news for people like themselves from angels. I am not sure about that part but St. Luke was very fond of angels. One story says they went to Nazareth and settled down. Another says that they were visited by magicians who brought them presents. This visit aroused the suspicion of King Herod who was told that Jesus was somehow his rival. Jesus, Mary and Joseph became asylum seekers in a hostile land." The children and some of their teachers looked puzzled. "Then," Perpetua continued, "Jesus My Brother preached peace and love in a fiercely competitive and violent world; and he was given a show trial, tortured, beaten up…" "Stop!" shouted one of the teachers, "you are upsetting the children!" "It is a bit like sex education," said Perpetua, "somebody has to tell them. And he was judicially murdered. And then," unusually the boys were much more interested than the girls in this story "and then he broke apart everything everybody had ever known, like a scientist discovering for the first time how the universe works but bigger; like the biggest bang there has ever been because Jesus My Brother was not dead after all. He still lives and we celebrate his birth next week because he is the most loving person there has ever been; and he loves all of us, even when we are unkind. As long as we are honestly sorry, He goes on loving us."

The teachers were much more shocked than the children who seemed to take in their stride the idea that Mary was Perpetua's Auntie. As for people living again after horrible deaths, there were numerous examples in stories and everybody knew that when you were killed in a computer game you went back to the beginning, alive. As Perpetua said to Bill Midway later: "It seems to me that the adults need the snow, the cosy stable, the colourful shepherds and kings, more than the children." On that basis it was not surprising that Bill received complaints from teachers and parents that Perpetua had upset the class and put back its Christmas preparations.

"This is Bad Morning with Rod Stirrer and me, Owen Grumpy. The headlines: a new report says that our children are the unhappiest in the 'Developed World'; Hypo sales are up by more than 5%; we are working longer hours than at any time since the Second World War; and obesity is on the increase. Norma, what's the reaction in political circles?" "Well, Owen, this is all very bad news for the Government. The report on unhappiness is a damning indictment of all its supposedly 'family friendly' policies; it can't get through its policy on working hours because Brussels supports it; and it can't get a grip on what people eat." "And what about the talk of an excess profits tax on supermarkets?" "As that would feed straight through into higher prices nobody is considering it seriously. The fact of the matter is that when it comes to fundamental conflicts between what people want and what governments want, the people always win." "You might have

said something important there, Norma."

Perpetua spent time in the week before Christmas talking to and help-ing harassed mothers. The gift scheme with Hypo had helped the poorest and most affected by the recent disturbances but wherever she went everybody seemed to be short of what they needed: presents they could not afford; time they did not have; family who would not turn up; children who would not help out. "This is not a good time to change," said Perpetua (practically) "but next October we must try to remember what this week felt like. Do the children want presents or do they really want us but get the presents instead? Do we really dare to face that question?"

As she was standing at the gate of Grunge Park Primary with some moth-ers, a woman walked past. They turned their backs. "Disgusting!" said one. "She dares to walk past the gates of her child's school touting for business!" Perpetua signalled to the woman, pointing at a coffee bar. "There is no point complain-ing about her." "But she is a disgrace!" "No. When I speak up for the poor I am often confused with radical feminists but that is a mistake. The real problem is not the woman's behaviour but the men—our men—who will pay money for what she offers. They are our husbands, partners, sons. Secondly, going on from there, why do our men want to pay for what they should enjoy in loving relationships? What are we, as women, doing about loving relationships? The popular wisdom is that there are noble, brave, feisty, determined women who have been let down by feckless men who have sowed their wild oats and run away from responsibility; but we are not passive furrows to be sown at will. What were you thinking when you lay under a man you hardly knew? Were you really thinking that when it was all over you would form a permanent re-lationship as a prelude to getting married; or were you planning to be a single parent, bringing up a child without a man? How true is it that our children do not have fathers because we got it wrong? Some men are violent and reckless and feckless and just want to get their rocks off and run away but we cannot leave it at that. Where are we in this?"

The women looked stony. "So much for your support," said one. "You needn't bother to come around again with your pretty ways," said another. "You try to live with one of them, little virgin!" said a third. Perpetua only said: "Think about it and, if you have a few minutes, pray about it; pray to that baby, Jesus My Brother, who is causing so much fuss this week."

She crossed the road with Heather to the coffee bar where the woman was waiting for her, sitting at a table as far back as she could go. "It is all right," said Perpetua. "Thank you for staying. There is no need to be frightened. I am not going to tell you off. What made you do this?" "It's the presents. I am trapped. I have to work longer hours to afford the presents, so I see the children less, so I work longer hours to get better presents to make up for it." "At least you recognise the problem you are facing; that is better than most people ever do. It would be impossible to change it for this year so Heather will make sure that you get some help to buy presents without any more attempts at prostitution. It was only attempted?" "Yes, I was frightened and would have been hopeless." "After this Christmas, however, you must think again. Talk to Georgie and Sam about seeing you more in exchange for smaller presents. You will be pleasantly surprised. Children know what love is; and when they are deprived of it they manipulate to get as much compensation as they can."

When they came out, the school gate area was deserted except for one child standing alone, crying. "Come on," said Perpetua, "I know who you are." "What about regulations?" said Heather. "You tell the school and I will text his mother," said Perpetua. "There is no need to cry." "I want some sweets," said the child. "Sweets or a cuddle?" asked Perpetua. "A cuddle".

15.

Reviewing the Perpetua file after her (heroic) role in the Grunge Park disturbances there was a move to downgrade her surveillance or remove it altogether but this was opposed by the SU (Surveillance Unit) because it liked being kept busy with interesting cases and the alternative was analysing ministerial traffic which (everybody knew) was tedious, mainly consisting of outraged and over-worked politicians trying to manage stubborn and over-worked civil servants. The fact that Perpetua knew that she was being watched—and encouraged it as a form of outreach—and that she knew who the mole was made no difference. SAD continued to collect masses of data for no apparent reason.

On Christmas Eve the *god4u* group went to Bill Midway's church again. "It's purple this week," said Kylie. "Yes, that man thing." "And he said it isn't Christmas Eve, it's Advent Four; but it is Christmas Eve." "Mmm! But if it was only Christmas Eve my Auntie Mary would miss out on her really big day, so there is some point to the device."

Perpetua had a long talk with Bill while the church was being transformed for Christmas. "I know this is difficult," she said, "but we really do not have any choice. This is a lovely old church and people feel so comfortable here; but that is part of the trouble. I think that churches should be for celebrations but people cannot celebrate every week. I think we will need fewer big churches for these occasional celebrations. It is not sensible to go on with a church life that ignores the invention of the motor car; we can learn a lot from Hypo. The objection to losing churches is that they are the centre of community life; but for all the hard work you have done, Bill, this church is not the centre of the community, it is the centre of a community; that is why we have to go out to talk to the rest of the community."

After visiting the huge crib at Hypo, the group fanned out through the poorest areas to invite people to an act of worship at the Civic Centre. They assembled an amazing collection of people whose habitual hostility to others was usually only tempered by a desperate indifference. There were problems with the Duty Manager because people were bringing in food and drink which was strictly forbidden. Perpetua asked whether this included bread and wine for a Eucharist and he said not; and she then asked whether it included any other elements which might be used in an act of worship and he said not; and she said that what people were bringing in would all be involved in her kind of Eucharist. "As it's Christmas," he said (decently).

Before the service, Perpetua stood at the door greeting the most diverse imaginable throng of (socially problematic) people. It was strangely moving to see how they greeted her and each other and smiled as if they were old friends.

After the (supposedly rather unorthodox) service, famously beamed on all channels because of an unsolved technical problem, Perpetua relaxed with the people. The Duty Manager said they could stay until 2 a.m. as long as everything was tidy by then as he needed some sleep before the morning service for *The Dot*, a church-free Christian group. "Very interesting," said Perpetua. "They understand how forbidding church buildings are so they break free but their Christian outlook is so forbidding; how can they think that God Our Parent is vengeful? How can they think that Jesus My Brother was deliberately murdered by His Parent as the only way of atoning for human sin? It does not show God Our Parent in a particularly inventive light. There are any number of ways in which God could have put right what human imperfection got wrong; but the importance of Jesus for us is that He was human and that humanity killed Him. The mysteries of the Incarnation, Crucifixion and Resurrection are like a plait or, better, an alloy; they fit together. But all we can try to understand is why; it is impossible to penetrate how.

"Now, Goran, tell us why the Serbs and Croats, who both love God Our Parent, want to kill each other? And you, Patrick, come and listen and share your experience of the troubles in Northern Ireland. What is most distressing is people using violence, or even violent language, as a way of 'promoting' Jesus My Brother in His world. It is this terrible need to control everything when Jesus deliberately emptied himself and chose to control nothing. We need to go on with these discussions. Wayne, make sure our friends are assigned to house groups if they want to be and give them some educational materials; they are much more literate than society thinks they are."

Nobody in SAD should have been surprised by what happened the next day as it had been (frequently and honestly) telegraphed by Perpetua. She launched a social experiment in community cohesion by taking the bulk of Bill Midway and Father O'Helly's congregations and allocating them to house groups to be sited with poor people. As they came out of church they had clearly been inspired by what they had heard because they were singing carols as they went. Trina said it was the first time that Perpetua's face was transformed from serene benevolence to absolute joy; she almost danced down the street with her followers and all the new recruits. Bill Midway was doing his best to be cheerful but Father O'Helly was furious, shouting at Perpetua: "This is an outrage! You are turning people against God." "God came before the Church, Father," she said. "We are the church; but for your sake I am sorry it had to be this way. Let us pray for each other. Wayne, see if you can cheer up the poor Father."

She stopped in front of a shabby front door. "May this house," she said, "be a house of peace like the house of my Auntie Mary, Uncle Joseph and Jesus My

Brother. There will be hard times ahead as we learn to understand each other but the hardest time is over, the time when you were brave enough to face what we had to do to bring the good news of God Our Parent to all the people; and you were also very brave to agree to be hosts to people you do not know. There are two thousand years of Christian tradition but in many ways it would be good to start from scratch, reading the Bible and trying to work out what it tells us, without the influence of historical power and the exercise of personal preference. Some of it is very difficult but the bits we need most, the stories of Jesus, are almost the easiest. Fortunately for us, Jesus was not a theologian but unfortunately for us the people who wrote down the Gospels were theologians so we have to see through their 'spin'; just as you have to work out what is going on when people talk to you in code as I know they do: social workers, councillors, politicians, advertisers, journalists, all have their codes." "Are you saying that the Evangelists were not honest?" asked the puzzled host. "No, I am not saying that they were not honest, I am saying that they were human. They saw the life of My Brother from a certain standpoint and wrote down what they saw as true. They were filled with power by My Sister The Spirit but they were still very human people who made mistakes. The bit I like best is where Matthew has Jesus riding on two donkeys at the same time; Matthew seemed to have a kind of double vision, he was always seeing things in twos." That made people laugh and they were more comfortable. When they settled down to working out how they would function, the Excelsior Gardens people were surprised to find that the person best qualified to assist Heather as leader of one group was a Grunge Park lady who had been a Sunday School teacher.

The Christmas meal at Perpetua's house was quiet but joyful. Before the meal Jim played his flute and they sang carols. Then they prayed round the crib. Bob was puzzled. "I know we have holly at Christmas but why is it making a kind of fringe round the straw?" "Because Jesus My Brother was wounded with thorns and blinded by His own blood; it reminds us of the connection between Christmas and Easter. It is in the old carols but the holly seems to have migrated from the manger. If you look, you will also see a tiny wooden cross tucked away in the corner." "And there is a big stone just outside the crib," said Brian. "Yes; just as Jesus was born in a cave he left an empty cave which the women found on Easter morning." "I suppose that is why I can smell lamb," said Brian. "Yes. I have never liked the turkey tradition. I suppose chicken might be all right but I prefer to remember the liberation from slavery in Exodus not just at Easter but on all big occasions. My Brother was a Jew; we must never forget that; He rejoiced in the freedom that God endowed through Moses; and My Brother's birth is, in an even more significant way, the birth of freedom. We have celebrated that freedom today by beginning to bring good news to the poor so that they will all know God Our Parent and discover the meaning of creation." "It was hard going, though," said Wayne, "particularly Father O'Helly." "It will be to start with, but that is for another day. There is a time to work and a time to play."

After the meal was ended she took pitta bread, broke it, dipped each piece in oil and gave it to them saying: "Take this bread which is the true body of Jesus My Brother made present through the oil of My Sister the Spirit." Then she took a jug of wine and put small pieces of fruit into it, blessed it and gave it to them saying: "This fruit is the creation of God Our Parent, mixed with the blood of Jesus My Brother. This is to remind us of how creation was made new in His sacrifice."

Afterwards they watched television, drank wine and ate chocolate. "Funny, those Evangelists, they were so fired up that there is no record of My Brother and His Disciples having a good time, except at a wedding, and they are so embarrassed by the wine! Jesus brought so much joy to so many people but His closest friends do not seem to have shared in it. I suppose by the time the Gospels were written the men were all busy becoming bosses, even the saintliest of them just could not resist. So here are some frivolous presents that I picked up from Hypo after we prayed at its crib. It was so sad and funny watching people with their shopping not knowing what to do, whether they should pretend it was not there or stop for a moment. I was tempted to ask them about the meaning of Christmas but that would be unfair. As long as they are hoarding in order to be generous to others I should not complain. Here is a big bag of stuff with nothing even vaguely religious in it."

16.

"Well, Minister, it would help the listeners if you were prepared to be honest."
"Well, Owen, it would also help them if your certainties and your doubts were not equally synthetic."

"Just to reassure you," said Perpetua on the morning of the first full house group sessions, "we are only recording my introductory talks so that they can be shared on the *god4u* Channel; once I have finished we will shut everything down and you can speak in complete confidence. We need to establish trust so that people can ask whatever questions or make whatever comments they want, no matter how simple or stupid they might seem. Usually the questions which we think are the most naïve are the most telling. And you will find out near the end of my talk that I think that in this area seriousness is vastly over-rated.

"Doubt is the companion of belief. You might be surprised that I want to start by talking about doubt as it is possibly the most misunderstood aspect of being a Christian. Separated from belief, doubt is rather empty; if an atheist doubts the reality of God Or Parent it does not amount to much but if a Christian doubts then that has true value. How could there be belief without doubt, given the mysterious nature of the topic we are thinking about? Indeed, the mistake we often make is not doubting enough, of thinking we know it all, have got it all sewn up.

"There are many Christians of all kinds, Petran and Toran, who talk of religious certainties as if there is no mystery at all and that whoever disagrees with these certainties must be wrong. But in creating us to think, God created doubt.

"Believing means pressing inwards towards the core of doubt, it means braving discomfort; it means leaving the fairy story of Jesus My Brother which begins joyfully, goes through a bad patch, as all fairy stories will, and ends happily ever after. But if learning about God does not make us flinch, what is it for? Where are the sharp edges of commitment?

"Too many Christians exchange the discomfort of doubt for the comfort of doctrine, for the formulae that become a mental and social ritual. But My Brother Jesus might have doubted as he hung on the cross just before his death; he might even, in a moment of blinding despair and pain, have lost His faith altogether. As a human being, He had denied Himself the knowledge that He enjoyed as part of the Godhead. He knew that what He was dying for was to absorb, as God's vessel—as I am also God's Sacred Vessel—the pain and wrong choices, the choices not to love. He knew the will of God but He did not know, as we put it, 'the mind of God.'

"Humanity was meant to live with uncertainty, created to choose, to confront extremities of belief and doubt instead of living in the soft centre. Only when we have faced the prospect that our lives are shallow, that we will disappear without trace, can we learn to understand our position of humble creatureliness. Only then can we see that all we think about, all we do, including all we do as Christians, does not produce a set of answers but a set of questions. The whole of life, including our spiritual life, is a question; churches are questions.

"There is no such thing as risk-free commitment; to take no risk is to deny the possibility of belief. We are too obsessed with comfort and control; these deny mystery and make belief more difficult.

"Looked at the other way round, belief is not the opposite of doubt it is the fragile flower that grows out of the rich soil of doubt. The soil will always be there but our flower of belief will bloom and die and bloom again. Churches may claim 'The Faith' but belief is an individual experience which benefits from the mutual presence of others asking similar questions. We are all in the garden of God Our Parent but we are different kinds of flowers: we bloom at different times of the year; we are different colours; we are simple or complex; sometimes we go through a whole painful cycle of growth and decline and do not bloom at all. Some of us like rain, others like sunlight; some are big and decorative, others are small and medicinal. It is this fragility and delicacy, variety and vulnerability, which make us so dependent upon Jesus My Brother as our gardener. But we crave other gardeners, we are jealous of other flowers, we want a hermetically sealed greenhouse or we want to grow wild outside the garden.

"Yet in spite of the obvious frailty of belief, there are many Christians who say that it is robust and uniform. They think that we are not delicate flowers but rather ugly and utilitarian cabbages; as long as we are given enough divinely authorised but humanly manufactured fertiliser we can be forced into a dull but safe conformity. We start with Baptism and go through life and end up in the cemetery or crematorium and they know whether we will go to what people call 'heaven' or 'hell'. Yet this is to deny our delicacy and vulnerability, living in ground that is too dry or wet, living under sun that is pale or scorching, living in need of constant care; we are not flowers of chance but, rather, flowers of mystery because God is in us and that makes us fundamentally unaccountable to each other in matters of belief. The corporate church, established by Jesus My Brother, is a mechanism for support not accountability.

"The ultimate act of belief is to doubt, to doubt our worthiness, to doubt our destination. It is so easy to move from the questioning of youth to the comfort of middle age, to the answer that is 'good enough', but then we grow desperate, wondering whether our belief will carry us to God Our Parent. The problem with faith is that it is reflexive, we have to have faith in faith. Just as wisdom is knowing what we do not know, so faith is knowing that we have not fully abandoned ourselves to God. We cannot get away from the idea that there is a deal to be made with God which matches our worldly virtue with divine judgment. This does not mean we must not try to imitate the life of Jesus My Brother, it simply means that we cannot measure our earthly behaviour and predict our 'heavenly' reward. Yet with belief we can be courageous. Jesus My Brother does not ask us to be prudent, or correct, or even pious; He calls upon us to be brave, to take risks, to contemplate being unpopular or even wrong; and sometimes this means staying still.

"Stillness is perhaps the most difficult of all states to achieve in a world full of restless virtue and frenetic vice. Instead of being satisfied with the ground in which we are planted we long for a programme of forced flourishing; we want to be fat with grace, shiny with virtue, bursting with advice, rich in learning; but the danger is that all this ripeness and richness makes us think that we are entitled to judge others; and we pick on the flowers that are limp and bedraggled in our eyes, as if they were not as much in the care of the loving gardener as we are.

"How easily we are moved by the rich and the colourful, the perfumed and the pretty; how easily we value the aesthetic over the healing. One reason why we are so attracted to the pretty and the perfumed is that there are so many people more powerful than us who want to make us like the cabbages I talked about earlier. It is very strange how, in what we call a democracy, there is actually so little freedom to be free, to choose, to be unorthodox; this unfortunate reality includes the sacred democracy of belief which is ruined by orthodoxy and control. As we were created to choose to love or not to love and as the nature of God Our Parent is the supreme mystery, no two ways of loving and believing can be the same and to pretend that they can is a dangerous illusion. Ever since the death of Jesus My Brother men—and it mostly has been men—have recognised that belief endangers social control and so they have corrupted belief by using it as a method of social control.

"Finally, I want to say a few words about teaching. This house group, like all the others, has a leader but the leader is not here to tell you what to think or how to think. The leader is here to help you to learn wider and deeper ways of thinking so that you can draw your own conclusions. In many ways you will do better if you think of learning about God Our Parent as a game or a dance; thinking of it as theology or philosophy tends to make people exaggerate their own genius, their own ability to articulate the sacred mystery of God. At least if you think of this as a dance or a game, as creating patterns that are always changing and often disappear, you might grasp the ephemeral nature of what you are doing. It is no less valuable for being ephemeral; stability is the enemy of growth; the longer you are trapped in one set of words or images, the more difficult it becomes to find the next words and the next images. If we think back through our lives I am sorry to say that almost all our images of God have come to us through solemn people, solemn ceremonies and solemn books; the sacred fool has long departed. Creatures were made to choose to worship or not worship the Creator but where did the social controllers get the idea that worship should be solemn? Occasionally we are 'allowed' to take part in worship that is joyful but have you noticed how much easier we find it to be solemn than joyful? It is as if our culture has had the joy beaten out of it by two thousand years of solemnity. So, as you embark upon this great and treacherous journey, make the risk enjoyable."

17.

"Forgiveness is the foundation of hope but it only becomes alive if we recognise the evil in the world, not just collective evil out there, but personal wrong choices. I know many people find words like 'sin', 'wickedness' and 'evil' difficult when they are individually applied; but we have to find some way of thinking about how we fail to choose to love.

"Although I think that it is really important that we do not fudge the issue of personal responsibility for wrong choices, I am not very attracted to the idea of Satan with horns and a tail, stoking up the fires of hell, as this is a distraction from the main point of tension which is not between Satan and God Our Parent with humanity caught in the middle but between us and God Our Parent. I say tension because there is a tendency for us to pull away from God which causes the tension. There are two ways to God: the first is directly through our obligation to worship as creatures of the Creator; the second is more complex as it involves seeing God in all creation and treating it accordingly. So rather than thinking about Satan and hell fire, think of the stress of pulling away from God and the absolute disaster of an irreversible falling away if our denial is so absolute and deliberate that the tension becomes so unbearable that our line to God snaps. I am not sure that it ever does. We are all children of God and were born to be receivers of God's self-communication. I do not see how such a parent who is the essence of love could cast away children; but there is the possibility—only in my view a very faint possibility—that children can cast themselves away. I take this to mean that life is not a terrible struggle to please God but is the space in which we can choose to love. This makes life sound too easy which is why many reject this view of God; but it is difficult enough being made imperfect.

"We must therefore remember that part of our freedom to choose involves wrong choices and the core, the essence of wrong, is choosing not to love. The danger is that we see this in terms of outcomes, in terms of the external act, when what matters is motive. There are many apparently good people who are captivated by their own goodness and there are others who struggle with desperately difficult problems where they can only choose the better of two evils.

"But there are many Christians of all kinds who talk of good and evil as if they know who is a sinner and who is 'saved', but this is a disastrous caricature of God's purpose. Nobody but God knows what we choose and how; people only know what it looks like. Yet we must do more than face up to wickedness in an intellectual way, telling ourselves that 'society is to blame', we need to feel our pain and the pain of Jesus My Brother who died that we might understand forgiveness. Let me be clear, particularly as I know that some of you have been misled; Jesus did not die because God Our Parent decided that that was the only way that some sort of slate could be wiped clean. How foolish it is to think that we know the workings of God and how foolish to think that there was a set of options; and how even more foolish to think that God only had this one, gruesome option of arranging for the murder of Jesus in order to make forgiveness possible. It is, incidentally, very unhelpful to think of God being 'angry' or 'demanding justice' of the kind we dispense in in our imperfect world when God lives in a state of eternal perfection.

"Jesus died so that we could understand our own weakness in killing Him and our own strength in God's forgiveness, under-written for all time by the Resurrection. Jesus forgave His persecutors but as all of humanity, through wrong choices, is part of that persecution, all have been offered forgiveness; what we must do is to accept it. And, just as words like 'anger' when used of God, are useless, so it is useless to think of God's forgiveness as similar in any way to our forgiveness which is often cramped and duty-driven, full of mitigation, a settling of accounts, a drawing of lines, an embarrassment. I often think that the reason why we find this so pain-free is that we have God's forgiveness at the back of our minds as some kind of safety net, but to think that God will put right all that we do wrong is another piece of human folly; only we, with God's loving support, can put right what we have done wrong. As Jesus came so have I come to be a vessel for the absorption of wrong and an encouragement to love but when I have gone it will be like it was when Jesus went; God will, in the words of Theresa of Avila, have no body now but yours. As God's creatures, then, we should forgive unconditionally, knowing that we can only forgive in the sense that we have nothing to forgive, knowing that we are not worthy.

"And yet, having grasped how we choose wrongly and forgive incompletely, we are able to hope. Hope is the recognition that our journey towards God—or at least the struggle not to get any further away, to increase the tension—is not simply a personal matter; that the very God from whom we pull away is also helping us to become closer. We are not doomed to an endless and pointless struggle, rolling a stone uphill only to lose strength and see it push us backwards down the hill again. Because of forgiveness, we may hope one day to see the full, heavenly light but we see it now if only faintly, like seeing the sun in the moon; it is what helps us to survive in a muddled and threatening world. Without it we would live in a permanent state of fear of the unknown, of each other, of God. Hope is our entitlement as children of God to aspire, with God's help, to live in the heavenly light to be, as a theologian might put it, insubstantiated with God; that is, to become part of God again as we were part of God before we were created as ourselves.

"Yet there are Christians who go about with tariffs for heavenly light, who think they know the price, as if we can buy our way to God through behaving in a certain way. This is perhaps a natural reaction because hope is not an easy idea; it is much less clear cut than the transactional model of 'doing good equals going to heaven'; but that model is corrupt because it debases God's love by representing it as a set of power relations where some claim to know the 'mind of God' so well that they can impose their ideas on other people. The more important flaw, however, in this understanding is that God's mercy is more profound and generous than anything humans can imagine.

"Once we see that hope is not related to power we need not be frightened of the earth. Instead of seeing our lives through the limitations of an earthly perspective which makes us frightened of other people, we can live in the innocence of heavenly light. We are not here to be competitive, to be stronger, richer, more beautiful, but to strive, individually and together, to reach the heavenly light; and even though that light is faint here, whereas it will be inhumanly bright in heaven, there is no earthly place it cannot penetrate: no walls too thick, no scheme too dense, no evil too great. Our weakness is not in thinking we are not worthy but in thinking that God's mercy is so shallow.

"So much of what passes for religion is no more than filing a prudential insurance policy. Have you noticed how people tend to become more interested in God Our Parent as they get older? There is a great deal of self-delusion in all of this; and so I want us to make a different kind of start, to adopt a different kind of approach. The starting point for everything we think about in connection with God Our Parent is that love, not anger, vengeance or justice, is at the centre of everything, is everything; that Jesus My Brother came to earth, broke into history, to show solidarity with suffering and imperfect humanity, to show that He was prepared to suffer and die in order to help us recognise ourselves and our relationship to God Our Parent. The death of Jesus was the most powerful indicator in human history that God, in Jesus, recognises and forgives the imperfection that is part of what we are. It is, if you like, divine solidarity with divinely created imperfection. But all that would be nothing, would be a strange, truncated intervention, without the completing of the cycle, without the hope given to us of being illumined by the heavenly light through the Resurrection when Jesus My Brother who was killed by humanity broke, for a second time, into human history and under-wrote the promise of God Our Parent that all may be saved.

"How sad that so many people cannot bring themselves to believe in the reality of the Resurrection and resort to constructing a human power structure on which they impose their own version of God. I suspect that the reason for this is honourable, that such people think they are not worthy of God's love; but that is to misunderstand the purpose of creation. Humanity was created to strive towards worthiness, not to be worthy. Humanity, unlike angels, can choose to love of its own free will.

"As you think about these ideas, many of you will quite properly want to think about the Cross and even wear a cross to remind you of the suffering and death of Jesus My Brother; but never forget that the Cross is only a signpost to the Resurrection. You cannot carry a tomb about (nor a crib, for that matter), so a cross is very handy; but there is so much more to Christianity than the Cross. Never look at the Cross without seeing the dawn of the Resurrection behind it."

18.

"Dependence is the kernel of love; we cannot really love until we know what it means to depend on God Our Parent and on each other; yet in our society it is a dirty word; we are so caught up with ideas of independence, pleasing ourselves, choice. We think of growing too old to help ourselves, of people in wheelchairs, the blind and the deaf; and we link with these scroungers and misfits, the poor and the poorly, the bruised and the battered, the helpless and hopeless; and we say: 'there but for the Grace of God go I.'

"When Jesus My Brother was hanging on the Cross he was sick, disabled, bruised, battered, despised, outcast, poor and alone. He had to ask for a drink and when it was brought it was so horrible that He could not drink it. That is what it is like for people in wheelchairs, people who watch as the rain does not come or too much comes. And it happens here where people feel trapped in welfare, surrounded by barbarity and violence. There are hundreds of millions of people, knowingly or unknowingly, living in imitation of Jesus, who are the special care of Jesus who suffered when He lived on earth and suffers with us now. But the world does not see it this way; it is proud of its independence, it worships what it calls freedom and choice: free to choose from almost countless kinds of ice cream, diamonds, whiskey, lovers, motor cars, olive oils, friends, shoes, speciality breads, places to live, CDs, sparkling water, clothes, chocolate, hair styles, house plants, holidays, breast size, exotic vegetables, mobile phones, toothpaste, jobs, television channels, potato chips, perfume, tables, moral codes, pasta, cameras, chewing gum, condoms, avatars and tatoos. These are incidental choices; what is essential is the choice of whether to love or not love.

"Yet there are many Christians who see worldly prosperity and independence as marks of the special blessing of God Our Parent which means that somehow the poor are less favoured. But Jesus My Brother was born in poverty, worked hard physically and walked through Palestine preaching, dependent on others for His food and drink; in today's terms He was a loser and a scrounger and He spent so much of His time warning that the independent and powerful were in serious danger of not reaching the only true goal of oneness with God. It does not matter how often Jesus is claimed by the rich and the powerful; He cannot be bought.

"Our human dependence is only a reflection of our Divine dependence; and so we must not only learn to depend on God, the human consequence is that we must learn to depend on each other, to take as well as to give. The powerful are in the habit of constructing virtuous tables of what they give and what they have denied themselves; it might make them feel better but it is not love. The poor, on the other hand, need to see that often what is given is well meant and might even mean hardship for others. We may be trapped in the welfare system but other people, whom we think are much better off than us, are trapped in paying for it. Part of being properly dependent, worthy imitators of Jesus, is to see the best in what others try to do for us instead of seeing the worst and resenting it. But in the end the whole discussion is rather shallow because we are all dependent on God Our Parent; our independence is a gift of creation which we need to see as a means of love.

"Love. There is no word more abused than love; it is the human talent for corrupting the divine that can take its most sacred word and turn it into selfishness. I love chocolate means I want chocolate; I love a girl means I lust after a girl; I love you means I want something you have; I am doing this out of love means I want to force you to be more like me. We have got it completely wrong; if ever a word has been turned upside down and inside out it is love; if ever a glass has been broken, a picture blurred, a melody twisted, a smile distorted, a candle blown out, it is love.

"Love is not what we do, even with the best intentions, to other people. Love is creating the space which allows others to behave unconditionally, to exercise their freedom to choose. It is that simple and that difficult.

"We are born to choose to love or not to love; we perform a variety of acts of preference and denial; we form friendships and break them; we marry and divorce and marry again; we try to love our children but sometimes we are speechless and indifferent; sometimes we cannot express how deeply we feel and sometimes we too readily say how deeply we feel when it would be better to say nothing; and yet, through all of this thicket of small torments and triumphs, Jesus loves us.

"And do we really think that Jesus loves us for what we have done or not done? How can our actions and words, our restraint and silence, be worthy of the love of Jesus My Brother? How can we think that there is some correspondence between what we do and how Jesus relates to us? There is no correspondence. There is no way of describing the relationship between the love of Jesus and the way we behave; they are not relational in any way we understand; and for that reason, for that state of being, we live in a judgment-free space, a space of love, which God has created for us and in which we live and move and have our being. Jesus meets us in this space which God has made; He meets us on earthly ground which God has made; He meets us by a lake and in the city; He meets us on a mountain and in a market town; He meets us, most of all, amid squalor and despair, amid the urban jungle where we try to lead decent lives. He finds us wherever we are but He never pushes or pulls, He never makes a face or drops a hint; He never passes a comment on what we have done or on what we intend to do. He inhabits our space when we let Him and sometimes when we do not, thanks to the zeal of My Sister the Spirit. But He lets us know that it is our space. We are not living in His space; for God lives in God's own kind of space quite separate from ours.

"And yet there are Christians who believe that love is a form of obedience. They carry lists of what love requires, of actions, words and attitudes which will indicate whether we are loving or not loving. They have rules for who can love who and who cannot; they have rules for what is good love and not good love; they have honed love down to a set of proofs that Euclid would recognise; there are propositions, working out and proof statements; there is a whole sub-culture of love theorems which have been devised to circumscribe, to keep people in confined spaces, to ensure that love does not get out of control. In an act of supreme arrogance, divine love is modelled in human love, divine enterprise is modelled in human enterprise; but, worst of all, divine space is cramped into human ecologies. There are supreme moments in our lives when we know how to love outside the walls but we grow frightened; we do not flex, we wither.

"Jesus My Brother was a terrible disappointment to the religious authorities and He still is. He sits with sinners and enjoys a meal and He says nothing about their bad behaviour. He disrupts a perfectly proper trial of a prostitute and sends the prosecution packing. He forgives sins without ever wanting to know what the sins were. He spends a lot of his time telling the law makers that their laws are not divine at all but a human invention. He seems to like the outcast Samaritans, He has a soft spot for the Prodigal Son, He empathises with the Publican at the back who thinks Himself not worthy to pray, He tells Peter that he will deny Him but seems to think that recognition of the denial by Peter will be punishment enough; He even seems to have no complaint against Pilate.

"Looked at objectively, Jesus is a discredit to contemporary Christianity; He refuses to judge, all He wants to do is to love.

"The question is, where do we stand in the argument between love and judgment? Are we prepared to take the risk of love, of creating space where others might do things we would prefer them not to do, or are we content to be Pharisees, defining everything that must happen and must not happen in earthly space? Are we prepared to take the risk of love and then ask Jesus for the strength, when we have taken that first step, not to judge when we feel that the space we have created has been violated, that we have been let down? It is the supreme mission of the Christian to make space knowing that others will want to violate it.

"What we so often mean when we think about love in a conditional way is that our love has not been returned; that we are, in love terms, in debit. But if we think that love is a matter of debit and credit we have misunderstood.

Love is a valve; it is one way; it is not a boomerang; it goes and it goes and it goes, for its own sake. That is why parents who expect their children to return love are sadly deluded. It goes and it goes and it goes; and yet the more of it we give away the more of it we have; the more space we make the more capacity we have for making space. No wonder people worry about love and the space it creates; love is the greatest risk of all; but that risk is under-written by the 'King of Love', Jesus My Brother.

"The mystery of love is that the closer we come to Jesus, the more space we have.

"Love is what I came down to earth to put right. Together we can put it right.

"Our Media Correspondent, Ivor Slogan has joined us in the studio. Ivor, people are saying that god4u *is the most boring channel ever." "Yes, Rod, its unremitting serious-ness is certainly off-putting..."*

19.

When Perpetua returned with her followers from a few quiet days, she again found Grunge Park in its customary state of fear. The pirate stations were on air, street lights had been systematically smashed, gangs and fragments of gangs were looking for trouble and, on the night before she arrived, there had been yet another skirmish between Roy and potential rivals but instead of the usual injuries not reported to the police, a fourteen-year-old boy had been stabbed to death. Everybody knew who was to blame. Nobody said anything. SAD and the local Council, which also knew, called the customary special meeting at the Civic Centre so that people could let off steam and go through the motions, save face. There would be plenty of calls for more effective policing (even though most people, on balance, supported a policy of almost complete non-intervention), more male role models (even though there was majority resistance to family rearing partnerships and a fear of men in primary schools) and more regeneration funding (even though the major problem was absorbing this to produce positive results). In other words, the whole predictable response had nothing to do with the known causes of the problem.

A number of officials and officially sponsored 'leaders' said what they had to say, followed by Father O'Helly and (reluctantly) by Miles. Then the mother of the dead boy (courageously) called upon Perpetua to say something.

"It is so hard to talk at this time," she said. "While I am standing here we all know that Roy's gang members are waiting threateningly outside, only kept off because my people, through my power, have got them under control, but we all know that this will not last. It is hard to speak because we all know how this murder came about and we know the people responsible for it. So what do we expect everybody else to do? Do we expect the police to collect evidence while we keep quiet? Do we expect justice to be done while we say nothing? Do we expect the underlying conditions to get better while we turn a blind eye to our children becoming addicted to and dealing in drugs? Do we expect this place to become re-generated if we leave outsiders to make all the effort?

"How can we live together and improve ourselves when there is so much mistrust? We do not trust the police when they come here and we do not trust them when they stay away. They do not trust us because we complain about violence but close ranks against them when they investigate. We do not trust the social services when they come to see what is happening and we attack them when they want to take action. We blame them for the neglect and murder of our children but we do not even confront the murderers in our midst. We do not trust them because they come from outside, they do not trust us because we will do nothing inside. Perhaps, too, they do not trust black people and we do not trust white people."

Then the mother said just loud enough for everybody to hear: "But this fine talk will not bring back my son. I tried so hard." "I know you tried and this is no time to say how it might have been different; we should all behave differently and why should the shortcomings of any individual be a matter of public discussion." "But if you want to, you can bring him back to life, I know you can." "No, it is not like that. What matters is your belief not my action. Look, I can always use power but it is a short term kind of game. All of you who have radios, switch them on to pirate Head-Jam; all right, I hereby put it off air." There was a gasp but the surprise did not last; people had experienced this kind of power before. "Now, I say to all of you, that when you look for signs as if God is a magician you are wrong; it is only your faith that will save you."

Perpetua took the mother by the arm and gently led her out while attention was turned to wording a petition for more support for the community. "I will come with you to the morgue," she said. "When I said I know you can bring my son back to life I did not mean it theoretically, intellectually. I know in my heart."

Perpetua called Andy and Heather and the four met in the hospital reception. Perpetua did not trouble the people at the desk. "That will only cause bureaucratic muddle," she said. They went, as if invisible, down corridors and through security doors until they came to the morgue. Without seeming to look, Perpetua opened a drawer and said: "Help me to lift him out." She breathed on his chilled face and his eyelids flickered. "Now," she said, "may God Our Parent renew earthly life in you, as the Spirit breaths her spiritual gifts into you and as I, in memory of Jesus My Brother, absorb your past trouble, weariness, desperation and wrong choices, so that you may enjoy a new life. Andy, give his mother the money. Heather will make sure you have all the necessary papers to comply with regulations. Go away and make a new life, in every way. Say nothing about this, any of you, the time is not yet right." The five of them passed through the hospital again as if they were invisible.

This (apparently improbable) story was put on the SAD files shortly after the fuss over the missing body of the murder victim died down. Hospital records were innocent of the body's admission and the tussle about who had lost it only lasted a few days as the news agenda moved on.

Perpetua and Trina went to see Miles. "I know we disagree," said Perpetua, "about some rather silly man things—what you call the theology of penal substitution and what I call human presumption—but we need your bravery and determination now. I can calm things down but I am not the local policeman nor miracle worker. I am relying on you to go on being brave and to encourage Father O'Helly." Trina stayed behind to talk to Miles and Perpetua went to see Roy. "You have got away with it this time but that should not make you feel any better. It is not the law but your own conscience which will catch up with you. I have nothing to say to you that you do not already know. You were once weak, you were once lonely, you were once desperate and instead of learning from that you exploit it in others; and you know that. Say nothing that you will regret. I know you know."

"This is Bad Morning with Craig Knocker and with me, Owen Grumpy. And the main news today is that journalists and politicians are joint bottom of a poll on trust. Minister, why do you think that politicians are so untrustworthy?" "Well, Owen, it might just be that what they say and do is reported by journalists who are equally mistrusted." "So what are you going to do about this?" "It would hardly be viable to exercise any political control on news, even if we wanted to—which we do not—but there comes a point at which cynicism makes good government impossible. A substantial part of our community does not trust the police, our social workers are routinely denigrated, doctors are perceived as greedy, banks are exposed as unscrupulous; and no matter how good they are at what they do, Owen, society can't be run by nurses, vicars and lollipop ladies." "No Minister, I suppose not, but it can't get any worse than it is." "Yes it can and it will. It is much easier to erode trust than it is to grow it but the people in the best position to know how to discriminate between honesty, spin, duplicity and corruption are the very people who are so cynical that they think that honesty is impossible." "Thank you Minister. Well, there you have it, the Government has thought about media control and has only turned it down because it wouldn't work. Craig." "The other major story of the day is that vital workers, including nurses, cannot afford to buy houses. I have with me a representative of the opposition. Mr. Stickler, who do you blame for this crisis?" "First of all, I blame the Prime Minster, Mr. Blair. He has had ten years to sort out our housing crisis so that nurses and other vital workers can get on the property ladder and he has done absolutely nothing about it." "But isn't it true that your party is against state planning of the economy and in favour of market forces?" "Yes, of course we are; we can't have government telling people where to live so of course we support market forces." "So how does that help nurses? You seem to be saying that you want market forces except in housing." "Nurses need a substantial pay increase to put them on a level with junior doctors so that they can deal in the housing market." "If the Government proposed that measure would you support it?" "Well, that is a slightly different matter." "You see what I mean by trust, Owen! Finally, Mr. Stickler, there are reports that you have been opposing the construction of small, low cost houses for people like nurses, behind your own rather large mansion." "Well, not precisely; but we do have to preserve our rural heritage."

Next day Perpetua went to talk to the people in Excelsior Gardens. "For you," she said, "events in Grunge Park are entertainment; how close do you come to enjoying the frisson of fear as you choose the most lurid newspaper headline? How much do you think about the reality of fear and violence and how much does it feel like fiction?

"All I can say is that you are more responsible for what is going on in

Grunge Park than even the poor people themselves. You refuse to become involved with your neighbour. Once, when this suburb was built, it shared everything with Grunge Park but arrangements have been made: you do not share the same churches, the same schools, the same shops, the same social amenities; the only thing you have in common is support for Grunge Park United. In every other aspect of your lives, your only contact with the poor is through your under-paid cleaners. When you go to hospital you do not notice the porters and cleaners, they are not real people; you do not notice your office cleaners; you do not care how dirty jobs get done.

"It is so easy to condemn those who resort to drugs in their desperation, because they see no way of improving their lives. Thinking that good advice or, even worse, bullying, will solve this problem is foolishness. Meanwhile, you gain hundreds of thousands of pounds simply by sitting where you are and watching the value of your houses rise. But this selfishness cannot go on forever; selfishness brings terrible misfortune. You may wonder why the poor and the oppressed resort to drugs but why are your children taking them and dealing in them? Why are your peaceful streets the object of criminal desire? What is it about your lifestyle that makes your children so alienated in spite of wealth?"

She could see Dexter edging towards Rory Varnish and Oliver O'Helly. "Nobody is perfect. There is no point in making a public exhibition of the shortcomings of other people." Dexter, reluctantly, took the hint. "I want you all to think very carefully about our responsibility for each other so that you can learn how other people live and how they can learn that it is possible to trust white people, to trust wealthy people, to trust strangers. The crisis of our culture is mistrust, the crisis of our being is that we think that love is conditional. People think that contracts cultivate trust—and to a certain extent they do, as an imperfect expression of mutuality—but the main source of trust is unconditional love, so that people can rely upon us to do what we say without imposition or judgment.

"Last time I came here you gave generously and I am most grateful, we really needed money to launch our movement for God but now we need your personal commitment to your neighbours. Give time, give care, give love, not to get anything back, not to to keep the threats from Grunge Park at bay but because it is the extra responsibility of the rich to care for the poor and to love them.

As they left, Dexter took another long look at Rory and his small cluster of followers. "No," said Perpetua. "You are to go nowhere near them. They will cause havoc but we are not to use human—and certainly not violent—means to prevent it. (She said this because she seemed to have some idea of what might happen to her.)

20.

Undeterred by the strange happening with the material for his private recreation, Father O'Helly was still determined to undermine Perpetua's growing hold on the community. She had taken most of his congregation and with it his purpose in life. This made him spend even more time thinking about his personal dilemma which she knew about. He gathered the remnant: those who had stayed faithful, as he saw it, to Church and Pope. Much against his nature—he was at his happiest in his sanctuary—he organised a demonstration at the Plaza outside the Civic Centre where Perpetua was celebrating God's Carnival, a pre Lenten festival. He stood grimly as he heard the beating of steel pans and the high notes of Jim's flute within; and, almost masochistically, he imagined dancing. He had reluctantly given way to new developments in liturgy, grimly obedient to the Pope, and he was beginning to feel relieved now that Vatican II was finally and decisively being overturned; and so this raucous music was particularly offensive.

As the audience came out—he refused to call it a congregation—his followers handed out leaflets saying: "Return to God who lives in His Church". Perpetua came down the steps shouting and smiling: "Oh what lovely banners you have made for my Auntie Mary! You do love her so, Father; but she would be upset if attention to her in any way detracted from the adoration of Jesus My Brother." "You are doing a disservice to what you call your 'Brother' by dismantling the Church." "O Father, you know only too well that the church is not the buildings but the people. I have led many of them out into a new place; they would love you to be with them as they test the boundaries of their renewed spiritual lives. You have such a lovely pastoral manner with the poor and the distressed even though you have such a crusty surface when you are standing on your dignity. All your parishioners tell me how wonderful you are."

Father O'Helly's faithful followers began to sing a hymn to Mary. Perpetua went inside the Centre and shortly afterwards Jim and some of the others came out and joined the singing group. "I cannot resist a song or two about my Auntie Mary," whispered Perpetua to Father O'Helly. "But I thought you were against us." "No, I am not against you; I am against the followers of Jesus My Brother locking themselves away inside their grim churches. Now you have come out into the street, even if the idea was to compete with *god4u*, at least you are here and that is where Jesus My Brother wants you to be."

Perpetua gathered her followers around her as she stood on the stone dais at the end of the Plaza, facing the Civic Centre. Father O'Helly found himself, reluctantly, pushed by his singing followers into the middle of the crowd as the steel band came outside. Perpetua was getting ready to speak when the strains of a bugle and drums could be heard in the distance. "It's the WWJD Corps" said Trina. "Look down the hill," said Perpetua, "and watch as the WWJD Corps comes toward us. Anybody would think that we are about to have a fight; that is how so much religion looks from the outside." She raised her voice: "Welcome, it is so rewarding to see the Petrans, *god4u* and the WWJD Corps all mingling together."

"We don't want to mingle with you," said Miles, standing with a human sized wooden cross at the front of the Corps. "It's a nasty accident." "What would you like us to do?" "For a start, stop that riotous music." "King David danced before the Lord, when did the dancing stop?" "And tell that young man to throw that can of beer away." "The Jewish people drank wine and beer, when did the drinking stop?" "And that couple over there are behaving disgracefully." "When did the need for human loving stop?" "But that kind of intimacy should only be within marriage." "So you are saying that because they are so much in love they must necessarily not be married. Oh dear, Miles; if that is true what is marriage for? But they are married." Trina signalled furtively, then openly, to Miles to stop but, as usual, he was driven by the demons within. "How can you claim to follow Jesus when your lives are so publicly wicked?" "Oh Miles, do calm down and think about the concept of wickedness just a little more carefully. Perhaps calling people wicked without knowing how they came to do what they are doing is wicked."

As with the Petrans, the Corps seemed less suspicious than their leader and pressed towards the dais. "Let us all sing a hymn we can agree upon," said Perpetua. It took almost five minutes of wrangling to settle: the Petrans would not have anything about personal contact with God; WWJD would not have anything about Mary or the Eucharist; and *god4u* would not have anything with masculine gender overtones in it or references to soldiers and fighting for God. They settled, out of grudging respect for her, on Perpetua's favourite song: It's The Sign That Counts, sung by her followers, and then Jerusalem (which is not strictly a hymn at all) sung by everybody, and then dispersed.

As she was leaving, Perpetua saw a WWJD follower handing out forms. "What are those?" The follower pulled away, slightly embarrassed. "A gift commitment form." "And who receives the gifts?" "The Corps." "For the poor?" "Well, not really. It is very expensive to keep the Corps going with all the costs." "Pastor Plumtree does have a very nice house in Excelsior Gardens." "Yes, he needs the peace and quiet so that he can write uplifting sermons." "I will not judge because I depend on my followers to live; but think about the poor."

Later, Perpetua had the idea of building on the gathering by asking Bill Midway to host and chair an inter-faith forum. Bill was delighted, not least because his role would spare him the problem of trying to put the Church of England point of view.

The forum was keenly anticipated by the various factions which saw it as a great opportunity for point scoring. Perpetua had to stop her followers 'collecting ammunition' to fire at the others. "We have to stay positive about our own message and not attack other people because of what they believe. Belief is very difficult."

Bill Midway began: "Jesus is confronted by a known sinner, what would He do?" "Send him to a priest," replied O'Helly. "Tell Him that God's wrath will overwhelm him," said Miles. "Forgive him and tell him to sin no more," said Perpetua.

"Jesus is in a dispute with the Pharisees over a point of law, what would He do?" "Send for a Canon Lawyer." "Consult the Scriptures." "Say that love is above the law."

"Jesus is asked to include women in His followers." "Look to the traditions of the Church." "Remember male headship." "Act within His culture."

"Jesus is called upon to condemn war." "Consult his Spiritual Director." "Support good over evil." "Share the suffering of the soldiers."

Bill thought that Perpetua's answers were by far the nearest to the truth, if it was possible in any way to guess what Jesus would do; but he thanked everybody for taking part so enthusiastically.

Perpetua seemed downhearted as she reviewed the evening with her followers. "It is so depressing that we have come into Lent, when we are supposed to turn back to God Our Parent, and it seems that many who call themselves Christians will turn anywhere else but to God. They are so confused about the Church and the Bible that they have ended up worshipping them instead of worshipping God. No wonder people turn away from organised religion. Who would ever want to worship a self-perpetuating group of white, middle-aged men or a book? You only have to listen to what happened tonight to see why the Christian Church is dying. We must dedicate ourselves in Lent to explaining to people how the things that Christians have grown used to are tools not idols."

The next morning Perpetua came to the SAD sub-office. "I am so pleased that you are spending so much time and money collecting and sorting what I say and do; but would it not be better if you spent the resources on helping the poor?" "Well, strictly speaking you are not supposed to know that you are under surveillance. It rather goes against the idea of your doing something that we know about that you don't know that we know about, something that is self-incriminating." "But it seems rather pointless, even though I am grateful for your assistance with our mission, for people who have estranged themselves from God Our Parent to be using public money to record public discussions which I put on our *god4u* Channel anyway." "It's the fine detail in between appearances that we care about." "When the time comes, your surveillance will not catch me saying anything subversive and it will not preserve me from the violence, born of oppression, which you supposedly exist to ameliorate."

SAD (perversely) increased its surveillance and occasionally (just for fun) Perpetua made the recording and archiving systems malfunction. "I am not even sure they understand this," said Perpetua, "but there are still six weeks to go." "To what?" "Easter." "Why is that important?" "You should know."

21.

After the Ash Wednesday solemnities, Perpetua and her followers embarked on a major tour of the country whose aim was, according to the press release: "To call on people to take responsibility for their lives and turn back to God." At the press briefing before she set out, Perpetua (in a truly admirable summary) said: "As a culture we are in deep denial about our collective and individual selfishness; we are apt to blame other people for everything and cast ourselves as victims. We call for improvements and when these happen we discount them instead of being grateful and we turn to our next desire. We have lost the power to rank concerns so that we concentrate on what we need most as a community; instead, we make our demands almost at random, like tiny children; we want everything at once; and we want it now! We are beyond contentment.

"The only genuine way of dealing with this problem is to see ourselves as God's Creatures, grateful and striving, living in a state of imperfection which requires constant self-awareness, repentance and re-dedication."

The tour was based round the *god4u* bus. Each time they arrived at a new city or town, they would park the bus discreetly and be welcomed by the local *god4u* group. They would then walk quietly through the commercial area, led by Perpetua carrying a large, light weight, wooden cross. They would stop and talk to people as they passed along and would hold an act of worship at an open-air site. By this time the steady, low level national publicity, good and bad, about Perpetua and *god4u* was being supplemented by local coverage, so that the processions and gatherings had their complement of opponents as well as supporters.

The following is a sample of short reports from SAD regional files:

A woman burst out of a crowd of people dragging her son behind her; he was cursing and trying to get away and she needed all her strength to move him. He tried to get his knife so that he could injure his own mother but she held him with even more determination. "You are my last resort," she gasped. "I don't believe in religion; it's never done us any good; just lectures about what a privilege it is to be poor and obedient. But you're different; they've told me about you." The boy broke free but his forward momentum made him cannon straight into Perpetua and then crumple. "What do you want me to do?" she asked, stroking the top of his head. "Why, it's obvious that he needs to be cured. He's mad with desperation and drugs." "Why do you not take him to a rehabilitation centre?" "There are no places; you have to commit a serious crime to get into drug rehabilitation; that's the way the system works. My boy has never committed a crime, I have used all the family savings and pawned all our goods to feed his habit but now it is desperate. If I let him steal and he is caught he might be given rehabilitation; this is a stupid world! But I know that you can get past all that and help him." "How do you know I can help him? Am I not just, as you say, a 'last resort', a final throw of the dice?" "No; you misunderstand me. I know that you are the Daughter of God sent to save us all." "What wonderful belief this woman has. I have not heard myself described this way even by many who have followed me day after day. What is your name?" "Sol." "Such a nice name for wisdom and for sunshine. Solomon, because your lovely mother has faith in God Our Parent and in me," (she touched his head with the Cross) "stand up like a man. For the time being you are cured but you have to take responsibility for yourself. You are strong, athletic and handsome; do not spoil that with indulgence and foolishness. And you; it is easy to say that you believe in God but you do not believe in religion. You need religion as a sharing way of giving you support and strength from fellow believers and from My Sister the Spirit. There are a few hermits; but most of us cannot be committed believers while we stay away from worshipping God together. Go in peace as you journey towards God. It is not over; it is beginning."

There were some demonstrators standing by with placards and one of them said: "You are claiming to be God but you are wicked; you are a blasphemer." "O please do not resort to such foolish slogans," said Perpetua. "I have just done a little, temporary good and you know that I have. How can it be wicked to cure somebody of a deep illness? And how can that kind of a cure be magic? How sad and strange that you cannot see God Our Parent in what I do. Spend a little more time listening and loving and a bit less time shouting and hating."

And she said to her followers: "Notice how faithful the woman was even though she was proud and even a little stubborn. Some of you have not been so forthright in recognising that I am the Sacred Vessel of God Our Parent."

Perpetua's small procession was suddenly blocked by a fracas. Stones and bottles were flying and people who had come to greet Perpetua were running away, shouting and screaming. "Stop!" she shouted, raising the Cross high above her head. There was complete silence and stillness. Later one of the combatants said that he felt as if his limbs had been frozen; he was then filled with a warm feeling as he looked at the Cross above Perpetua's head. He said he would never fight again (to date SAD records confirm the promise).

A man came up to Perpetua and said: "I want to be one of your followers. I will give all my money to *god4u*." "But will you give yourself?" "What does that mean?" "Will you affirm in humility that we are all creatures of the Creator, brothers and sisters of Jesus and in thrall to My Sister the Spirit." "I have to make decisions and control things; I will go on working so that I can give more money to the cause." "I do not wish to seem ungrateful but God Our Parent

needs your creatureliness in all its glorious imperfection, not your money."
But then she smiled and said: "This is too hard, too hard. Just try a little more
humility and a little less profit." (Afterwards he was approached both by the
Torans and Petrans for a contribution to their cause.)

Perpetua said to her followers: "See how difficult it is, what standards I set.
I know you have left your private concerns to follow me. Even when things look
at their worst, do not lose heart. You will not always succeed in being faithful;
but go on trying, repenting, seeking forgiveness and strength."

A clergyman came up to Perpetua and said: "You keep talking about love
but your kind of love seems to depend on letting everybody do what they
want." "That is exactly right," said Perpetua. "That is what love is. Love is like
fire and so it cannot be given to little children without lessons in self restraint
and openness but love is the ultimate freedom." "What does that mean?"

"There was a rich man: he was married to a beautiful woman; he gave
money to good causes; but he kept himself very private. And the woman was
unfaithful to him and he knew it but said nothing. He treated her in the way
he always had since he first met her. But his friends said: 'She is making a fool
of you. Everybody knows what she is doing but you just go on treating her the
same as you always have. This is making you look stupid.' 'It does not matter
what I look like,' he said, 'I love her and that means being the same no matter
what she does.' She left him once she had drained his wealth and went where he
could no longer reach her. He said nothing but when a close friend asked him
why he had been so passive he said it was not passivity at all: 'I promised to take
her for better or for worse, for richer or for poorer and it turned out worse
and poorer; and I still would love her but I cannot reach her.'

"He built up his income and he gave to good causes, particularly to those
which wanted to promote freedom of speech and action; and every time a new
space was created for speech or action it was invaded by people who tried to
limit freedom, for the sake of 'the good' and the bad. And his advisers said to
him: 'You need to take precautions to protect the free space you have created.'
'But if I take such precautions to protect free space,' he said, 'it will no longer
be free.'

"And when his money was completely finished, spent on his wife and the
good causes, he worked quietly to make just a little more; but he said nothing.
He had no complaint, he had given his love to the woman and his commitment
to unconditional freedom which is the longer phrase for love.

"Listen," said Perpetua, "so many people in the Christian churches cannot stand this kind of love. They must exercise power, they must have control,
they must judge. True love is having no control whatsoever; true love is making
space. The man did not make a deal with his wife or with those who wanted to
curtail freedom; he just went on quietly loving. When he had no more money

he still went on loving because he still held to the same values; his love did not depend on how much money he gave to the woman or the good causes."

"So," said a bystander, "who are we supposed to love?" "I understand," said Perpetua, "why people sponsor chickens and wells and goats and school books for poor countries but somehow that seems to be intermediate, not quite right. For me, the idea is that we should give people money so that they can choose what they need; and we should not think of giving money to people in distant lands as a substitute for exercising our faculty of love directly with our poor neighbours by giving our time. Look over there: to the north of the United ground there is poverty; to the south there is affluence. The people of the south have twin towns in France, Germany and Holland but they have no twinning arrangements with the people just to the north."

"But if you give poor people money instead of books and other worthwhile goods, they will spend it on cigarettes, alcohol, drugs and unhealthy food." "Apart from the practical argument that the more you give them the more likely they are to spend it, as you would term it 'sensibly', the main point is still that love is unconditional. You might want to make a social contract with these people out of generosity, so that they spend your gift in a certain way; but do not call it love."

"Are you saying, then, that divorce is wrong?" "No. When the woman took herself away from the reach of the man, he could create no more space for her unless she came near enough to him to allow him to do that. Only God knows when that happens and only the man could use his God-given gifts to make some sort of honest estimate. Divorce is wrong if we cease to love when we still have the opportunity to create space for the beloved. We cannot love in an abstract way as in: 'I love all the human race'. It is a pleasant idea but it does not really mean anything."

"Why do you spend so much time with bad people?" somebody asked. "Because 'bad' people need help to be 'good'; but be careful not to assume there is an easy distinction; we are all bad and we are all good." "Including you?" "As the Sacred Vessel of God Our Parent I have a special place in creation." "Jumped up!" "A strange expression which seems to indicate that some people are supposed to stay 'down' where they are kept by others."

The conversation was interrupted by a man who burst through the onlookers, shouting obscenities. "I know who you are, Perpetua Daughter of the Almighty. You are creating havoc. Go away and let us get on with our lives." As usual, Dexter was edging his way between Perpetua and trouble but she held out her arm to halt his progress. "Let me look straight at you," she said. "Why would you want to go on living this terrible life?" "Because it is better than facing the life I threw away and the life that is to come." "You are not really mad as you sometimes think you are, giving you the excuse to behave badly. I will take away all your sadness and regret and this will help you to remember what you have buried deep down, that you did your best. Whatever you have done wrong is forgiven. Go away now, smiling; remember to pray for you and me."

She said to her followers: "Remember never to go on appearances. He was neither truly mad nor very bad, just scary and irresponsible. People like him need our support but the long term solution is community support so that when we need to ease ourselves free, we are sure that the right people are in place. We cannot pick people up and put them down like chess pieces."

"Over to you Owen." "Thank you Craig. As you may have heard in the news, what we may call a 'spiritual evangelist' has been touring the country calling on people to turn back to God but, unlike conventional Christians, Perpetua has some very individual views on God and Christianity. Archdeacon Varnish, what do you think of Perpetua's view that there might be more than three persons in the Christian Godhead?" "I am not sure whether her views are simply ridiculous or harmful. The Bible and two thousand years of Church tradition have stuck to the doctrine of the Trinity?" "But why should God limit him/herself to three and what difference does it make? Perpetua seems to be calling on people to turn to God and behave better; isn't that what you want?" "Well, yes but we don't want people to be confused or disappointed by false doctrines." "But how much do you think people understand what you would term 'true doctrines'?" "Well, I have to admit, not much." "It seems to me that Perpetua is taking the Christian tradition, making it contemporary and simplifying it." "Well, that's the trouble, it is not reverent to simplify ideas of God." "Because it dispenses with the need for clergy. Thank you Archdeacon. Craig." "A new report says that there is a strong link between anti social behaviour and poverty. I have with me a senior and influential opposition backbencher. Mr. Niggler, what do you think of this idea?" "Plain rubbish. There are plenty of very poor people who behave beautifully; and rich people who behave badly." "So you don't accept a general correlation. No. All this nonsense about love will get us nowhere."

Near the end of the tour Perpetua was heckled by a small band of Empiricans. "God is a dangerous delusion," said one. "Not so dangerous as the delusion that God is a delusion." "That is just clever talk. There is no proof." "All talk which involves God's creatures saying that the Creator does not exist is often characterised as 'clever' talk but it is empty talk. Ask yourself: why is there something rather than nothing? And if you find an answer in science, come and tell me; and be careful. The question was not how there is something rather than nothing; but why?"

Perpetua said to her followers: "You will meet many people who talk like that but what you will face that hurts most is indifference. Meet challenge with firmness but with the smile of Jesus My Brother; and when you meet indifference, pray to My Sister the Spirit. Never forget the beauty of what God Our Parent has made."

22

At what turned out to be their last quiet day together, Perpetua focused on the qualities needed for a successful *god4u* movement.

"I know if I ask you to make suggestions you will all say 'love', so that is a given. Let us look at the idea in more detail. And for once, smile!"

Here is what they agreed and posted on the web site:

1. In an institutional setting, like a church or religious movement, the most important feature is empowerment over power; the movement exists to serve, not to control.

2. Neither hierarchy nor democracy can guarantee that the will of God Our Parent will be honoured: neither hierarchies nor majorities necessarily reflect the guidance of Our Sister the Spirit.

3. Good order depends upon self-discipline and tolerance not on strict rules.

4. Organisations seeking to live in the will of God need an ethic not a code. The ethic will stay the same but the way it is lived will change. God gave us brains to assist with the exercise of free will; we must use our intellectual gifts, under the power of prayer, to live out our ethic of love as the creation of unconditional freedom.

5. Collective and individual worship of God Our Parent, Jesus Our Brother and Our Sister the Spirit, is not optional for believers, it is an integral part of our being which emerges from the Royal Priesthood of all the people of God. In collective worship we should be generous to the ideas of others and never allow the ritual to obscure the object of worship.

6. Listening is more than hearing words. Listening is calling upon the assistance of Our Sister the Spirit when we, as part of the Royal Priesthood, are exercising pastoral care.

7. The Christian doctrine of 'Original Sin' or 'The Fall' misunderstands the reason for human existence. Humility is the recognition of our intrinsic imperfection into which we were deliberately created in order to exercise the freedom to love. Humour is the best expression of our imperfection.

At the end of the day Perpetua warned her followers (yet again, without being understood) that she would not be with them much longer. "You already know of the accusations about to come out in the press that I have been a drug dealer. It may even be that some of you have been involved but it does not matter now. I came to live out God Our Parent's solidarity with humanity and part of that is to suffer and die. Unlike the impact on His followers of the death of

Jesus My Brother, this should not shock you; you know how Jesus was treated and what happened afterwards; but you will still be shocked."

"But if we know what's coming, why can't we stop it?" asked Wayne. "Because the events have been set in train and will come to their logical end. This is what I came to accomplish and this is what will happen. I also want you to think carefully about what happened to Jesus because His followers swore not to betray and abandon Him but that is what they did. I think that I am about to be thrown to the media and then killed. The important thing to remember is that no matter what you do or do not do, no matter what happens, I will still love you, as will God Our Parent and Jesus My Brother; and although My Sister the Spirit will not become alive in quite the spectacular way in which she erupted into the lives of the followers of Jesus, Her steady presence will be with you. This is not going to be the story of the reality of God bursting upon an unsuspecting world; what you will have to do will be hard and unspectacular. The Church occasionally thinks that it has come to new life with contrived initiatives but it has grown hard; the wood of the Cross has turned to stone.

"However, we do need to leave some tangible joy that you can look back upon, so we need to plan our London spectacular to round off the national tour."

They all went to (what turned out to be a farewell) a meeting at Grunge Park youth club and then Perpetua left them to spend the night alone in Bill Midway's church. The next morning the streets leading into central London were lined with followers, well wishers and people who were merely curious. When Perpetua was passing through the gates of Royal Park she was given a huge cheer by her most loyal followers. They chanted:

"Sister and God!"

(It looked as if she was uncertain whether to thank them or to discourage them. She looked very pleased but slightly embarrassed. Trina kept signalling to her to stand at the front of the open-topped bus and wave and smile; but she bent down as she came through the gates and raised her lightweight wooden cross.)

The service was televised nationally and so everybody knows what happened but afterwards London was taken completely by surprise. After an exit procession from Royal Park down one of the major shopping streets, Perpetua plunged into Gogo where there were tramps, addicts and rough sleepers. Every time she found somebody in distress she put her hands on their head and made them better. Text messages brought ever more desperate and broken people to where she was as she made her way through the streets with the crowds pressing in. There was panic on the part of the police and DISC (The Directorate for Internal Security and Control). As Heather had lost some of her enthusiasm, no permit had been granted for a celebration which involved impromptu music, dancing and healing. The traffic was grid-locked but nobody minded as long as ailing passengers could be brought to Perpetua. Through the afternoon she headed steadily eastwards, greeted by waves of joy and relief. The police and DISC gave up the struggle as their officers went home for relatives and friends or simply joined in the festivities. (For one day) Perpetua was the Queen of London.

In the late afternoon she reached the river and got into a small boat which was packed with sound equipment. Thousands of people stood on the bank. (For the first time SAD noted a substantial number of placards calling for various social justice measures). Brian and Kylie had worked wonders to provide extension audio and large screens in Mammon Square.

"Rejoice and be glad!" she said, "Because the love of God Our Parent for all of you is like the river's water. It might look different depending on the seasons and it might look dirty because of all the things we do to spoil its clarity; but it flows among us always, carrying us, supporting us, cheering us. This is the river of life. Long ago people needed it more than they do now. Today we build bridges because it gets in the way of what we want to do. The way we think about God and about ourselves changes through time; we would not be human if it did not; if we tried to stay the same we would be something else that we cannot imagine. And so some people will still think of God as water but others might more readily think of Jesus as bridges. But what does not change is God among us, flowing like the river, shining and smiling, ever different, ever the same."

As the sun began to set Andy said: "Many of those you have helped are still poor and hungry." "Have any of you got any food or drink to share?" she asked. An onlooker brought a hamper he had been carrying to a nearby boat; a girl brought an untouched bottle of water. Perpetua stepped off the boat and put the gifts down behind the bank of speakers, prayed, and then began to hand items out of the basket to her followers. The food and drink was passed along a human chain; everyone was so happy and relaxed that the people at the very furthest points were supplied first. It took more than half an hour for those at the front to be given food and drink but when everybody had what they needed, Perpetua appeared on the big screens and said: "Thank God for these gifts given through me as the Daughter of the Almighty sent to absorb the world's sin and sorrow as The Sacred Vessel. You have seen the unlimited power of God working through me." Then she smiled and told them to enjoy the rest of the party. She asked her followers to join her at Bleak Villas when everything had been cleared up, then she slipped away to the south side of the river before heading west, giving herself a little time to pray.

"This is Bad Morning with Janet Burns and me, Rod Stirrer. Yesterday there was an extraordinary event in London which was a kind of religious party. There are reports

that some people say they were cured of chronic illness and even one report that there was a miraculous food and drink distribution by the event's centrepiece, Perpetua. We are joined now by our new Social Affairs Correspondent, Patsy Downhill. Patsy, what do you make of yesterday's unusual events?" "Well, Rod, all the latest survey data shows that people are becoming less and less able to enjoy themselves, whether it's the problem of nuts in chocolate bars, food colouring, candles, the perils of tight trousers, loud music, slippery dance floors, broken glass, twisted ankles, blinding champagne corks, burning cafetieres, choking fish bones, boats on water, make-up poisoning, strangulation by halter top, or just the ordinary dangers of eating, drinking and dancing, there is certainly greater private and public risk aversion." "And what about these remarkable stories that Perpetua cured people of serious illnesses?" "Nobody is taking them seriously, not even church leaders who are sometimes a bit prone to being carried away—you will be aware of the need in the Roman Catholic Church for the late Pope to grab a miracle—are not giving any credibility to the claims." "What about the bizarre rumours about the source of the food and drink which seemed to appear out of nowhere?" "A god4u spokesperson said that this was a mass miracle but nobody is taking this seriously either. It is well known that Christian movements get tangled up with major companies in all kinds of murky ways and this seems to be one of those episodes." "Finally, Patsy, what about this quite extraordinary claim by Perpetua that she is God in some not very defined way?" "Well, Rod, as you say, the claim is rather vague and so nobody is taking it seriously. One leading church commentator I talked to said that he had seen no evidence but he would be interested in a claim if it was clearly set out." "Thank you Patsy. Janet." "The Government is considering regulations to limit the number of candles allowed on birthday cakes with a maximum of eighteen, nine for tens and nine for units..."

23.

Given Heather's long record with SAD, it was rash of her to break ranks with Perpetua and resume her connections with criminal elements in Grunge park and Excelsior Gardens. She had had a stormy relationship with Roy, exercising great (sexual) power over him at a time when he was just beginning to think about life after Dexter. He resented her power but loved to be seen with her. Until Perpetua came along to break things up, it had suited them both.

On the Monday evening after Palm Sunday, Heather, Jo, Roy, Rory and Oliver, met to discuss developments at the youth club (and for the forthcoming weekend). Miles was very angry and wanted to throw them out after the last incident with Roy but he had no choice. He retreated into a corner. "What if he says something?" asked Jo. "No chance," said Roy. "He knows what will happen. In fact, Miles, you better leave." "But we are discussing my club." "Not yours any longer. Get out." He had been so faithful for so long but something snapped, and Miles left, defeated.

"Let's lay all the pieces out logically," said Heather, "so we know where we are. Rory, Olly and some of his RIF friends want to have a genuine drinking, drug taking and violence experience in an exclusive location. This will bring Roy immediate cash and offer the possibility of extending his territory into Excelsior Gardens." "And we want to get our own back on Perpetua," said Rory. "We'll come to that," said Heather. "Calm down. I know from my experience in Grunge Park as a dealer and as Perpetua's agent for regulatory matters—what a laugh!—that if there is a red violence warning SAD and all the other grasping public agencies will pull out—not that they are ever around late on a Friday night when they are 'most wanted' according to their own rules—and it is not difficult to ensure a police pull-out. As long as we promise to stay in, they will stay out and keep other people out. This minimises the problem for them so that they can leave 'no go' areas and get on with arresting all kinds of misfits to reach their targets.

"Now for the spice. For reasons which we will come to in a moment, Rory and Olly have something against Perpetua and want to give her a hard time. Well, the fancy little bitch deserves it, taking on celebrity airs and oppressing her loyal followers. This would be interesting enough but Rory's dad's friend's shiny little girl, Poppy Smoother, wants to make a television programme about gang violence; and she rather likes the idea of a RIF element. She would prefer to have pictures of nice white boys with attitude rather than the usual—begging your pardon, Roy—run-of-the-mill black thugs. She will cover whatever happens live in a Good Friday programme, taking the risk that the delayer will pick up anything so gross it isn't in the public interest. DIM says that it isn't a censor and can only condemn programmes after they have been aired, so no problem there. We just have to be quiet this week because CEC has done a confidentiality deal with the the TT and we won't get our cut if the word gets out. As agreed, the centrepiece will be pictures of little miss purity out of her head.

"Which leads to you two. Why are you so interested in Perpetua?" "When I was a kid," said Olly, "my dad died and my uncle Joe, Father O'Helly to you, sent me to a Catholic boarding school where we were given lousy food, beaten and not taught much except for the Catechism. When I came home for holidays the beatings went on and he also wanted to interfere with me but I was stronger than him. In the end I didn't come home and he stopped paying the fees. Still, I won a scholarship to theological college as I couldn't think of anything else to do; but then I met Rory and we started working on porno computer games and managed to sell a couple of winners to a production company in Minsk. After that we came down here, knowing that if we got short again we could always design some more games; they're all the same, really; there's only a limited number of things—begging your pardon, Heather—that you can do with a girl." "But O'Helly doesn't like Perpetua, so why aren't you on her side against him?" "He's so unhappy, left on his own, needing a boy but not allowed to talk about it, that he isn't worth the effort. But every time I see Perpetua she's so smug, always telling people what to do." "No she isn't," said Heather, (automatically). "She never tells people what to do." "I'm not arguing, that's how it looks to me; and then there's Dexter always snooping around, trying to pick a fight." "Yes," said Roy. "And you're frightened of him," said Heather. "Look, just shut up, will you." "All right," said Heather, "I'm sorry, let's get on. You, Olly, why are you so worked up?"

"My father was a really good dad when he was a parish priest. But as he got promoted he became more distant and when at last he became an Archdeacon, just about the time I was ready to go to theological college, he lost interest in mother and me altogether. I wouldn't have cared if he had climbed the ladder to be a Bishop, trying to look after people, or to be a senior parish priest, even; or if he'd became a Chaplain or a social worker; anything but buildings!" "So as Perpetua is against buildings and in favour of people, why are you against Perpetua?" asked Heather. "Because, in a strange way, she will kill the church, just leave it with the buildings; which would be all right if she could hold onto what she takes; but she will lose it. People need those buildings as a framework to be inside. My dad was wrong but in a really horrible way she's even worse. He worries too much about buildings and not enough about people; she just doesn't know what she's doing. She will wreck the church and offer nothing in its place. Look, I know I don't go to church any more and that I'm mixed up in porn, drugs and crime; but I suppose I'm like millions of people who don't care about the church but couldn't bear it not to be there."

"So you are going to drug Perpetua by force just to get your own back on your uncle and your dad?" "Yes," they said. "It seems pretty stupid to me," said Heather. "I don't care," said Roy (suddenly angry) "That's the deal. It might seem pointless to a clever little girl like you but what is there that's pointful?" (Heather seemed rather confused but she soon gained her composure). "Perpetua must take her chance. She claims to have supernatural powers; she has even said she is going to be killed; so if she wants to get out of this she can and will; if she doesn't, that's her business."

When they had tied up minor details they left, barely noticing Miles who had crept back in although nobody knew when. He texted Trina who was already on her way. "You know I don't really like Perpetua all that much but something very nasty is going to happen to her." "It already is. Somebody has told the papers that she used to be a drug dealer and it's about to be splashed over tomorrow morning's papers, so soon after her wonderful London triumph." "I suppose that's Heather," said Miles. "I thought so; but how do you know?" "She has been here with Jo, talking to Roy and those Excelsior Gardens show-offs Rory and Olly, about kidnapping Perpetua and humiliating her; but Heather says if Perpetua wants to get out of it she has the power." "But she won't use it, Miles. You know the story of Jesus; she wants to go exactly the same way; in fact, she thinks that, in a very peculiar way, she's identical with Jesus; that's the bit you can't stand but that is what is happening." "Kiss me," said Miles (with a rush of courage). "Don't be stupid Miles, when we're discussing something as serious as this. I'm sorry, that came out wrong. I mean, let's try to take the question of kissing as separate from Perpetua." "According to her," said Miles (settling back to his usual screwed-down calm), "They are very much part of the same thing, living a holy life and kissing." "You have been listening, haven't you?" "Well, I am not stupid and I have been listening and watching. What really got me was the meeting outside the Civic Centre. I mean, she never said a hard word; she was so constructive."

They were just locking up to go when Perpetua arrived. "I am sorry Miles, it will not take more than a minute but we are in the middle of a little bit of trouble. I have been accused of being a drug dealer and Trina thinks that I ought to make a statement and hold a news conference. All I came to ask was how rough are they likely to be. I feel confident inside all of the time but I just have those moments when the way the world works makes me so depressed that I want to crumple."

"Don't worry," said Trina. "To them it's a case of a bit of celebrity scandal but none of them really believes most of what they write; it's just part of a big make-believe game. And if they ask you questions about religion they will be pretty basic, or even silly." She looked at Trina but said, "Thank you Miles, I am sorry to have disturbed you both." And before Trina could say anything else, she had gone.

She went back to Bill Midway's church for the night. "I know," she said, looking at the cross above the altar, "I have taken people away from here to try to love you in a fuller way outside; but I come here myself. I am sure that others will come to pray and to celebrate; I just wanted them to stop being routine about their worship and indifferent about their community responsibility; and I could be wrong; but it is too late now. It is not pride that stops me going back; I have run out of time. I pray that I have done the right thing with Your help but if it is wrong it is all my responsibility." "No," she heard a voice say, "we are responsible together, we in the Godhead and we in the alloy of the divine and the human in You and in Our covenant with the created, We are responsible for everything." "Even the things that go wrong," "Even the things that go wrong. The Creator and the Created, the Redeemer and the Redeemed, the Sanctifier and the Sanctified, the Vessel and the Contained, we are all responsible."

(We were all responsible. A senior SAD official who had been following the Perpetua case with increasing sympathy requested an adjustment to policy but her superiors ruled that the Red Warning procedure for withdrawal should be retained.)

24.

"The time is ten past eight and you are listening to Bad Morning with Janet Burns and me, Owen Grumpy. In recent days stories of Perpetua have proliferated. On Sunday she was the centre of the largest London rally since the Iraq War protest and the Save Foxes for England march; there are claims that she has healed incurably sick people; and even one claim that she conjured up a banquet for thousands out of thin air; but now her star is waning because the long-running accusation that her followers are really a criminal gang has been capped by reports that she herself was a drug dealer. Perpetua, what do you say to the accusation that your followers are a pretty bad lot?" "When I found them, many of them were, as you put it, 'a pretty bad lot' but that is the point. It is those in our society who are most in need of help who should receive it from those who want to improve society." "But as a self proclaimed spiritual leader, surely your job is to set a good example, to provide moral leadership, by upholding traditional religious values?" "I am upholding what I call 'traditional religious values'. I suppose what you have in mind when you use that phrase are the people who stick to the Ten Commandments, go to church regularly and, as far as outward appearances go, are a credit to their Church; but the real traditional Christian values are the call to repentance and loving forgiveness for the weak." "But many people say that you have brought religion into disrepute by being seen in the company of criminals." "Who are these 'many people' you talk about?" "Well, a number of church leaders, for example, have expressed doubt about the way you conduct your mission." "That is a quite different point. I suspect your 'many people' amount to nothing more than your researcher and the editor who put your script together. As for church leaders, what they have to say about my mission is widely recorded; of course they do not want their traditional power base to be eroded." "Worse still, however, you are now exposed as a drug dealer." "You would be a more credible public broadcaster if you named your source. One newspaper, the Toxic Times, a highly partial source, has published an accusation, apparently from one of my followers, that I was a drug dealer. I was brought up to believe that journalists, particularly public service broadcasters, were supposed to check their sources. What is more, it has become your habit to give coverage to 'stories'—a good word—no matter how far-fetched. Instead of dealing in probability you deal in possibility, no matter how distant and uncritical." "We are not here to discuss the BBC, we are here to discuss your conduct." "Only a minute ago you asked for 'moral leadership' and that is what you are getting. It is irresponsible for a public broadcaster to be an uncritical conduit for any trash that comes your way; you cannot ask society to be well conducted if you suspend your critical judgment for the sake of headlines. Your uncritical cynicism damages society; so you are not reporting on, but negatively transforming, society." "That is just evading the accusation that you were a drug dealer." "I will come to that but you, more than anybody, should know that what matters is the source of an accusation. I am prepared to admit that it is likely that one of my followers has accused me of being a drug dealer; I do not know why. The TT has published the accusation without any corroboration—how convenient the confidentiality of sources can be—and you have just repeated the charge." "So you deny the charge?" "It is sad that I have to; but I do; and I forgive my accusers." "But why should we take your word for it?" "To which the only logical reply is why should your listeners take your word for it? It is my word against yours; listeners can make up their own mind. In any case, I was told when I was asked to appear on the programme that I would be questioned about my beliefs not some silly story in a tabloid newspaper." "Listeners are hardly likely to be interested in your religious beliefs if you are shown to be a criminal leading a gang of criminals." "We have been round this circuit once; it is a game. You want me to admit that I am a criminal so that you can maintain your reputation for making the news instead of reporting it and I deny the charge. Either we go on to new territory or you might as well stop." "I am not used to being told how to conduct interviews." (Awkward pause) "Owen, why are you so defensive?" "It is my job to ask the questions." "There you go again; why are you so defensive? I suspect it is because you know that you are cheapening yourself by getting involved in silly stories instead of pursuing your earlier ambition to be a great journalist and a seeker after truth. You have stopped seeking, you are the creature of a system that thinks it is above reporting news; that is far too dull." "I am not prepared to go on listening to this." "Relax; it would be so funny—and make news—if you were to walk out of your own interview. So ask me a question worthy of your vitally important calling."

"Do you have anything to say about the well-supported reports that something unusual happened on Sunday when you distributed food and drink to thousands of people?" "To save you saying it, some people have said that I have made a deal with a retailer. Everybody knows that I am well connected with the major supermarkets because many of my followers have been drawn from them; but I have never accepted anything from them without being totally open. On this occasion I received some food and drink from the public and, through the power of God Our Parent, who sent me as the Sacred Vessel of the Godhead, I was able to turn this generosity into a feast for all. My faith in God combined with the faith of the crowd so that a special, sacred event took place." "Many listeners will be out of their depth with this kind of talk." "That is a pity." "Are you telling me that you performed the kind of miracle that Jesus is supposed to have performed?" "I am pleased to say that God has given me powers like those of Jesus My Brother." "But listeners will want proof." "Of what?" "That you performed a miracle." "If they want proof, then they do not understand the nature of miracles; miracles, as they are traditionally called, depend not only upon the power of the Godhead but also the faith of the people." "I'm losing patience with this evasive language." "Yes. I can tell." (Another awkward pause).

"Why have you spent so much of your time attacking traditional Christianity?" "I have spent some of my time trying to suggest constructive alternatives to contemporary Christian sclerosis but we have to be careful with the word 'traditional' it usually means the way things were when we were children. For centuries Christians went to church because they were awestruck by a god whose power depended on the iconography of hell and scientific ignorance; then they went to church because they were frightened of an angry god; then later still they went as a matter of social uniformity. Today Christianity is changing from conforming to affirming and I am trying to help people to recognise that Christianity is based on love not judgment or fear. An affirming church built on love needs very different dynamics from a conforming church based on fear and judgment." "That sounds like a clever way of explaining the steep decline in the fortunes of the church." "How would you know, simply from numbers, whether the church is declining or not?" "Well if you think that Christianity is so important, it is necessary that as many people as possible make contact with it." "That is a fair point but building an affirming church is far more difficult than sustaining a conforming church. My Sister the Spirit does not work in a human way, counting scalps. The Church should not panic, it should trust in the Spirit and not worry about the numbers. Numbers are a human phenomenon; the Spirit is God's good guide to Christian witness." "So are you saying that Christianity could survive without the Church?" "No; the Church is the corporate expression of the human desire to worship the Creator; only a very few of us, such as hermits, can survive without the mutual support of a church; but that does not mean that the Church has to be the one we grew up with. Indeed, because of the terrible afflictions of our world, the Church has an immense responsibility to reach out. Which brings me back to where I began; we need to reach out to the weak and the indulgent. This does not only mean people who are poor and criminal, it also means those who are rich and selfish; in fact, they are more in danger of not being united with God in the Kingdom of Eternal Light than those who are desperate."

"Are you therefore excusing criminal behaviour?" "No; but our society, aided and abetted by people like you who actually know better, is prepared to do anything but care for the poor. You will give them anything but money; you will accuse them of crime and drug abuse but you will not take the fundamental steps to improve the situation. Society treats these people like animals so they behave like animals. Hundreds of reports, paid for out of taxes, and hundreds of others from 'think tanks' all agree that crime is associated with poverty and that the cure for poverty is money. I would add that what my afflicted brothers and sisters need are love and money; money without love will help a little but self respect cannot be built on money alone; it depends on being loved and knowing that we are being loved which gives us the confidence to love." "Isn't that rather romantic?" "No; it is to ask us to give to others what we would want for ourselves. This stubborn, selfish denial of reality will have a catastrophic effect on all of us." "Well, so it might; but I am afraid we will have to stop it there for the sport. Barry, news of yet another England disaster."

25.

On the morning of Maundy Thursday Perpetua and her core followers again went into the heart of London, this time making their way to the City. At the boundary security barrier she took up huge sacks of coins which made her stagger as she braced herself to bear the load; and so she came, bent-backed to the nerve centre of the financial system. People came out of banks and other financial institutions. She said: "Look how money can weigh us down; look how difficult it is to travel towards the Kingdom of Heavenly light. Take these coins and put them into bags that people can carry away; make my burden their joy. But make the occasion even more joyful by topping up these gift bags with your own money; and then, when you have given, bring out the next level of management so that it can top up what you have given; and so on to the managing directors and chairmen."

It was an unusual (fascinating and moving) sight to see the junior clerks escorting their seniors, then middle management and finally the major figures in the City. When these came out Perpetua said: "Usually, you like to sit on donating bodies, Guilds and Trusts, but today I want you to spend your lunch hour finding poor people and handing these gifts to them; no name, no business card, just thank them for being, for trying to be good citizens, for cleaning offices, for cleaning toilets, for unloading lorries. And if you find somebody who looks idle and depressed, no judgment, just ask them to try to be happy with themselves and to pray to God; and ask yourself why they are idle. Is it really because they do not want work or because the gap between wanting and having has become so desperately wide that their weak imaginations fail."

"Did you come here to condemn capitalism?" asked one of the office workers. "No; there is no point in making wholesale condemnations of complex systems; that is the danger of political extremism." "But what about Jesus overturning the tables in the temple?" "The point is that trading was going on in the most sacred place for the Jews, the Temple, around which all their spiritual lives revolved. What Jesus attacked was not trade but a kind of idolatry. Even so, be careful; today it would be wonderful if our forbidding churches could be opened up to modest, honest trade." "So how do we survive in this greedy place?" asked another. "All I ask is that everyone tries to be honest with themselves. The more you have, the more difficult it is to stay honest. So here are some questions: in your company, how often do you reward bad and selfish behaviour and take advantage of the meek and well behaved? How often do you buy off trouble instead of confronting it? If there are two people, one a lazy worker who disrupts your work place and the other a quiet and faithful worker who makes up for the shortcomings of others without even admitting to it, let alone complaining; how often does the first one get the pay rise while the second one is left? Do you regard apologising as a sign of weakness? Do you punish the admission of human error and reward those who hide it? You need to think; but to do that you need time. Find a little time every day for yourselves and for God Our Parent; just a little time."

"The time is ten to nine and we are ending Bad Morning today with a discussion of the refusal of the Minister at the Information Directorate to apologise for an error in his statement to Parliament. Norma." "Well, Craig, people at Westminster are very angry that the Minister has refused to apologise. He says that he has to rely on the advice of civil servants whom he neither hires nor can fire; so why should he take the rap for their error. He says that saying sorry would be meaningless when everybody really knows that it was not his mistake at all; but his call for civil servants to take responsibility for their own errors has been met with outrage." "And what about his political career?" "Well, he might just save himself if he apologises, the House of Commons and the public have great respect for a Minister who admits wrong doing." "Norma! There is a news agency report that the Minister has apologised for his error. In a brief statement he says that he recognises that he must take full responsibility for his Directorate no matter what." "Well, Craig, I would say that will finish him. Nobody respects a politician who is too weak to stand up for what he believes. No doubt this huge admission of weakness will be exploited by the opposition, the media and some on his own side jockeying for position; so I think he's finished." "Thank you Norma. That's all for today. Next we have a special programme for Maundy Thursday on Jesus The Victim."

After all the money had been divided and augmented and handed out for distribution, Perpetua stood at the top of a large flight of steps at the front of an unused church. For the first time at a Perpetua meeting there was a definite air of protest with a huge variety of banners calling for all kinds of social justice measures. (There was a major panic at SAD which particularly wanted to keep faith groups and social justice apart and this explains why an emergency alert was triggered.)

"We live in a culture of deep division, of very rich and very poor people whose worlds increasingly do not even touch; but today I want to emphasise something else: that we live in a culture of public generosity but only private penitence. Should we try to do things the other way round? What about private generosity and public penitence? The private generosity would be a start, at least; but public penitence would take so much of the fear and worry out of society. If nobody admits that they are wrong then the result is concealment; and the result of concealment is the fear of being found out; and when we are found out the pretence is gone through that we are unusual, perhaps even unique; and that while everybody else is getting on with their virtuous lives, there are a few people who can be picked out for their bad behaviour. This makes us take sides; we end up being good or bad. There are 'respectable working families' and there are 'anti-social families' who need tough measures. But who is really going to admit that they are in the second group and not the first? If recognising our weakness is the first step to combatting it, surely we need to help people to recognise their weakness and that means admitting our own so that, as a society, we can own up to the mass of individual and collective weakness that we all share as part of our state of imperfection."

She took her wooden cross from Dexter and blessed the people. They seemed bewildered. "There is nothing that you need to do at this moment; do not be puzzled; just think, over the coming weekend, about what I have said; as you remember the suffering, death and Resurrection of Jesus My Brother, think of how we can admit our weakness because we live in the forgiveness of the Crucifixion and the hope of the Resurrection. Some of you might have seen my Christmas broadcast, how I reminded us all to remember Easter. It is now upon us. When you go home this afternoon, think of the Cross; and think of Easter."

She told her followers that she would see them in the evening and slipped away. She texted Jo (her mobile phone survived her death and the SIM card was intact and recovered) and Heather saying that it did not matter if they had given the false stories to the press, they were to come to the big evening celebration. Then she went with Jim to have tea with Bill Midway (although Perpetua seems not to have known it, Jim barely left her during the next thirty hours). "I know I have turned your life upside-down, Bill, but I am afraid I am going to do it again. I think I am being set up for some kind of horrible event. I can feel my own death coming on. I know that it has been impossible for you to follow me like the other core people in *god4u* but I count you as core. You have been with me every painful step of the way since before Christmas and although there are aspects of conventional, contemporary Christianity that I have spoken out against, I have not judged individuals and I have not condemned those who work hard for God Our Parent. The little band of followers I assembled is faithful but fragile; it will need your quiet strength as guide and counsellor. Please look after them for me if things go as I think they will. I know Easter is your busy time but do what you can."

Bill said nothing; he rarely did, accustomed as he was to almost interminable listening. He just nodded and said: "That's all right; you can trust me; I will." Perpetua went home.

After Jim's departure, the remaining *god4u* followers were restless. Dexter decided to confront Roy and he had almost reached Grunge park when Trina somehow divined his intention and intercepted him. "Where are you going? No, don't answer. I don't want you to lie. I know where you are going. And I suppose you have a weapon. No; don't answer that either, just hand it over. At the moment when Perpetua needs you more than ever you are playing your old gang games, deadly games. What would we have done if you had been injured or killed by Roy or, even worse, if you had injured or killed him? Be strong and self disciplined for her now. She needs you."

Andy toyed with the idea of blowing the money but Wayne persuaded him to hang on. Bob was tempted to break into a luxury car and have some fun but Kylie talked him out of it. Brian said he was going into an internet cafe to play games but Bob told him to grow up. Using their phones, they converged and discovered that sticking together was the only way they could stay loyal. Dexter had got his nerve back and said everything would be all right; but Trina found it hard to hide her nervousness.

(She was right to be nervous. Late in the afternoon there was a discussion between SAD and the police on the Perpetua issue at which the police mentioned the CEC television proposal. There were rumours that Perpetua would be involved in some way and it was agreed that to broadcast Perpetua confirming her drug connections would be helpful to both parties: SAD would have one less worry; and the police red violence alert policy would be justified; and it could all be sold as an example of media freedom. Immediate clearance was received from the ROD (The Respect and Order Directorate) and Roy, in effect, had become a state agent as well as a gang leader.)

26.

It was a (strange kind of) sombre celebration. When her followers arrived, Perpetua made them feel embarrassed as she insisted on cleaning their shoes, so they sat, awkwardly, watching her, dangling their socked feet. "I have told you that what I am doing is showing you that you must serve people as well as teaching them and praying for them; but as you sit there, imagine what it is like for people without shoes who contemplate walking the stony road, as Jesus My Brother walked the stony road. You are sitting there because you feel strange without your shoes but you could walk across the floor without harming yourself."

Although they tried to be cheerful they ate the highly varied takeaway meal which Perpetua had ordered in almost complete silence. They would rouse themselves to life and then Perpetua would say something about the gloom she felt over her future, that they would soon be left alone, that she had asked Bill to be their spiritual counsellor. It all seemed highly concrete when it came down to arrangements for Bill to be with them.

The atmosphere was helped a little when Heather and Jo left. Everybody suspected them of starting the rumours about Perpetua and not only Perpetua, but perhaps Trina, suspected worse to come. They had all exercised a good deal of self control in saying nothing offensive to the two girls, and trying to smile. Now they had gone there was a general discussion about them and how they had betrayed the group. "Be careful," said Perpetua. "You are in danger of thinking that you are better than them. Have you not heard anything I have said in the past eight months? How often have I warned you against appearances and reminded you that we cannot know what is inside the heart of another, that only God Our Parent knows and is in a position to judge if, indeed, judgment is the issue, which I doubt."

"But we have stuck with you since the beginning," said Brian. "Yes you have; and for that I am sure God Our Parent will give you a just reward but it does not mean that other people will not receive the same reward.

"There was a man who was very rich but he was so pestered by relatives, friends and local good causes, that he left his large city house, sold everything he had, put the money into a bank and moved to a tiny cottage in the country. He gave modestly but regularly to good causes, determined to reduce his wealth for the good of others. Now there was a man in the same village who lived in what had been the Squire's house and who worked in the city. He was double-crossed in business by a man he had thought was his friend and he had lost most of his money; but he kept the big house because it was in the family and because his wife loved it; and he scraped by as best he could, planning for the day when he would be fully solvent again. But the people in the village thought the first man was immensely self-sacrificing whereas the second man was niggardly; and they made unkind comparisons which upset both men. At last the two bumped into each other as they took their evening walks and they exchanged stories. The rich man with the tiny cottage made a deal with the poor man in the big house. Neither said anything and so the rich man, who had diverted most of his liquid assets to the poor man, fell in the estimation of the village while the poor man, his fortune partly restored, rose in popularity. I am telling you this story at such length at this time because if you only remember one thing other than the primacy of love it is the presumption of judgment. We all share the hope that we will be enfolded into the Kingdom of Eternal Light and then our knowledge of God Our Parent will be way beyond anything we can imagine or we think we deserve; and there will be no hierarchy in the Light; it will not be like a light that is bright but radiates more weakly the further away you are from it. All those are unhelpful images. This Light is indissoluble with no gradations or ranks.

"Now," she said, "each of you take a piece of fruit that represents one of the countries; together you are the world at this celebration, the world that has remembered Jesus My Brother for two thousand years. It is a slightly unusual proceeding but I have brought special bread with olives and two bottles of champagne." She set the bread and wine on the table and called upon the blessing of Her Sister the Spirit. Then she took the bread and blessed it and broke it and, after dipping each piece in oil, she gave it to each of them saying: "This is my body given for the whole world so that all of God's children, filled with this immortal food, may learn to love." And taking the bottles of Champagne, she poured them into a large, glass jug; she blessed the wine and gave it to them saying: "This is my blood, renewed in the Third Testament for the Third Millennium, shed for all the world, to be carried into every street and every home. Whenever you sacrifice this bread and wine remember Jesus My Brother. Never shroud that blood in gold and silver but make it clear for the eyes of all people; in the light and clarity of the glass which bears the blood of My Brother, remember me."

"Can we really do what you have done?" asked Bob. "After all, I am a rough and ready sort of man, you know, who likes mechanics and that sort of thing; I like to get my hands dirty." "Sadly there have been too few peasant and labourer priests but not only can you do what I have done, you must do it; you must have faith in the Spirit that you have been called to do it. Not everybody can do what I have done because it can only be done in the Spirit. But I know you are in the Spirit and so I dipped the bread in oil to ordain you in the Spirit. When I have gone you will know that you are in the Spirit." "Does that mean that we are like clergy?" "Yes but you will not be recognised as such by the established churches. They have established a massively difficult and complex superstructure that people must overcome to be a member of the clergy; and the automatic assumption is that the calling of My Sister the Spirit must be tested. How people think they can test the will of My Sister I do not know; but that is how it is. Offer bread and wine or other food and drink, offer love and care in the house groups, and the Spirit will guide you as to what you must do. For all his weaknesses—and we all know them all, including himself—I leave my leadership to Dexter; but I want you to know now, definitely, that this is not because he is male but because he is the best fitted person at this time to lead you through the difficult days to come."

(Not that Perpetua's confidence seemed that well founded.) When the meal finished she asked a few of her followers, including Dexter, to stay and pray with her; but they were overcome with food, wine and emotion; and she kept having to rouse them. So much had happened in the past few days that they had grown confused; they could hardly think straight; and the meal and the wine and the ceremony had overcome them. She said goodbye to them sadly and shut the door.

Outside, there was still a SAD presence and Miles was loitering, as if he just happened to be in the rather distant area of Bleak Villas. Reluctantly Trina acknowledged him as the group made its way homewards. Trina wanted to know whether there were any more developments in Roy's camp but Miles had been too frightened to visit the area since Monday.

Roy was making final preparations and checking them with Poppy who had the exclusive rights to cover the RIF event at the Grunge Park Hollow. There had been a little tussle with DIM but it was very difficult for officials to argue against the public interest, particularly when the survival of a marginal television channel was involved. The police had been squared, SAD (in spite of a vigourous protest from a Perpetua admirer) had decided to stick to its Red procedure.

Perpetua (according to Jim), closed the doors and began to cry. "They have been with me all this time and they still do not understand," she said. "Of course, I knew how it would be but it somehow does not dull the pain. They have tried to be such good friends but the engagement is so sporadic. On the other hand, if I had been more intellectual or if they had been more intellectual it would not have worked. It is raw but when it works it is vital."

There was a knock. She was usually reluctant to go to the door at night but the knock was soft. "Jim, what are you doing?" "I thought you might like a little music to help you doze off." "You are so kind. I knew I was right about the rawness and vitality. You play and let yourself out when you are ready. I like to sleep in the chair." "What shall I play?" "I have never asked you what kinds of things you can play; you always come up with new music." "I will play some

Tenebrae music; it's the right night for that, for the candles going out one by one." "Yes; the candles going out one by one."

27.

On Good Friday morning as Perpetua and Bill led a procession of witness from The Hollow, through Grunge Park and Excelsior Gardens to St. Simple the Lesser, she told Trina that she was almost overcome with mixed emotions. She was amazed by the commitment of the new followers she and Bill had gained for God; without any grasp of the traditional rituals they were intently focused on the cross which led them, they were serious and silent in spite of what was going on around them and perhaps partly out of that defensiveness which breeds defiance, they sang the hymns with true commitment. On the other hand, she said, re-living the Passion of Jesus was like going to her own death. She had prayed to be spared and she had prayed to be helped through the trauma and she was as certain as she could be of anything that she had to accept what was coming to her but that she would be helped in a way she could not yet understand. At the half-way point, at the plaza outside the Civic Centre, Bill asked if she wanted to talk but she said she would rather listen but she would be happy to read. As she had done at Christmas, she read Luke's account of the Nativity and Passion consecutively without a break and as she reached the climax she almost cried when she saw Miles and Father O'Helly out of the corner of her eye, pretending not to be part of what was going on but seemingly drawn in. Bill said: "You will remember how Perpetua told us all that we could not enjoy the birth of the Baby Jesus unless we remembered why He came, what His becoming human meant for us all; so now we are thinking of the same story from its other, its sad climax. If the birth was the first act of a drama and His mission of teaching and healing the second, this is the third; but there will be a fourth to come; and no matter how grim the reality of the death of Jesus on the Cross, we should not try to see this as completely dark, the light of Jesus rising from the dead is just over the horizon, the new dawn in which we live as followers of Jesus. For those who were there at the time there was only fear and darkness; not even Jesus knew that He was going to rise from the dead; He only knew that He was doing what God Our Parent wanted Him to do."

Perpetua was even more happy and moved when Miles and Father O'Helly followed them on the second half of the procession and went into St. Simple's. Like her, they sat at the back; but they were there. That was more than she could have asked for.

As the cross was brought into the church by Bill during the most solemn service, the world outside went mad. There was a huge thunderstorm over London which brought torrential rain and, at its heart, a tornado tore through the capital from the South to the North, wiping out supermarkets, tearing the huge doors from London Minster and wrecking media organisations. (It was as if it had been divinely directed.) Miraculously there were no casualties. All the major channels switched to disaster reporting until just before three o'clock when, without explanation, there was a short meditation by Perpetua on the death of Jesus. When she heard about it later, it reminded Trina of what had happened on Christmas night when Perpetua's worship had somehow replaced the worship in the BBC schedule.

Rory and Olly had wanted to wreck the procession but Roy had told them to lie low as they did not want to risk their evening entertainment by being arrested; the police might not care what happened in Grunge Park but they were certainly sensitive to any disorder in Excelsior Gardens where the up-and-coming Mr. Niggler was the MP. Now they were nervous about the fierceness of the storm and whether it would ruin their evening. Meanwhile, Miles and Trina had gone to the Youth Club. "Look Miles," said Trina, "I wish you would just leave yourself open to Perpetua's message and stop resisting it. I can see your struggle and I can see that it hurts; but your religion of discipline and judgment is so defensive and you don't need to be." "If you keep going on about it I won't see you again," said Miles. "But Miles, it's you that has been piling on the pressure to see me. I really like you, you know that, but, as usually happens with these things, it's the man that makes the running and you have surely been doing that; so don't threaten something unless you can carry it out."

Suddenly, something broke in Miles and in a way he could not possibly have imagined, he fell into Trina's arms, crying uncontrollably. "I have tried so hard for this God who seemed to grant me a place alongside Him as a soldier for the righteous," he said, "but it has been a god fashioned in the image of my own weakness. I needed a strict God with rules I could follow and impose; I needed a frightening God who would keep me from my own weaknesses; I needed a father figure although I am not sure whether this was a reaction or a reinforcement of my own father who was harsh and irresponsible by turns and who finally left us. I have been holding back because I don't want to make the same mistake again with Perpetua. I keep seeing my mother in her and I am tempted to model my new God on her." "Miles, Miles, we are not here to model God on anything, we are simply to listen and learn from those who work so hard that some hint of God passes through them to us. In a way that it's difficult to understand but which I have learned following Perpetua, you have to switch off the human brain, let God find a way in and then switch it back on again. I heard you talking the other day about the 'wrath of God' as if this was real, like human anger." "But if we can't use the word 'wrath' of God how can we use the word 'love'?" "Oh Miles, that's the point; that's the point! Just as what you call the 'wrath of God' must be infinitely different, if it exists at all, from human anger, so God's love is unimaginably different from anything we know of love; but whereas there's only misery in trying to model what kind of anger

God may possess—the word 'feel' seems all wrong to me—the exact opposite is true when we try to model love, it can do nothing but good, no matter how incomplete in conception and disjointed in action, no matter how often we go wrong, as long as love is at the centre of our being, radiating through us and out to people, living on this sad earth makes sense."

Again, in a way that he could not possibly have imagined, she kissed him.

After all her followers had left Bill's church with varying degrees of reluctance, Perpetua lay on the marble in front of the altar but Jim, who had been the last to leave, could not break away. He came quietly back in using Bill's vestry key which was in a pot by the door. She seemed to be struggling with herself and he wanted to comfort her but she seemed to calm down and become like a corpse, so he stayed where he was, well out of her sight. She got up and went to the back of the church where she found her large, lightweight cross and came down the aisle dancing, holding the cross as if it was her lover. "Give me strength now," she said. "For a few more hours let the strength from God Our Parent pass through You on the Cross to me. I know how close You came to despair but You hung on then and for the sake of the world I must hang on now. Give me strength. Believe me, Jesus, it is not the pain that frightens me, it is the cruelty, it is the feeling that everything I have said and done has changed nothing, has come to nothing. So far I have kept faith with You and God Our Parent with the support of Our Sister the Spirit but it is so hard to say what I say, day after day, and to see the world going on being cruel and selfish; or, even worse, indifferent. With all the media people have today they have never been in a better position to know about God's love but as I walked through the city today, so many people looked bewildered when they saw Your cross; they did not know what it was for."

She danced in front of the altar, her face drawn but lively, as if she could hear a tune in her head. Then she and the cross she embraced were bathed in red light so bright that Jim had to look past it to see its reflection on the high altar behind her; and then, as it faded, the lights came on as power was restored.

Jim heard the ring tone for a text message on her phone. Perpetua looked at it, kissed the cross, turned out the lights and left.

28.

"This is Bad Morning on Good Friday with Owen Grumpy and me, Janet Burns, where the main story is that teenage violence continues. No Minister was available to discuss the on-going crisis but we have with us a community leader from one of the worst affected areas. What is the solution?" "Well, we have to adopt a holistic approach with all the different agencies working together." "But isn't that a bit theoretical?" "Well, yes, but you have to have the vision." "But what about the approach at the grass roots?" "We need good role models." "Such as who? The footballer Sol Brookham?" "He's a decent bloke but he only plays football." "The industrialist Lord Blue?" "Look at his severance package." "Tony Blair?" "Out of touch with real people." "Jim Bruiser?" "Just negative rap." "Melanie?" "Vacuous." "Perpetua?" "Too idealistic?" "Jesus?" "Dead."

There was a substantial but dispersed reception committee for Perpetua as she came into Grunge Park: the police monitored her arrival and made some final checks before evacuating their under-cover investigators; a senior SAD Duty Officer performed a similar routine, pulling people out; Roy and his people provided an invisible guard of honour; Poppy gave a signal and the CEC television crew took a number of long distance shots before zooming in on the meeting between Perpetua, Heather and Jo. As they made their exit Perpetua put a hand on their heads and appeared to bless them. The Duty Officer for ROD signed off all remaining procedures and the police sealed the cordon. Roy's gang emerged from the shadows, the RIFs started to shout and the cameras focused on the waste ground that was to become the stage; everything was ready for the evening's entertainment.

"Who are you," said Rory, "to go around slagging off the church which my dad and Olly's uncle have spent so much time helping to preserve?" "I have not attacked the church as such; it tries hard; but it is failing, particularly in areas like this. People where you come from have enough financial and intellectual resources to work things out; your problem is that you are cold and heartless; but people round here are being failed by the church..." Oliver hit her in the face. "So you're admitting that little slum rats like you can't behave properly. And you come over all pious. Heaven knows what you have got up to as well as drug dealing. We know you've denied it by saying you've never had anything to do with drugs but some of your own people say otherwise. It doesn't really matter. What does matter is that you go round making people feel small by telling them off, telling them what to do." "Strange," said Perpetua, "because that is one of the very few things I do not do; but it is one of the things which conventional churches find it very hard to resist." "There you go again, slagging off churches." "Trying to have a rational argument is fruitless. Denial is fruitless. I commend all of you and myself to God Our Parent. I came to absorb the wickedness of the world; now, in my weakness, I wonder whether there is enough of me to absorb it. It would be foolishness to deny fear; that is what you smell; that is what arouses you. I am so sorry that it has come to this, for you, so sorry for you..."

"Anyway," Rory said, "we were going to give you a mega drugs cocktail but we thought you would enjoy something different to start with."

She would not cry, she would hardly speak but she said, just loud enough for them to hear: "The worst of it is, you do not know what you want; you are so lost. I sometimes wonder whether some of those God has created are beyond the reach of God. I should not think that; but now, I know I will see the worst of humanity. Sometimes people think the worst is in places of despair where driven people, turning into cannibals, eat their own children to survive; but such wickedness and obsession, such power and anger among those who are prosperous, is so difficult to take. Father, I have tried, let me know Your way."

Oliver pulled her down from behind and, as they formed a circle, he claimed the right to be the first to "Show her what enjoyment was all about." She, knowing what was about to happen said: "Father, how has this happened, that the act of love, praised in so many words of love, should be so corrupted into power and hate? I believe that love is making space and so I know that rape is invading space, using power to force and violate space. And I thought I was in some ways a Sacred Vessel for the sins of humanity but I am going to be a real, physical vessel, polluted by the seed of hate; forgive them; sustain me."

As Oliver pulled off her jeans she said: "Mothers, how did you come to rear such sons?" Then he raped her, clinically, joylessly, as an expression of power; not of love frustrated but of hate frustrated. Then each one of them, Rory and the rest, followed, to the accompaniment of a tuneless, obscene chant.

When they had finished Roy took a syringe and was about to inject her when Oliver said: "Make sure it's not pure joy in that needle, she needs a bit of contamination." Roy said nothing, he just looked hard, signalled for them to hold her down and injected her brutally, just above the bikini line.

She lay, deathly still, as the celebration turned sour. They were trapped in their failure to create anything (which is, perhaps, the essence of evil) and could only stand about, waiting for their own fixes to take hold. They knew they were doomed; this is why they were here in the first place; but all the spark had gone out. They were indifferent, even disgusted, by Perpetua, as she lay there. They veered off into the gloom but Roy and his followers steered them back into focus. He knew that the lull was temporary, that things would soon pick up.

Heather and Jo, who had hidden out of sight, left as soon as they saw what was happening. They had thought that there might be some threatening behaviour, some drug taking, but they had not been prepared for the rape. They had not thought it through. They had not thought. A temporary bout of jealousy and a sentimentalised view of their past had driven them away from Perpetua. Now she was about to be raped. For them this was not a moral issue, the subject of debate, it was the ever present threat of violation under which they had lived from childhood. Heather had been raped by her dealer 'boyfriend', Jo had been raped by her drunken father. Both of them knew that what had happened to them, and what was happening to Perpetua as they ran away, was the perversion of all their dreams, all the songs, all the books, all the pictures; all the smiles and the long, lingering looks into the distance. It had come to this. They had betrayed a woman. They had betrayed a woman who had tried to protect them.

They went to a top floor flat to which Heather had a key. They were partly stoned but they drank by turns from a bottle of vodka. They started in denial, in sorrow, but they steadily turned to pain and blame, to accusation, to violent regret. Somehow they started to fight (Heather's mobile "record" function was accidentally switched on). They somehow got out onto the balcony and Heather flipped over (the railings were broken) and fell to her death (the inquest reached an open verdict). Jo texted Dexter then followed her (her verdict was suicide).

Dexter sent a text to Trina and reached the police cordon in minutes. The police knew who he was but still went through the routine. Under repeated questioning, he (stupidly) denied his own identity and said he did not know Perpetua; but as this was all rather pointless, and as the police still classified him as a Grunge Park gang leader, he was allowed through.

He got to the edge of the waste ground. He was sure that She saw him; and part of that sureness was because She knew he was pretending not to know Her. He could not return Her look, half love, half pleading for help. He was broken and he did not know if he would ever be mended; but a tiny part of him knew the paradox that She, whom he had denied, would find the means to mend him. He had to get out.

Trina left Miles sleeping and went towards the Hollow. She evaded the police cordon and soon found the bodies, turned off Heather's phone recorder, checked the history and began sending frantic messages as she went towards the waste ground. She was blocked by Roy. He was holding a gun. Still, she argued with him until he came deliberately forward and put the gun in her mouth. Slowly she stepped back half a pace, turned, and walked, deliberately, slowly, away, until she felt safe to run. After a while she stopped and sent text messages to everybody she could think of but it was as if the whole official world had gone dead. Weeping desperately, she flung herself at Miles and said: "I've let Her down. She is being killed." Miles did his best to calm her down.

He did not argue. He did not tell her that she was being stupid, that she was over-reacting. He took everything she said calmly and seriously. He (sensibly) suggested that they should contact Father Bill as he was one of the few people who really knew the area. They found him and told him what they knew. Trina wanted to go with him back to The Hollow but both Miles and Father Bill insisted that that would just be punishing herself. Miles took her home and Bill set off.

As Roy had predicted, when the drugs and alcohol violently kicked in, the group coalesced into collective madness. They stamped on her, threw up over her, pissed on her, burned her arms with cigarettes, pushed broken glass into her face. They tossed a coin for her *god4u* top. "Somebody has to pay for all the evil in the world," said Oliver, "and the world has chosen you." "I know," said Perpetua faintly, "I always knew. From the moment God opened my eyes I knew that I would have to suffer like Jesus My Brother." They had momentarily stopped shouting and stamping. Rory felt ill, Roy was feeling slightly edgy. Oliver was getting bored. Somehow the evening had gone wrong. She lay there, the broken toy of deeply unhappy children.

Roy's text messager chimed. He stepped away from the cameras. "Yes" he texted back to Father Bill. This was the perfect solution. He told them it was time to go. "I love you," said Perpetua as they turned their backs. "I love the world in spite of everything; it is God's world and I love it; and I love you."

29.

Max Silver was born in the East End of poor, hard working immigrants from Eastern Europe. Determination and good luck had combined to make him one of the world's most prominent bankers. Then one day when he was just about to get into his chauffeur-driven Rolls Royce to seal the world's biggest bank takeover deal, he received a text message: "Bank deal ok; u out." Almost simultaneously the chauffeur received a message and promptly drove off, leaving Max frozen to the spot. He later learned that in a deal that sailed very close to the wind his bank had been re-registered under Pitcairn law; he had no rights, no severance package; nothing. Naturally, he had lived on his prospects rather than his means and although many friends were sympathetic he found that a lot of previous hospitality went only a little way now. The cause of his misfortunes did not matter; he was tainted. His wife left him during a draconian bout of domestic down-sizing for a rising banker. By the time he had sorted everything out he had a small flat on the cusp of Excelsior Gardens and Grunge Park and enough money for a year. Then the vodka kicked in. As time went by his lucid moments were fewer but when he was lucid his brain worked in the way it had at the bank, with absolute precision. (the SAD de-briefing record shows that he recovered and became a *god4u* back room organiser). As he came across the sodden waste ground his major preoccupation was to shut up his unwelcome companion. Ever since he had heard that he was a failed banker Brod Croker had stuck to him because he thought that one day Max would get lucky. Brod had been mercilessly beaten by his drunken father until his mother ran away from him; then Brod ran away from her.

"Shut up, Brod," said Max, quietly, "I'm concentrating on what's going on over there." "Just some nasty business that's got nastier. Look, she's stoned; or dead." He poked her and tried to turn her over. "She's got nothing, damn it!" "Poor girl," said Max. "She doesn't deserve it the way we do. I know her; she tried to put me on my feet. Marta.

"All I could do was feel sorry for myself. I wish even we could help a bit. It's only when you see somebody like this that you realise that being too rich and being too poor cuts you off from the rest."

He could not help thinking of being very rich and being very poor; when you were one, only television told you about the other. He remembered the bank's annual charity dinner with the Chairman's wife preening herself as a parade of well dressed and pliant supplicants and their organisations were paraded and honoured; but there was nothing to spoil the general atmosphere of decorousness and self-congratulation. And when you were poor you looked at them as if they were on another planet. But Marta.

"Damn it!" "Brod, please." "You hardly know how you will be rewarded for what you have said," Perpetua whispered. "God Our Parent has seen your love." Then she said: "I am thirsty." Max, feeling ashamed, handed her his can of lager. She took a sip and dropped it, splashing Brod who cursed. "Thank you for trying," she said. "You do not know but this is the best thing you have ever done." Her voice almost faded away so that Max had to go closer. "You have spent too much time trying to forget," she said, "but now do some remembering. Remember tonight. Remember Jesus My Brother. Remember me. Remember Marta. Remember."

He could see that she was in great pain. Whatever she had been given was wearing off. It was a helpless gesture but he kissed a cigarette wound on her cheek. "Jesus, look down on Your Sister and forgive the world. I know You have forgiven this poor man. Forgive those children; forgive." "Even us?" "Yes you; but also the other," (Brod growled) "and the poor and weak; those who do not know what they are doing". "I knew," said Max. "Not really. I recognise your face; on the television as you mingled with the rich and powerful you glowed with not knowing. I remember Marta."

She lost consciousness. Brod went away; Max stayed. He fought to stay lucid. He threw away half a bottle of vodka so that it smashed on a block of concrete. He knew that he had to stay there and concentrate so that he could tell the story.

Poppy Smoother stopped filming. She had been totally focused on the filming but now she was in a panic; she needed to get out before the police got in. The lightweight kit was packed away and she barely looked at Perpetua as the team headed off. Somebody had told the police; they were getting ready to move in. She told them vaguely that something had gone wrong. When they reached the OB van she cued the material; the camera memory was empty. She phoned the producer, trying to stay calm. It took him a while to answer. None of her feed was in the studio memory; and the output recorder was also blank. She had to tell him that she had no trace. Her dreams of a career were in ruins. The live coverage would not be enough. (In spite of appeals, nobody could produce a recording of the broadcast; and no item ever came onto *eLot*.)

When Max saw Father Bill and Jim walking towards the girl a natural reticence, reinforced by recent shame, caused him to withdraw a little way. He saw the priest exchange a few words with Roy whose people then all left. There were other figures hovering in the background. Bill knelt down. "I have come to help." "Just being here helps. I will never move from here alive; it is almost over. I do not want to die in a church or a hospital. Just here. There are so many people who die here. Their bodies live but they die so young. They die years before the knives and the guns and the drugs and the lashing out trying to find something. I should die here.

"Bill, I am sorry if I have been harsh to you, seeming to take what you love." "It's all right, I came to know what you were doing; it wasn't easy at first but I know now." "I know you are a good man. Love Jim for me; and Jim, Father Bill will need all the love you can give him."

Bill leaned over to hear her and Max, out of his eye-line, crept closer. Jim looked at him but, to Max's surprise, did not flinch or look away; he just looked straight at him. "I am going to God Our Parent to be re-united with Jesus My Brother." Bill began to shake. "Do not cry. I am going home but you will never be alone". She raised her head. "I believe in the God of love." She sank back so that her head was supported on Bill's knee: "I am full. There is no more to carry. Thank You for my mission, for my strength. For me it is over; for the world it is beginning again." She smiled; and died.

Max offered to help but Bill said gently: "Remember what has happened. Do you have a home?" "Yes." "Go there and sit quietly. I need to do some work; you need to absorb what you have seen and heard. Come and see me on Monday."

Jim and Bill gently picked her up and just before they disappeared from view Max saw Bill talking to Roy. Then they disappeared. Roy watched the body disappear. It had not meant to end like this. In spite of the usual arrangements he felt in danger.

Bill had said to Roy: "It's best for all concerned if we move the body. You can let the police back in a few minutes," but they were already moving in. He was finished. A police car came round the corner; he disappeared into the gloom.

Bill, Jim and the others hurried down a passage between two tower blocks and put Perpetua into the back of Bill's car. Bill texted Trina.

When they arrived at St. Simple's they took Perpetua into the vestry. They cleaned her up as best they could and wrapped her in some old red choir robes. Trina arrived in tears with Miles protectively in the background. She wanted to see the body but Bill refused. "The reality is bad enough without the detail," he said. "What we need to do now is to pray." The four knelt round the body and prayed in silence. Then Bill looked at Miles who gently but purposefully steered Trina away. Outside she said: "I was a coward, I abandoned her." "You could not have known; and, if you had known, you could not have done anything," Bill said. "Remember Jesus. She, like Him, knew it was inevitable."

Bill locked the door.

Next morning Bill went to the church early to say some prayers in peace before the invasion of the bickering flower ladies. The 'old guard' were determined to use the Easter morning service to reverse the house group tide rather than seeing it as the kind of celebration which would give strength to all the new house groups. Great festivals brought their stresses.

Perpetua's body was not there.

Jim appeared. "I suppose somebody could have stolen it, though it would have been difficult to get in." "Nobody came," said Jim, "I slipped back in before you closed the door." "What happened, then?" "There was a light like the one I saw on Thursday but then it was red and this time it was white and when it faded she was not there."

Bill reported Perpetua to the police as missing. (She was an adult who had spent the last few months travelling. The paperwork was simple enough to complete. People went missing all the time.) Bill, thinking about Jesus, had a strange feeling. Could lightning strike twice? So many things about Perpetua echoed Jesus; that is what had convinced him.

During the day the bedraggled *god4u* followers, except for Jim who did not want to leave St. Simple's, gradually assembled at Bleak Villas. They were ashamed and bewildered. Dexter was broken, Trina was remorseful, the rest could not look each other in the eye; but Bill never gave up trying to bring hope.

30.

On Sunday morning after a restless night when praying had been difficult, the remainder of the *god4u* core group sat together listlessly, not knowing what to do. Dexter was still wrestling with himself, wondering how he could have been so unfaithful. Trina could not forgive herself and, what was worse, she could not get Miles out of her head when she was supposed to be concentrating on her guilt. They were temporarily lifted when Jim arrived, followed by Father Bill, but the atmosphere was still sour. They were on the verge of recrimination and only Bill's persistent gentleness kept them from a dangerous outburst.

Then Jim said: "Perpetua is alive again; it says so in the TT; but I know anyway." They were incredulous. "There's something in what Jim has told you," said Bill. "I don't place much faith in the TT but the situation is very strange and so similar to what happened to Jesus."

Brian was fiddling with the computer. "Stop it," said Bob. "It's so irritating." "I just want to look at our own channel," said Brian who clicked on the g4u-TV webcast and saw the logo and a picture of Perpetua.

He thought he saw her eyes move.

The usually rather serious face smiled.

Perpetua said:

"I promised that I would never leave you. God Our Parent and Jesus My Brother want you to know that everything they have done has been re-confirmed in me as their Vessel.

"You do not need to do anything drastic. Remember what we learned together. You must now go out and practice what you have learned. It says in the Gospel that there were fifty days between the Resurrection of Jesus My Brother, His return to God Our Parent and the sending of My Sister the Spirit; but the world does not work like that any more. Be ready at noon today to receive further help for what you have to do."

Dexter said: "Where are you? It looks like the top of some tall building."

"I am alive but not in the way I was when we were together. I am taking this earthly shape so that we can talk. If you think back to all the things that I told you, it will become clear."

Perpetua reminded them what she had said about her death and return to life; and their mission. They could not understand. When Perpetua had gone they realised that She had been able to hear Dexter even though there was no feedback facility. Brian went on fiddling but he was back with the logo and the picture.

"I told you," Jim said but they were still arguing when the screen came to life (DIM was later forced to report that all broadcasting media under its remit had lost control of their output and had simultaneously carried Perpetua broadcasts.)

Perpetua said: "I have taken the highly unusual step of speaking to you all on every media channel on planet earth in your own language because I want you to know that God Our Parent loves all of you. That love was shown when Jesus My Brother was sent to demonstrate God's love on earth; and it was shown again when I was sent as a witness, as the Sacred Vessel of God's fullness. I was killed but I have returned to proclaim God's love afresh to all the world...."

Miles burst into the room brandishing his media communicator: "Perpetua has risen!" He shouted. "Why are you looking so serious. Alleluia! Rejoice! Perpetua has risen!"

Trina jumped to her feet and threw her arms around him: "Why have we been so stupid? How wonderful that you saw it first, Miles. Jim told us but you put it into simple words!"

"...In matters concerning God, forget complexity, hierarchy, tidiness, cleverness and calculation; these are simply human attributes for human situations.

"When you think of the divine love of God for everyone, think only of returning God's faith in you, expressed in creation, with faith in God; God's hope in you, expressed in the Resurrection, with your hope in God; and return God's love for you, expressed in my space, through your love of God; and in all three, recognise the constancy of My Sister The Spirit."

The screen went back to the G4U-TV logo. For a few moments there was complete silence. Then Bill said: "Let us pray. God Our Parent, Jesus Our Brother, Our Sister the Spirit and Our Beloved Sister Perpetua, God's Sacred Vessel, we thank You for giving us Perpetua as our own special incarnation of the Godhead for the Third Millennium. We thank You for Her suffering and Her Death, for obeying Your collective will in making Her the Sacred Vessel to contain our sins. We thank you that Perpetua has risen to be with us and has now returned to be enfolded into the Godhead. May we be inspired by Her life to follow You anew and to ensure that we do not fall away as the followers of Jesus fell away in the First and Second Millennia. We make this prayer to the Four In One, Parent, Brother and Sisters. Amen. Alleluia! Perpetua has risen!"

"Alleluia!" they shouted and, as if moved by an invisible force, they rushed out into the street and down towards the Easter Market.

"Perpetua has risen!" they shouted to bewildered shoppers and stall holders. They marched around like a small knot of football supporters but then Brian and Kylie, whose absence they had not noticed, appeared with the portable sound gear. They found a clear space at the edge of the market and Bill and

Trina pushed Dexter forward.

"You will remember," said Dexter, "how Perpetua Our Sister was condemned last week as a drug dealer; and some of you will have seen the disgraceful way in which she was humiliated and murdered, callously broadcast on television, with the connivance of all the public authorities" (a brave and fully justified statement). "I am here to tell you that She has risen from the dead, spoken to us and the world, and has now ascended to the Godhead." "You must be mad," said a listener. "That kind of thing was a superstition of simple fishermen." "No, brother, I am not mad. Just as Jesus Our Brother rose from the dead as an act of the Godhead, so Perpetua was given to us as a third chance for the Third Millennium: we got it wrong when we were first thinking beings; we got it wrong in the two thousand years after the witness of Jesus; but now we have a chance to do better in the Third Millennium. We are here to preach the Word of Perpetua, to encourage you all to turn back to God."

"We need to continue what Perpetua began. To reform the argumentative and self-serving Christian Churches, to fling open the doors of established religion so that the poor and the weak, the destitute and the desperate, can be brought in; not just allowed to come in, not just encouraged to come in, but carried in shoulder high in celebration as the specially favoured of God. We must never betray Perpetua the way we have betrayed Jesus."

Poppy Smoother, strangely moved by the idea of Resurrection, smiled as she stood at the back of the crowd. Oliver O'Helly and Rory Varnish, still looking the worse for wear, felt new life. Their respective uncle and father, taking the air after an unusually emotional Easter, felt new hope. Max Silver, looking almost healthy in cheap new clothes, walked with Marta, carrying her baby. He tapped Andy on the shoulder and offered help. Baby Perpetua and her mother were intensely involved in each other.

Bill, feeling strong and sure, noticed that all kinds of people, even Japanese tourists, were listening intently. He thought of Pentecost and smiled.

"There is no such thing as cost free faithfulness. We have to put an end to comfortable Christianity. A little generosity, giving what we can spare, is not enough. There is so much suffering and instead of acting, we watch it; we watch it on television. Worse, instead of acting, we turn away; not just from the television but from people who are so close to us geographically but so far apart in every other way. Perpetua, like Jesus, came to save the poor. How long do we need to be told what we must do before we act? Perpetua has risen from the Dead, praise to God, the Four In One, Alleluia!"

Scores of people came up to the group when Dexter had finished. Wayne handed out stickers and the few leaflets he had left.

They agreed to meet during the evening when Dexter would preside at a thanksgiving.

Miles and Trina slipped away together to buy a few essentials. The first thing they wanted was a teapot. They asked a stall holder whether they could see a smaller pot than those on display. She went behind a screen; and Perpetua returned with the pot in her hand. "I promised not to leave you," she said. "Rejoice! alleluia!"

This account of Perpetua is taken from SAD files and associated sources. It is submitted as a confidential, personal report with one recommendation: that the followers of Perpetua be encouraged and not hampered by official action. Comments in brackets are personal—Claire.

BETH

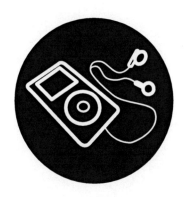

Grunge Park Community College
Department of Diversity Studies

Creative Writing Course: Coursework Summary Form

Student's Name:

Beth "Laser" Lesar

Submission Date:

July 2007

Creative Writing Module:

Chapters 1-3 5-7 9-11 part of 13 14-15

Creative integration of Resources:

Chapters 4 8 Carols in 9 12 part of 13

Plagiarism Decleration:

Own work except attributed articles Carols in 9
and It's The Sign That Counts in 13

Notes:

Will set lyrics in module on multi ethnic composition.

Supervisor's Comments:

It is difficult to know what is real and imagi-
nary in this script. You will need to keep a
tighter control of your sense of reality. The
use of lyrics, at first creative, became hack-
neyed. Grammar and spelling much improved but
you must learn the use of the comma and dashes
to free you from the inappropriate use of the
semicolon.

One

She was God's own Daughter and we killed Her
we ran when they captured Her and killed Her
She had been so kind
She had won our hearts and minds
but we left that all behind when we killed Her.
But She came in a blaze of glory
yes, She came in a blaze of glory
the sacred babe in Her own love story
in a blaze of glory She came.
Such an end, such an end
when we said She was a friend
such a deep betrayal of a sacred heart
such a waste of space, we were soldiers in disgrace
when we promised Her that we would never part.
But She came in a blaze of glory
yes, She came in a blaze of glory
the sacred babe in Her own love story
in a blaze of glory She came.

We lived in the blackness of the night
with its hard and heavy beat
in the harsh, barbaric light of anticipated pain
with the sound of running feet and the smell of danger in the
    street
and yet when She promised to save us, we blew it.
But She came in a blaze of glory
yes, She came in a blaze of glory
the sacred babe in Her own love story
in a blaze of glory She came.
She was God's own Daughter and we killed Her
we ran when they captured Her and killed Her.
We left it all behind when we lost our hearts and minds
we left it all behind when we killed Her.

The only stars we saw were sparks from riots in the street
or the cocaine burst behind our eyes
but Her eyes were like candles
so much nearer than stars
so much warmer than stars
and Her voice sang just enough off the beat
and She knelt in the broken glass and prayed
and collected what everybody said
and would not believe the cries of victimhood
and would not believe that we could do no good
and She knelt in the broken glass.

We did this in media studies. So I can analyse the pictures in the albums. The faces and bones make up the same superficial patterns of features; but everything else is different. Then there were just straight-backed figures in pictures that could almost have been taken at any time in a hundred years; the background was plain so you couldn't tell whether the pictures were before or after the boat. Now there is a litter of props. Then they dressed what they called 'smart' in clothes that were only for Church, not the smart that people wear for parties. Being analogue pictures, they had to reserve them for big occasions, so there is evidence of the Christening robe passed down from one generation to another; and they carried hymn books they didn't need to use. And you know they have just come in and are going through this important ritual of self consciously historicising their lives before the rice and peas. A strange tribute they make to Western clothes and the Western church which captured them and took them into slavery; a tribute at that moment in time, for a very brief moment in time, more formal from them than it was from almost all of their white neighbours; the whites had given up ties for church and the passed-on Christening robe, if not Church altogether.

Yes, the bones and the skin are the same but everything else is different. The stiff backs and straight faces have gone; the pride has gone from the old and respect has gone from the young; the old slightly stoop and don't look straight at the camera and the young slouch and try not to be a part of the picture. You suspect that if it's a First Communion picture the kids are more bothered about what's in the envelopes than what was in the silver chalice. Looking at pictures from the mid 1980's you can see the children less framed and formal, pulling away from the focus of the picture, pulling away from the family cohesion, pulling faces that ruin the gravity of the picture without the charm of candour; this is the self destructive, self referential sneer. And the ties are loose and the skirts are tight; and the pants get baggy and the tops get skimpy. The pride goes, to be replaced by props; but that pride was inside;

and the props are outside; and you can see that the props are a bit cheap and tacky and we have less of them than other people; so there's no real pride in the props; they tell of how poor we are and not how rich.

> The 'Iron Lady' was told
> She was told in Toxteth and Brixton.
> She was told that she was asking too high a price
> for the kind of self reliance she believed in
> in an abstract sort of way.
> She was told the price was too high
> as we stupidly burned our own property
> instead of going somewhere to pick on the rich
> as if we were so ashamed of ourselves
> we reacted violently to ourselves.
> What poor, sad, stupid people.
> Broken people.

But when she was told, she persisted with a theory that ignored people; she was in favour of self sufficiency not welfare; the kind of self sufficiency possessed by men who ran the slave trade and the cane fields. The self sufficiency that needs slaves. Then it was slaves in the ships to provide profit on the Westerly run, slaves in the cane fields to make sugar viable, slaves in the go-downs, slaves in the kitchens, slaves under the stairs, slaves under the Master. Now it is slaves in the factories, slaves in the warehouses, slaves in the canteens, slaves in the brothels; and a nice big pool of unemployed slaves to keep down the price of labour for the rest of the slaves; and for those who are in that pool and can't or won't be slaves, there is the slavery of the narcotic and the knife. And she called that self sufficiency?

> She was told.
> Now everybody is angry with us because we are out of control
> we have lost our cohesion
> we have lost our self respect
> we have lost what we ever had of being families
> we have lost our soul.

Perhaps we needed the photographs to glue us together. Of course there are things we should have done; and things we should do; but I wonder as she fades away towards death whether she still thinks of the price. After all, she might think it was a price worth paying but she never paid it; like politicians who send soldiers (more and more black soldiers) to war, she didn't have to pay the price; we pay it; and our victims pay it; and our neighbours pay it; and honest taxpayers pay it.

She called it progress; And the kids saw through it; and saw through those they were supposed to respect. And church and the 'Three W's' went into the shade and there was Marley and ganja.

But She came in a blaze of glory.

Of course She was Christened in the usual way because Her mother was almost the last of her kind around. It didn't matter that the father had gone away, everything was going to be formal. Strangely, too, nobody seemed to blame the mother for getting involved in a relationship which was bound to be risky; it was so short lived that nobody saw him come; and nobody saw him go; and she never talked about him. She got some kind of public attention over an inner city media gimmick just after Thatcher won her third election but all that was left were pictures of the baby in Her Christening robe with Her mother in silly Western formal clothes that didn't go with her ample figure; and a hat that looked forty years out of date; and a Vicar who looked as if he wished he was somewhere else, only just not looking at his big watch. And you can tell that taking pictures was lazier than it had been; the composition is not so formal and the people are not so cleanly and symmetrically framed.

Of course She was Christened, but that can't account for what She did. The first time anybody noticed anything was in the early '90s when there was a bit of a riot in Grunge Park. Parents took their children off the streets and left the gangs to it. Mothers worried about their teenage boys but knew there was nothing they could do. Girl friends had long since given up protesting in case they were ill treated or dropped. Horrified, Ruby saw Perpetua walking real calm towards The Hollow which was the hottest spot in the fighting which careered around within a few blocks. Nobody knew where Her mother was. She walked towards the cursing and violence holding a bunch of flowers. Everybody else stopped as if they had seen a ghost but She went on walking and as the noise died down people could hear Her singing a song:

"It's the sign that counts".

She went right to where the boys were still looking at each other and She took a flower from Her bunch and gave it to the leader of the biggest, best established gang; and then She gave another of her flowers to the estate's big pretender who had been de-stabilising the area.

Then She divided the rest of Her flowers into four tiny clumps and dropped them on the ground in two spaced pairs and said "Play football". They began to laugh in a forced and harsh way; as if they were laughing at Her. Then they laughed at each other; then they laughed at themselves. "It's a cliche" one of them said "like what I read that they did in the First World War; but it made no difference."

"It's the sign that counts" She sang; and walked away.

Of course it didn't stop the violence but nobody forgot it; and nobody forgot the song. It became a kind of theme tune.

What people noticed about Her, other than Her extraordinary behaviour, was Her calm. She walked with loose but graceful movements; unhurried. Her gaze was calm when it wasn't engaged with people and things; but when it was, the animation seemed to quieten rather than quicken; it was like She wanted to slow everything down because it was all too fast. Some of the old men said that it was like the great fast bowlers who never seemed to be pounding and jerking but just ran in real smooth and let the ball go; you never noticed the speed; only the batters did. And in Her case you never noticed Her coming; She was just there; and then everything slowed down, the frame rate just slowed without the picture going jumpy.

As She grew up, She was marked out by teachers as a strange girl who was either docile or a trouble maker; they could never make it out. She went through most of Her lessons real quiet, without too much trouble but without any signs of real cleverness; but when She thought that there was injustice She became stubborn without ever losing her calm. They would have preferred Her to be naughty but She never was. She was calm; ultra polite without being sarcastic. They found it hard to pin anything on Her but She was such a challenge to authority.

It was a small thing but typical. One day just before She left primary school, somebody stole some money from a coat pocket and the whole class was told it would have to stay in on a beautiful Summer day until somebody owned up. Perpetua said it was unreasonable for 26 children to be punished for the supposed offence of one person; and, in any case, how did they know it was one of the 26 children? Was it true that adults had never been known to steal anything? Was it only children that stole? Why were there so many adults in prison? She had not taken the money but if people wanted to think She had, She could live with that; then everybody else could go home. They objected that there was no point detaining Her when She maintained She had not taken the money; so She said that was 26 times more sensible than detaining 26 people who hadn't done it. In any case, the person who had done it was punished by knowing he or she had done it; the essence of punishment was what happened inside you, not what other people did to you. If that was not so, if you did not feel the pain of what you had done, you were in desperate need of help. People who knew their wrong hurt themselves; people who did not know their wrong needed help. There was nothing more to say. Worn down, the teachers agreed to let everybody out; but She planted Herself in a corner and would not be moved until the appointed detention time had run out. When She was asked why She was so stubborn She said it wasn't stubborn, She was simply letting them feel a little what they had imposed on others.

At secondary school the same pattern of moderate achievement and religious controversy continued. For some reason She got hung up on what Miss Dawkins called "The Blessed Trinity" which Perpetua said was a provisional, makeshift sort of thing that needed improving. We couldn't follow all this but the local Vicar, old "Liquorice" Comfort, was sent in to investigate. She gave as good as She got. It was something about human beings trying to tell God that there could only be three bits, what Comfort called "Persons" but She called "Manifestations". She said the number could be any number and that Comfort didn't know whether there had been "Manifestations" on other planets. We couldn't see the point of the dispute but it got Dawkins very annoyed.

The other thing that got Dawkins annoyed, without the same support from old Liquorice, was when She kept on saying people were naturally good and knew what God wanted. Dawkins said it was well known that the main purpose of religion was to provide people with a system of punishment and reward, with a proper sense of fear of doing wrong; without hell, Dawkins said, everybody would go mad and the whole planet would disintegrate into chaos. Perpetua said that fear destroyed people; like it was destroying people on housing estates; guilt cut people up and made them feel responsible for things they hadn't done. Love was the only thing. And every time She used the word "Love" you could see Dawkins wince and say that you had to put Jesus and His message of love into a proper context, starting with the Garden of Eden, and ending with the structures of Christianity which were essential for social regulation, not to mention The Last Judgment; sheep and goats.

She left school and nobody knew where She had gone but some people said She had gone to Jerusalem; others said it was Rwanda. As She became more famous the stories of where She had been became more outrageous; and ever more people claimed She had been with them. If you believed it all She must have had loads of money and been round the world. It was like this thing the English have about the bed of Queen Elizabeth I but a jet set thing. She told me one day that there were stories that the followers of Jesus had ended up in all kinds of places like India. Well it wasn't left to Her followers; Her picture spread all over the world from satellite television and the web and there were little shrines with Her picture all over the place. And somebody told me She had become the Patron Saint of sex workers in Sao Paulo.

When She came back She never said where She had been. After a while people forgot about Her altogether. She was just one more girl who had left school too early to get a proper education; but She didn't seem the sort who would have a fling with a man and get pregnant. She didn't seem to be a fling kind of person at all. She did bits of voluntary work and walked quietly through the streets listening to anyone who wanted to talk. For somebody in social work she was really strange because She never told people what to do; She never even gave any advice. She said if people thought about it enough; if they could stay quiet for long enough to 'hear'; then they would know what the right decision was even if they felt too weak to take it. To know what was right was a good start. Even if you went wrong you would know you had made a mistake and feel some remorse; and that was the beginning of wanting to do right and not wrong; to follow what you knew.

> *But She came in a blaze of glory:*
> *No snow.*
> *No snow.*
> *Not a star but a dull fire glow.*

There was a major fight between gangs; but it was more than that. Gangs are what happen when people are oppressed and frustrated. Sometimes politicians say "Don't throw money at it" but throwing money at it often cools people down; rich people don't go round fighting and burning each other's houses. So it looks like a gang thing but it might be an oppression thing; a survival thing; a fight for the scraps of social recognition that are left thing.

> *No snow.*

But it was like in the time of Jesus who was born among the soldiers of an occupied land. There were gangs called Zealots, or freedom fighters; who all seemed to be led by people called Judas. Well, it was a bit like that when the police came in. It would be stupid to ask them to show understanding or start a peace seminar or something; but they didn't come slowly and watch and wait; they weren't tactical or practical; they just came straight in; and as they pitched in, the core of fighting and fire exploded into pieces that flew all over the place so there were new fights and new fires.

> *No snow.*
> *But She came in a blaze of glory:*
> *No shepherds, no kings*

Just police and firemen too frightened to put out fires.
It was like when She was a little girl with the flowers but even more delib-

erate; more calm; no naive, childish gentleness now but adult, mature gentleness; like She had been formed naturally to do what was right; as if it wasn't a struggle. Still, like something from Her past, as She came She was singing It's The Sign That Counts. There was a cordon of police and She walked through it as if it wasn't there for Her and as if She was invisible to them. She walked towards a group of kids setting fire to a shed and silently shepherded them towards the middle of the chaos; and She went round the edges of the conflict like some kind of shepherd or sheep dog; I'm not sure about this farming stuff; and moved the people into the place where the fighting and fire had been most intense. She sang Her song now and again but said nothing. She didn't shout; or tell people what to do; or make angry faces; or even wave Her hands about. She just walked from place to place gathering the people together. Then She waved the firemen in and the police away as all these bewildered people stood there; silent. The firemen went the same way as Perpetua; they started at the outside and when that was sorted they moved steadily towards the middle; towards the people they were once frightened of.

At the centre She turned round slow like a dancer; like a dancer in slow motion—that slow motion thing again—and then She led a silent procession to The Hollow. And then:

She knelt in the broken glass.

She raised Her joined, pointed hands to the sky and there was a burst of light like a full moon but yellow; like a full, big, yellow moon; like that comet that was in the South all of one Summer, glowing yellow; but this was much more intense and overhead; making shadows; making patterns in the broken glass. "God Our Parent," She said, which sounded strange "I thank you for this blaze of glory which you have shown to Your children. Help Your children to remember that they are Your children. Help them to be free inside, to choose where they can choose. To keep their self respect even where they cannot choose."

She got up and took two pieces of slightly charred wood and put them across each other at rightangles to make a cross; and with Her bare hands She began to pick up bits of broken glass to surround it. People started to pick up glass and other bits of stuff and make patterns around the cross.

"It's getting late," She said. "It's getting late in the night and late in our souls but it is never too late. Bring all your sorrow to the cross."

And the boys came forward, with a strange calm, and put their knives and broken bottles and half-made Molotov cocktails and bits of wood with nails in them; and put them at the bottom end of the Cross. There was one gun and the leader put it right at the top of the cross near where the head of Jesus would have been; near that plaque thing they wrote in different languages.

"If there is anybody here with nowhere to stay for the night; if their house is too damaged, stand together. Now you who have violated and ransacked your own people, take one of these people you have made sad and take them to your house. There is no need to be afraid. The violent and the victim must pray together. I know you do not know how to pray very well but ask that the love of God Our Parent which is showered on all is clearer to you, so that you can see it better, just as you can see this terrible mess you have made because God's glory has blazed above it."

"If there are any people left unprotected they must come to me but I do not think there should be. I do not expect that such harmony will last—it never does—but we cannot possibly survive unless there are some moments of light between all the time we spend staggering around in the dark.

> No angels in the sky
> Just bewildered people in small groups
> the violent and the victims walking together.

Just as the Blaze Of Glory had come suddenly, it went. And left her kneeling at the foot of this cross in the broken glass.

> No snow
> no shepherds
> no kings
> no angels.
> Different signs for a different day
> but, still, it's the sign that counts.
> But She came in a blaze of glory
> yes, She came in a blaze of glory
> the sacred babe in Her own love story
> in a blaze of glory She came.
> She was God's own daughter and we killed Her.

Two

The Kingdom is here
it's freedom not fear
The Kingdom is here
The Kingdom is here.
Get up and dance, there's no time to wait
The Lord is with us now
it's a big space, there isn't a gate
focus on what not how.
The Kingdom is here
it's freedom not fear
The Kingdom is here
The Kingdom is here.
Get up and sing your praises out
To fill you up inside
The time is now to wave and shout
There's nothing left to hide.
The Kingdom is here
it's freedom not fear
The Kingdom is here
The Kingdom is here.
Gone are the lonely places
the walled up spaces
the struggle to get in
gone is the disapproving
the fear of loving
the tyranny of sin.

The Kingdom is here
it's freedom not fear
The Kingdom is here
The Kingdom is here.

The bruiser kept looking at me. Not at the shopping bags that weighed me down. There was all this confusion because something had gone wrong with the tills. The check-out girls were confused. Mine let me through with my stuff even though the beans hadn't registered. It was happening to loads of other people. At first I thought it was because I was black; but soon I realised it was my top or, well, what was inside it. Instead of worrying about the confusion and the beans he was looking at my cleavage. He didn't even do it, like sly, he just looked. Instead of trying to make sense of what was going on he just followed me as I tried to walk away calm; without looking back; without seeming to hurry; it was hard work not hurrying.

"You thieving black bitch!" he shouted. "You good for nothing black bitch!" I thought he was going to hit me but I couldn't run. "Well, you are just about good enough for something," he said taking me by the shoulder so it hurt and turning me round. "Promise to give me a good time and I'll let you off." Then, for no reason I could see, he took his hand off and I put my head down and walked; but that made me hurry; so I raised it and saw a cop; that must have been what had stopped him. Then like some piece of dance with me in the middle, the cop came forward, the bruiser came from behind, and Perpetua came from the left. "This young woman has stolen goods from Hypo," said the bruiser, in a silly, formal voice, like a bad actor. "Yes, I gather there have been some unaccountable incidents," said the cop, placid. "In some ways the incidents have been unaccountable," said Perpetua "but I think if we all stay calm we will be able to reach an amicable agreement." "Amicable!" said the bruiser, slipping out of actor mode. "There's evidence." "Very likely," said the cop, hesitating, looking round; but when he saw a couple more cop cars arrive he decided to go ahead. He looked a bit embarrassed as he fiddled with a pair of handcuffs. "There is no need for those," said Perpetua; calm; firm; like you wouldn't argue. "The guard can sit in the front with you and I will sit in the back with this young lady."

When we got to the police station the cop took us into a room full of paper and dirty cups. "I do not think you will need to go through all this procedure," said Perpetua. "That is my decision, madam," said the cop; a bit offended. "Do you wish to press charges?" The bruiser nodded and pushed a button on his mobile. "It's dead. I only charged it this morning. It's dead." "O dear," said the cop, half sarcastic. "Well, let us have an informal chat, then. What's your name?" "Beth." "Beth what?" "We are being informal," said Perpetua. "Well, Beth, what's in your bags?" "Shopping." "Did you pay for it all?" I looked at

Perpetua. "Tell him," She said. "There is nothing to fear." "When the stuff was put through, the four cans of beans registered zero." "A likely story," said the bruiser. "On the contrary," said Perpetua "a highly unlikely story." I thought She had changed sides. "Unlike the malfunction of this man's mobile phone. Technology. Such things happen all the time; but not to tills." "We were told something like that when you called, weren't we?" "Yes. I was asked to go to check-out because there was a problem with the tills." "So you admit there was a problem which is, as you say, why you called us?" "Yes," grudgingly. "So if there was a problem why did you choose to follow Beth?" "Because she was stealing." "But you have just admitted she wasn't stealing; or, even if she was, it was no different from scores of other customers." "Well, yes." "So why did you follow her?" "I suppose it was my professional instinct." "Sexual instinct," said Perpetua. "Now, gentlemen, you would both have to admit that Beth is a very pretty young lady. Still, that is no reason to victimise her. If you want a date there are usual ways of going about it." "I see," said the cop; sounding and looking as if he didn't. "I suppose I need to give her an informal caution." "I do not think you do, but if it makes you feel better, officer. Beth, would you mind if this professional gentleman made himself feel more comfortable by giving you an informal caution. It would be an act of kindness. He has a difficult job, particularly when officials in charge of protecting members of the public try to take advantage of them." "OK." "Consider it done," said the cop. "Beth and I are meeting for a drink later this evening at the Down & Out, so if you want to pursue your amorous intentions, I suggest you meet us there." "I hate the pig!" "Nobody is perfect—well, there are a couple of very special exceptions—so give him a break. He has made a bit of a fool of himself but I dare say you have, too." "Pig!" "We cannot limit our company, particularly in taverns, to people we like." "I don't believe I'm hearing this. Anyway, I probably won't come."

When we went out the guard stayed behind with the cop. I didn't trust them; but what can you do? "You are not to worry," She said. "We will go for a drink later with some people; and if he wants to say anything to you he will have to start with a lot of company. If you want to be alone with him that will be your choice but you will not be forced." "Pig! I hate him. He wanted to rape me." "There are many men who rape but there are many more who wish they could; and many more still who say they wish they could. It would be unwise to under-estimate this terrible problem of the misuse of power by people over each other, by men over women; but the way to deal with it is to socialise with those we do not like, those we are frightened of, so that familiarity and mutual-ity begin to grow. No means no to people with whom we can have a dialogue. It does not mean no to those who are using power and refusing dialogue; but dialogue is a learned habit, part of the process of learning naturally to become good. Being good should not be a terrible struggle as the Torans says it is; it should be natural, cultivated." "OK." "Go home now and work out why you wear what you wear. Is it to look pretty? Is it to look prettier than other girls to make them jealous? Is it to look prettier than other girls to attract men so that they want you when you want nobody? Or is it to attract men from whom you want to choose one?" "Just because I wear a skimpy top it doesn't mean I'm asking to be raped." "I know; I did not say it did. I want you to ask yourself, honestly, what it does mean. There is nothing more beautiful on this earth than young people full of life, looking for love; but love, too, is a dialogue where you give people space, not where you suck them in. The Kingdom is now, in your body and in your search for love."

The Kingdom is here
it's freedom not fear
The Kingdom is here
The Kingdom is here.

As we walked towards the Down & Out we saw that creep Miles walking towards us from the opposite direction. He was about to go in when he saw Perpetua; so he changed up a gear and went on past. "Not your usual haunt, Miles." "I was just going for a walk." "In the opposite direction from your nice little youth club, at this time of the evening?" "Well, if you really want to know, I was thinking of bringing The Word to those who are in danger of hell." "I know you were. I could tell. You are very brave. It is even more difficult than supervising those noisy boys who play table tennis to humour you and then make fun of you. Go on in. We are just going to the hole in the wall."

As we went round the corner, we almost bumped into Father O'Helly who was almost sliding along the wall, dressed in real weird clothes. "Father!" He flinched and turned as if to go away. "Father, what a nice evening for a drink away from your lonely Presbytery." "Just going for a walk." "And in such festive attire; I like the pink shirt; and the black jeans; what is the logo? It is nice to see you with your cassock off. Your legs are quite wasted in it, as I think you know." "Just a walk." "Break it with a drink. We are just going to the cash point; and see that young Miles does not get hurt. He is trying to save some rather difficult souls from hell."

At the hole in the wall She put in a card and pressed Her PIN. The display showed amounts up to a maximum of £250. "O dear," She said, as She keyed in £500. The money came out and She counted it. "Technology is so strange," She said "like the tills and the phone. God Our Parent looks after all of us; but in different ways." "But what will the bank do?" "It will be all right; it will not know; and it will not lose a penny. God Our Parent and technology; a truly fascinating subject."

When we went into the Down & Out it was packed even though it was barely eight. Miles was already red-faced, arguing with a group of three boys, trying to corner them even though they were all bigger than him. The biggest, Dexter, was finding it really difficult to keep his hands down; you could see that he wanted to give Miles a big push. O'Helly, far from looking after Miles, was looking furtively at a gay boy called Wayne.

Somebody was playing a guitar. "Can you play It's The Sign That Counts?" "I've heard you sing it. Hum it and I will try." After She had sung it as a solo She got other people to join in. "What are you doing here?" "I have come here for two reasons: first of all, to rejoice; secondly, to conduct preliminary interviews for some followers." "In here?" "Why not?" "But it's full of scum. "Including you?" "Well, no. I play a guitar." "For the scum?" "Well, I suppose they are all right, really." "So if you wanted to do a bit of good in the world, to make people happy and fulfilled, would you start here or in the Thumbs Up in Excelsior Gardens?" "Well, here, I suppose." "Which is why I am here."

She walked towards the corner. "Dexter, be careful with Miles; he is brave but fragile. He is the only person I know who has even tried to stand up to you. Respect it and buy him a drink."

"Orange juice. Alcohol is the work of the devil." "Miles, how can you say that? The devil could never have made anything so beautiful. Wine to gladden the hearts of people, it says in the Psalms. But, then, the devil probably could not make real orange juice; he could have made the bottled product in here which has never seen a tree." Dexter bought the drink but while he was taking his change he saw something in the mirror which made him stiffen. It was the Hypo bruiser. He had an instinct for those sorts of people. Perpetua followed his movements and said "Leave him to me. We are good friends." "I'll punch his face in if he makes trouble." "That is no way to celebrate." "We don't want him here." "You cannot simply have here the people you want; it is a public house. Now, Beth, you are not to back off like that. Make pleasant conversation, like practising your scales. You will not be a good lover if you have no conversation. By the way, I did not say how much I like that lacy top, very flattering. It makes you look happy with yourself instead of straining to impress.

She turned to the bruiser. "What is your name? We never did find out as we were only honoured with an informal caution." "Kronyer." "South African?" "Yes." "Beth, I think you chose Nelson Mandela as your media studies project. Tell Mr. Kronyer about it." I did. He got bored. After a while he overheard Miles saying that he didn't care about football but he liked cricket. Kronyer excused himself and went over. It was all right; Miles needed Kronyer more than anybody else needed him.

Perpetua went over to the guitarist again. "Would you mind if I taught us all a song?" "Suppose not." She started tapping and singing The Kingdom Is

Here. The guitarist was clearly embarrassed but wanted to please Her. Other people shuffled and pretended not to hear; but somehow could not help learning and joining in. The landlord was worried about the atmosphere that was building up. Under new rules he didn't have a music licence. "It is fine; My Sister The Spirit has just granted you one." "The police won't care about your sister." "I will take care of the police. Father, stop agonising; either talk to him or leave him alone for now. Have that drink."

> The Kingdom is here
> it's freedom not fear
> The Kingdom is here
> The Kingdom is here.
> Get up and dance, there's no time to wait
> The Lord is with us now
> it's a big space, there isn't a gate
> focus on what not how.

By half past nine the celebration was wavering; people were running out of money. The landlord was fretful. "Here's cash for a kitty," said Perpetua. "Ask for more if you need it." "But that is encouraging people to drink; and to drink to excess," objected Miles. "You are more or less sending them to hell." "I am sending them nowhere. I am living with my brothers and sisters where and how I find them. Now is my starting point." "But they will get drunk." "No doubt." "And that is sinful." "Whatever that means." "Excess." "But you argued that any alcohol was sinful." "It's the loss of control." "Yes, I thought it might be that, Miles. I know you disapprove but there is a massive gap between love and approval; they simply do not relate. Torans and Petrans are so wound up about whether or not they approve of people that they never get round to the loving." "But love involves helping people." "Yes, helping them now, where they are; not 'helping them' to improve so that they will be closer to what you want in the future. The problem for you, Miles, is that you are getting people ready to choose between heaven and hell some time in the future; but The Kingdom of God is here; it is now; you and I are standing together in it." "It does not feel like that to me. This atmosphere makes me feel embarrassed and almost sick." "Yes, love, living in The Kingdom now, is giddy, unpredictable, impossible to control; it is the emotional equivalent of alcohol; too much is good and overpowering; and then too much is bad. I often think that Christians are so concerned with the solidity of the bread in the Eucharist that they forget the risk of the wine. But it takes some getting used to, and if you feel uncomfortable you should go home now and try again another time."

The Kingdom is here
it's freedom not fear
The Kingdom is here
The Kingdom is here.
Get up and sing your praises out
To fill you up inside
The time is now to wave and shout
There's nothing left to hide.

"But what if they had been taking drugs instead of drinking beer? Those platitudes about wine are fine, all those old Toran monks making brandy; but what about heroin and cocaine?" "This is really difficult, Miles, but I would still fund a kitty and give people freedom of choice." "But they could not help themselves." "Nobody, nobody is wholly a victim. Where we can choose we must. Nobody but God Our Parent knows why people choose what they choose, why they think they need drugs, how they get into drugs, and out of drugs. People usually use that image of keeping matches away from a child; but we adults cannot treat our fellow creatures like children; that would be an assertion of power and an imposition of what we think is right. People will not be in the Kingdom for doing what we think is right."

Gone are the lonely places
the walled up spaces
the struggle to get in
gone is the disapproving
the fear of loving
the tyranny of sin.

Miles left. I started talking to a girl called Trina who seemed a bit posh but she was shy and listened to my answers when she asked about my media studies thing. Perpetua was going round the room talking to everybody. The only thing that got Her a bit rattled—well, not really rattled—was when somebody suggested that we should sing Blaze Of Glory. "No thank you," She said, a bit stiff compared with her usual calm. "There is a time and place and this is not the time for that. Stick to The Kingdom being now and not to blazes of glory."

Trina said she worked in Hypo because nobody made fun of her there. I asked about Dexter. She said that although he was tough on the outside he was very good to her. "But what is Dexter doing at Hypo stacking shelves? I mean he could just live off the gang revenue." "Everybody knows he could; but he's really mixed up. Part of him is bullying people and doing all that stuff and the other part of him wants to look after people; and the people he likes to look after are shelf stackers. He also likes to use his muscles and show off a bit." "Yes," said Perpetua, who must have been listening "people are mostly muddled, like that guard, Beth. Not 'A pig' at all."

Father O'Helly was clearly drowning his sorrows over the gay boy, drinking big whiskeys. "Poor man," said Perpetua. "I think the oblivion will be worth the headache. I hope he agrees. Dexter, could you and some of the boys help Father O'Helly home when he's ready. There, there, Father. This is no time to feel guilty or to wish for something that is not for now. Until you come to terms with yourself in those nice tight jeans you will always be chasing thin air and suffering for it."

She gave the landlord another bunch of notes and said goodbye. I did not know whether to stay or go. "Beth, you know how to establish a proper dialogue with Kronyer; you have earned his respect. Do not be afraid."

As She was going through the inner door you could see Her talking to a policeman but I only heard "It is a special celebration but impromptu, as all the best ones are, officer. Just a little singing and jumping up and down. Would it not be a better idea if we were to take a walk to see if there are any real criminals about?"

After She went, the party that had blazed began slowly to die; but instead of the usual friction of too much booze, things became more and more mellow. Dexter and Kronyer played darts and when Kronyer won easily Dexter even shook hands. The landlord was puzzled, not disappointed by the absence of the usual trouble; but puzzled. "Who was that girl, then? Some sort of guardian angel?" "Yes, some sort of angel," said Dexter. "She's a mixture of a social worker and a bit of a mad woman; never quite here; always a bit somewhere else; but never lectures like Miles or O'Helly over there, sliding off his stool. She's like a grown up who still has this big bit of child inside."

"Yellow Is The Promise," said a Downs Syndrome kid called Jim who shouldn't really have been in the pub. He liked to play his flute and the guitarist was always friendly. "All right; but only once, Jim."

We stayed for that and then dexter hauled O'Helly to his feet and I went out with Trina. You could just hear:

> *The Kingdom is here*
> *it's freedom not fear*
> *The Kingdom is here*
> *The Kingdom is here.*

Three

Love is the fruit of Grace.
Love is making space.
Make our words into a book
Words and notes into a song
make our clothes into a look
wonder as we go along:
make the space for our brother to love
have the calm in Our spirit to live
hear the truth of our sister's regret
feel the joy of our mission to give.
Love is the fruit of Grace
Love is making space.
Smooth a path for us to walk
help to make our choices clear,
listen while the others talk
step back when the time is near:
make the space for our brother to love
have the calm in Our spirit to live
hear the truth of our sister's regret
feel the joy of our mission to give.
Love is the fruit of Grace
Love is making space.
Leave judgment far behind
there's no love in a frown
see that no-one's left behind
and let nobody down.
We won't stand by when we hear hate
or turn our backs when times get tough
in a crisis we will act not wait
because when we give love, there's still enough:
make the space for our brother to love
have the calm in Our spirit to live
hear the truth of our sister's regret
feel the joy of our mission to give.
Love is the fruit of Grace
Love is making space.

Love is the fruit of Grace
Love is making space.
Love is making space.

Before Perpetua chose Her core followers She went away on Her own for a few days to pray. It was the worst time of Her life. Praying became impossible as She was inhabited by a series of vivid scenarios, like spot ads, She said, in which the options for Her future life were portrayed. She was not tempted by the prospect of cars, money, travel, houses, food or glamorous partners. The most difficult temptations were those which promised Her the power to bring about change; to do good; to put things right.

There was a scene of enormous devastation brought about by a tsunami with the slogan:

Take The Power
You can change the world.

In another scene, two factions in a civil war were using children as human shields in a vain attempt to protect them from their opponents, with the slogan:

Take The Power
You Can Make Peace

But the most difficult of all was a scene from Her own scruffy patch of Grunge Park with the slogan:

Take The Power
That They All May Be Happy

Love is the fruit of Grace.
Love is making space.

These images were highly disturbing because She knew that their opposites would be Her reality; the struggle; the pain' the vain attempts; the one step forward and two back; the things you could really do nothing about at all; the wasted promise; the broken promises. It was not the facile promises that tempted Her, nor the offer of power in itself, it was simply Her knowledge of their opposite; of what happens when people struggle to their own fulfillment; but, in the end, She thought, better something tiny from a struggle than a big present like a hamper dropped in your lap.

> *Make the space for our brother to love*
> *have the calm in Our spirit to live*
> *hear the truth of our sister's regret*
> *feel the joy of our mission to give.*
> *Love is the fruit of Grace*
> *Love is making space.*

In the the strange town where She was staying, She saw a man knocking on a door and watched as it was narrowly and frightenedly opened. She could tell immediately that he was a loan shark. As he turned away, the door was shut quickly. "Why are you doing that?" She asked him. "To earn an honest living for my wife and kids," he said. "You try to scrape together enough money for your pregnant wife and four between the ages of three and fourteen. It's not easy. These people spin all kinds of yarns about the good reasons they need to borrow money and then they just fritter it away and have no means of paying it back. Imagine how difficult my life is!" "I am not sure why you complain about your clients when you are spinning yarns yourself. You have abandoned a wife and a woman you lived with and the four children they have given you between them; and you will certainly run away again when your latest girl friend tells you she is pregnant. You have run away from your commitments, changed your name, and you are not paying any support costs for the two women or your four children." "How do you know so much about me?" "It does not matter. I have come to bring you much greater wealth than you can imagine." "I don't know about that. If you know me as well as you say, you will know that I can get through an awful lot of money very quickly, what with horses, women, jewels, holidays." "I know; and I also know that you are no happier now than you were when you bribed your first girl friend to have sex. You thought then, and you still think now, that money will do anything you want; but are you running towards something that you want or away from something that you are frightened of, something we might call truth? I have come to bring you all the wealth of the Heavenly Kingdom, to make you rich in My Sister the Spirit, to give you the wisdom that will help you to be happy, to bring you again the good news that Jesus My Brother brought." "It's not the sort of thing I would reckon on doing; but as you know so much about me, you ought to know if it will work. What about this collecting business?" "You know what I am going to say." "All right, I'll turn the books in. I'll help the worst off people on my books.

I'll start paying maintenance to the girls and the kids. I'll. . .". "I think those are quite sufficient undertakings for now." "the only problem is, how will I make a living?" "It is still difficult for you to realise how much I know about you. Remember what you were like, just before you became obsessed with money and thought it could get you anything you wanted which, you thought, would make you happy. Remember how good you were at calming people down, at smoothing things over. That is why you are so good at this job, you have never threatened people. You lure them into debt and into more debt. Turn this gift around, stop luring and start persuading, go and be a peace maker, resolve conflict. There is enough of it."

She had almost reached home when the car she was in, hitching a ride, had to stop suddenly to avoid adding to a pile-up. She found a woman clutching a dead child, her husband on the verge of violence, and a badly injured teenage boy who had obviously caused the accident by driving too fast. She went first to the boy and said "Sit still; right there; do not move; do not worry." She went to the father and said "Be still; have faith; do not worry." Then she went to the mother and said "I heard you calling upon God for help. Do you believe?" "Well, I would now if. . ." "Do not worry; this is not a doctrine class. Were you calling upon God or was it just a phrase?" "I was calling." "Your baby has had a bit of a knock on the head but she will be all right. Look, her eyes are opening. Get ready, she is about to scream; the nicest sound you will ever hear. What is her name?" "We are not really sure; we keep changing. What is your name?" "Perpetua." "It will be hers."

She went to the father "Your baby got a bit of a knock but she is now fine. Go and rejoice with your wife; her faith has saved your child." She went to the young man and said "You had drunk a little too much and were driving a little too fast. If the baby had died and you were found with too much alcohol, your life would be completely changed; it would be hard for you ever to get back to the lovely life you have been promised. I have taken away the taint of alcohol; you will still have to suffer something for the carelessness; but I know you will never do anything like this again."

Once they heard the sirens in the distance, Perpetua's lift drove away.

After She came back and chose Her core group, I was not included. When I asked Her why not, she said "It may sound a little strange to say this; in life people expect to be rewarded for being good; but my purpose is different. It would not be kind to say to them that the people in the core group are those who need most help, even though they know, and you know, that is true; and you are mature enough to keep it to yourself. I want you to work with Trina; I will never be far away; but my close followers need me to be there with them most of the time."

I was a little upset but I saw what Perpetua meant. I felt proud to be trusted and pleased that I would be near to the centre of events, using my media skills.

> *Make our words into a book*
> *words and notes into a song*
> *make our clothes into a look*
> *wonder as we go along:*
> *make the space for our brother to love*
> *have the calm in Our spirit to live*
> *hear the truth of our sister's regret*
> *feel the joy of our mission to give.*
> *Love is the fruit of Grace*
> *Love is making space.*

When they had finished most of their preparation to go out into the world to spread the Gospel, Perpetua drew the core group and all the other followers together and said

"It is very difficult to sum up all that we have been through together in the past few days, but I want to try to give you a mental manual.

"First, three ways of behaving: create, act and enable. By "create" we mean that we were not made simply to be consumers. The world we live in puts a huge amount of emphasis on consuming; we are judged according to what we can afford to consume; but we would be better estimated on the basis of what we make. There is the phrase 'added value' but this should be applied to what we do with other people, not to products. Wherever we go we must try to add value to the lives of people."

> *Smooth a path for us to walk*
> *Help to make our choices clear,*
> *Listen while the others talk*
> *Step back when the time is near:*

"To enable is the gift of the servant. It is tempting to do everything we can for everybody. There are times, when people are sick or desperate, when we must give them our help directly, when we must exercise power but the purpose of a child of God Our Parent is to enable all children to fulfill themselves through their own choices and actions. It is also very important not to confuse this duty of care with the over-riding obligation to love; care and love are very different but often muddled. Care is a necessary—and as often as possible, temporary—exercise of power in an unequal relationship; love only works in an environment where the lover accords complete equality to the beloved."

We won't stand by when we hear hate
or turn our backs when times get tough
in a crisis we will act not wait
because when we give love, there's still enough:

"Related to these is the capacity to act, to fight indifference, to do something. Most people feel helpless in the face of major events; many people feel helpless about every detail of their lives; but no person is devoid of all choices; even the choice that we want to choose when we cannot is better than giving in. We must act and, in enabling, we must revive the love of action in others so that they steadily expand their area of choice. This is not consumer choice, choosing to be according to what you buy, but taking life choices about loving and not loving. God Our Parent has made us all very complex and unique; but in spite of our seeming helplessness, none of us is only a victim and nothing else. It is very difficult to strike the proper balance between enabling and acting; but not at all difficult to establish the importance of being active over being passive and, even more critically, of avoiding turning ourselves into victims. To assert victimhood is what they call a paradox but it is one from which many here suffer. To claim victimhood is to insult God Our Parent who created us to choose.

"We must undertake these three activities of creating, enabling and acting with truth, joy and calm.

"Contrary to what most people, even very clever people, say, the idea of truth is not all that difficult. Be careful with this word, it means the opposite of what most people take it to mean. To think and act truthfully is to do so in accordance with our purposes as best we can, knowing what we know. Truth for a theologian will be different from truth for a manual labourer; what makes them equal is their obligation to think and act truthfully.

"Our purposes are those which flow from being children of God Our Parent; we exist to worship God and to love God and each other. Sometimes in desperate situations it is difficult to know where love is but we are still bound to look at ourselves and to act truthfully to show whatever love we can salvage from a situation.

"If we are faced, for example, with a set of complex issues surrounding the custody of a child, there is no such thing as objective 'truth'; the different people will see truth according to their experience and perceived obligations.

"We can only tell our own truth for ourselves which might help others but mostly will not. Advice is one of the most dangerous things because we think when we give it we are being kind; but the receiver must watch out. People who tell us that truth is easy or that they know what the truth is are confusing truth with their own individual version of it when two versions necessarily cannot be the same. Most often when people tell us how we can be truthful they are really telling us how we can be obedient to their wishes, fitting their pattern, gaining their approval.

"Freed by God Our Parent to live in truth, we must go out into the world filled with joy. If we can create, enable and act and if we can live our own truth, the world, in spite of all its difficulties, should be a place of joy. Jesus My Brother is so sad when He sees how miserable people are, thinking this is what He wants. The Church is very good at sad hymns and sad prayers and sad occasions but it does not seem to be so good at joy. Churches are full of the joy at the birth of Jesus but most people miss the big joy of the Resurrection, which is the main reason I am here, to live so that people can be made alive to the idea of Resurrection.

"I will be a kind of Resurrection.

"The root of our problem is that people forget that when Jesus My Brother rose from the Dead He rose physically, He was not a ghost. Christianity is plagued, chronically plagued, by what philosophers call 'dualism'; the men who took over the Church from the Apostles and the faithful women became frightened of women and in the end learned to hate them so that marriage and physical love were down-graded. Women were thought to be second best and sex was wicked; so that people came to believe that being a monk or being a celibate priest was a higher calling than being married. All that joy squeezed out of church life. How can we begin to think that the Kingdom is now if there is no joy in it?

"The third thing to think about is calm. this is not a matter of staying still and quiet; though these things in themselves are very good; what I mean is that we should not thrash about; we should be deliberate and purposeful; we should, therefore, be courageous but not boastful in our courage; we should just get on and do what we have to do without any drama. We all know how vulnerable we are; that is an integral part of loving; and we need to be calm in our vulnerability, too; but, above all, we need to be calm when we are in a crisis.

"In creating, enabling and acting, we should live a life of truth, joy and calm."

> *Leave judgment far behind*
> *there's no love in a frown*
> *see that no-one's left behind*
> *and let nobody down.*
> *We won't stand by when we hear hate*
> *or turn our backs when times get tough*

in a crisis we will act not wait
because when we give love, there's still enough:

"Some people will tell you that the truths that the Christian Church proclaims are timeless but I say that that is a misunderstanding of creation. God created time; and put humanity to live in time; and the relationship between humanity and God Our Parent changed through time, critically when Jesus My Brother became a member of humanity. Jesus lived in time; He rose from the dead in time; He and God Our Parent sent my Sister The Spirit to earth in time. Everything that is said about God is a metaphor; it is provisional; it changes through time. Time changes the meaning of words; time changes the meaning of ideas; time changes what we mean by meaning. Time shapes meaning and through these shapes we make moral decisions; when time changes the shape, the moral decisions change.

"As the Sacred Vessel of God Our Parent I have come to earth in time. If time does not change everything, what is it for? If doctrine stands still it means that the imagination is dead. God Our Parent wants humanity to try to grow, to be restless, to try new ways of understanding and of loving.

"There are many that say that understanding what God has 'said' to humanity is easy. I say to you that it is so difficult that no person or group or unanimity or hierarchy will ever know. God is a mystery and ways of understanding God in Scripture are vitally important but they are imperfect in the way that humanity is imperfect. Scripture is not simply God talking to humanity it is also humanity talking to God. My Sister the Spirit does not live in our individual hearts and collectively in the church to channel a monologue of God into humanity; she exists to enable a dialogue.

"When humanity calls upon Scripture to validate what it says it is not calling upon the 'pure Word of God', it is making reference to a dialogue between God and humanity enabled by the Holy Spirit. The human part of that dialogue is human, the divine part is divine. They cannot be separated and so when people claim the support of Scripture for their opinions they are not in harmony with the 'pure Word of God' but simply in harmony with a dialogue of which the human element is, necessarily, flawed. If humanity was not flawed it could not exercise the will to choose and the will to love. Because humanity is free to choose and because the truth for each of us is different, the ability to use language to forge agreements on meaning is severely limited. Doctrine is brave and beautiful but if it endangers love it is not worth keeping."

Make the space for our brother to love
have the calm in Our spirit to live
hear the truth of our sister's regret

feel the joy of our mission to give.
Love is the fruit of Grace
Love is making space.

"From all this it follows that in terms of what God wants; if God can be said to want anything other than the eternal love within the Godhead and the voluntary love of humanity; the idea of judgment is alien. Humanity needs to pass judgments to preserve order; that is the nature of God-created human difference and human free will; but it is wrong to bring God into the matter. No human being can make a judgment on behalf of God or claim God's support for it. A person might claim the support of Scripture for a human judgment but that is not the same as claiming the support of God. As I have said, Scripture is the Word of God flawed by the human endeavour to understand.

"It also follows from what I have said that the virtue above all virtues is love; that is what we are here for. There are many that say we have to be cruel to be kind; we are harsh out of love for someone. We are back with the image of the child with the box of matches. We love children unconditionally but we must also care for them as they grow so that they do not come to harm; the two things become more recognisably separate as children grow. When somebody becomes an adult the love and care are easy to separate but they are too often not separated so that adults have care imposed on them which is falsely designated as 'love.'"

Love is making space.

"Love is making unconditional space in which the beloved can exercise unconditionally the freedom to choose and the freedom to love.

"Unconditionally. That is the word that makes love so wonderful but so difficult. Wonderful because the openness of love reflects the openness of the Godhead; difficult because humanity rejoices in making meaning, in making patterns, in ordering and shaping; but to shape for ourselves or to be part of a mutual shaping is quite different from wishing to shape others. Shaping makes unlimited space more manageable; but, in the end, you cannot manage space and, equally, you cannot manage love; you cannot parcel it out or distribute it. When you have shaped something, individually or mutually, whatever it is, it is not love. Love will not be controlled because control is a specific and harmful kind of shaping. Once it is controlled it is not love, it is something else. Love is intensely counter intuitive but it is so often mixed up with the idea of feeling. Love is beyond feeling; so far beyond that it is not dependent on feeling."

As she finished, the sky went yellow like that time when She came in Her blaze of Glory; just for a moment. Everybody was still. She led them away, almost in a dance. Then the special light faded and the stars appeared.

Love is the fruit of Grace
Love is making space.

Four

Yellow is the promise
of a happy day
shining out between the threatening clouds of grey
the promise
of a friendly smile for a face that's down
the promise that the clouds will blow away.
Purple is the prospect
of our life journey
stretching out further than earthly eyes can see,
the prospect
of a struggle to the journey's happy end,
the prospect of a shared eternity.
Red is the experience
of a fatal pain
calling out for words of fellowship in vain,
the experience
of a threnody for a cause they say is lost
the experience that a chance will come again.
White is the Resurrection
of the faithful heart
reaching out to all who yearn for a new start
the Resurrection
of the hope that our new lives have now begun
The promise that God and man will never part.

Yellow for the promise
purple for the way
red for the sacrifice
and white for the new day.

Perpetua was saying Her night prayers when Her chime generator signalled that somebody wanted to see Her. "Who is there?" "Bill Midway." "Father Bill?" "Yes."

"Come in. You are out a bit late." "I have been trying to pray but it has become very difficult. I can't pray any more. I keep thinking about you. No, I don't mean in the usual way, though I think you are very lovely. No, I mean, perhaps you don't know but I was there that night when you made the Cross out of broken glass and I had a really strange experience when the light changed. It did change, didn't it? I have often wondered but didn't want to ask anybody in case it made me look stupid, people saying 'What do you mean? Of course it didn't!' or 'What do you mean? Of course it did!' I've tried to get you out of my head but I can't."

Yellow is the promise
of a happy day
shining out between the threatening clouds of grey
the promise
of a friendly smile for a face that's down
the promise that the clouds will blow away.

"I knew you were there and, yes, something did happen that night after I led the making of the Cross. Something happened to the light. It was God Our Parent giving me, and everybody, a sign both of God's special presence in me as the Sacred Vessel and a confirmation of my mission."

"I can just about understand you saying 'God Our Parent' rather than 'God the Father' but what is this idea of you as a 'Sacred Vessel'? Are you a different kind of vessel of God from me?"

"I do not want you to feel in any way embarrassed by what I am saying. I do not want you to feel different or smaller, but I am the Sacred Vessel of God Our Parent in a very different way from that in which all human beings are vessels of God. To put it in conventional theological terms that you used at College; I am the Fourth Person of the Godhead; although I think that is a rather clumsy way of putting it."

"But we learned at College; have held for two thousand years; that there are only three persons in the one true and living God."

"Just as the Chosen People thought that there was only one person in the one, true and living God. What scandalised the Jews was that Jesus My Brother said that He was the second person of the Godhead; the Son of God; equal to God. Then God Our Parent and Jesus My Brother sent My Sister the Spirit to live in the Church.

"Of course this idea of the Spirit is also a complicated piece of theological imagery. Jesus promised the Apostles that they would be specially helped by 'the Spirit of truth'; 'the comforter'. Christians have found it easier to use the word 'Person' for these three ideas of God combined in one Godhead although the meaning of 'person' has changed so much over 1500 years that I am not sure how helpful it is now. I use the term 'My Sister the Spirit' because it makes it easier for people to get some idea of the diversity within the unity of God but of course My Sister the Spirit is no more a woman than God Our Parent is a man. It just seems unfair; in the way humanity understands things; to have a 'Father' and a 'Son' and a genderless Spirit. The only human person in the Godhead until now is Jesus My Brother. The central idea of Christianity is incarnation not trinity."

"So where do you fit?" "

The Chosen People lost touch with their wild God of the 'burning bush' and got more bound up in the Temple; and so Jesus became human in order to help humanity become closer again to God; to help people to choose to love God and each other. Now the same problem has arisen two thousand years later. Humanity has lost touch with God again, the impact of the life of Jesus My Brother is ever more difficult for people to realise. People become very depressed and angry about this. They think that times are worse than they used to be; that God is loved less; as if love can be counted. They are too hard on themselves and on everybody else. If God is everywhere—which is one way of giving human expression to the idea of God—then, quite reasonably, people have believed that God can, so to speak, erupt into time and space as a human being. This is not such a radical development from God appearing to the Chosen People in some way that they could recognise and respond to. What is puzzling is that so many theologians think that God somehow was only allowed one throw of the dice, one incarnation, one deeply significant (as of a sign) way of human dying."

> *Purple is the prospect*
> *of our life journey*
> *stretching out further than earthly eyes can see,*
> *the prospect*
> *of a struggle to the journey's happy end,*
> *the prospect of a shared eternity.*

"The Church talks about the death of Jesus being 'The full and final sacrifice.'"

"Well, of course the sacrifice is full because Jesus as God as well as human could do nothing that was not perfect; that was not, in that sense, full. Yet it was an act in time of a timeless God. We do not suppose, do we, that nobody could be fully united with God until after the Resurrection? Would we put Isaiah and all the holy prophets in some kind of supernatural ante-room? People have been making their journeys towards God since the beginning of humanity. It has always been a difficult road; but it became too difficult for the Chosen People and so God intervened in history, in time. The idea of the journey contains space and time.

"There has always been divine Grace in the world to sustain people on this journey and there is still divine grace for all people; not just Christians. My Sister the Spirit is eternal or, rather, external, outside time; but Jesus made the Grace of God known in a concrete way through His life, death and Resurrection; and through leaving to humanity the eternal gift of Himself in Sacraments, signs..."

"...But where do you fit?"

"I am coming to that. The sacrifice was full; but, as I said, why should God be limited to any kind of finality? God cannot be bound by such rules; no matter how tidy they make the idea of the Godhead. As the Sacred Vessel—as the so-called 'Fourth Person'—I am here to live my life as a witness of God's love and goodness; helping people to recognise Jesus and to choose to participate in dialogue with God Our Parent through the 'good offices' of My Sister the Spirit. There are other ways of thinking of the Godhead. Created beings on other planets do not know about Jesus My Brother but they do know about other manifestations of the Godhead in forms identical to their own. These are different kinds of what you might call in-form-ations, as opposed to incarnations."

"Yes. I had never thought of that."

"This is why the current agonising in Christianity over what God might or might not demand of believers is so discouraging. At best it is an argument about metaphors; at worst it is just another form of power politics.

"Without common metaphors we cannot speak to each other; so metaphors are important; but we should not argue about metaphors; we should try to understand them together. As we are different we will find different individual and different mutually acceptable metaphors; our ways of making experience formal."

Yellow for the promise
purple for the way

*red for the sacrifice
and white for the new day.*

"I know we might think that it is a little boring but just for a moment let us think about the raging debate between Torans and Petrans on the one hand, and Amorans on the other, about gay people. The Torans and Petrans claim that God does not want gay people to be clergy. Put that way; as a simple proposition; it is surreal. What makes anybody think that God wanted clergy? But if, by any chance, they are correct in their assumption that God does want Christian clergy; what makes them think that God does not want gay clergy? For sure the Chosen People did not want gay clergy; but that had nothing to do with God any more than God would have minded whether they ate prawns. The trouble is that when powerful men; and it usually is men; say that God wants this or that people who want to do what God wants find it very difficult to argue with them. To the extent that God wants anything; to use another metaphor; God wants us to love each other and God freely.

"The sadness about the current dispute is that people want to keep closing down space for each other in the name of 'sound doctrine' instead of opening it up; making more room for love. Church critics say that there is so much concern about gay people that other bigger issues are being ignored. That is not the point. For a Church there is no bigger issue than its God and the mutuality of a Church means that people are bound to discuss what they understand by God and how they can best fulfil their role as creatures. This should be a joyful, exploratory, always travelling, mutual learning, never arriving experience. Some people want conclusions but being a searcher after God has always been a journey. Today some people, like Archbishop Hawthorn, call it (to use the language of business) a process and rightly think that this process is more important than product.

"Metaphors are tools. We use different tools for different things. We know that human beings were built to compete as well as collaborate so we like to answer questions like 'Is Wordsworth a better poet than Homer?' In a deep down way it is a foolish question because they are such different poets and most people would not be so extreme that they would want to promote one to such an extent that the other was never read. That should also be the case with discussions about God. People will be passionate about their metaphors; their theologies; their poetries; but they should not be to the extent that they want to drive other metaphors, theologies and poetries out of circulation. All humanity is equally entitled to be opinionated about God. The meaning of love is that we leave room for people to be opinionated, whatever we personally think. Signs allow people to have different opinions about the same phenomenon so that…"

"So where does that leave you as an idea in theology?"

"Like Jesus My Brother, I am both human and of the Godhead. I have to say that in human language because we are both human. What that might mean to you can only be worked out by you in the way you work things out. Some people read; some people think systematically; some people contemplate, trying to leave themselves open. No two people do things the same way. My mission is to help people to realise an idea of God in themselves so that they can better choose to love God and each other. I keep coming back to this but, however complex men (and it usually is men) make matters concerning God, they are ultimately simple, though never easy, and always a mystery."

> *Red is the experience*
> *of a fatal pain*
> *calling out for words of fellowship in vain,*
> *the experience*
> *of a threnody for a cause they say is lost*
> *the experience that a chance will come again.*

"You talked about sacrifice?"

"Yes. Just as Jesus My Brother was inevitably killed because what He had to say threatened vested interests, so I will also die in an unpleasant way. People understand the idea of dying for each other. If Jesus had preached and simply 'gone to heaven', nobody would have felt the impact of the incarnation. If my mission is simply easy and ends tidily, the impact will be tiny. It is the old saying that most people do not value something until it has gone. People needed to know that they, collectively, killed Jesus; that the ultimate consequence of freedom of choice was that humanity killed Jesus. That is the only way people can be persuaded to take choice seriously.

"Like Jesus, however, I will always be with humanity from now on; but, in the meantime, this will involve an unpleasant death experience. Without really understanding it, and often getting muddled with the metaphor, the only way humanity can understand God at all is to go through some death process. That is why Christians think of Baptism as a death process."

> *red for the sacrifice*
> *and white for the new day.*

"But will you really die and then come back in some way?"

"Yes; but this is not the time to talk about that, Bill. Will you sleep any better now?"

"After all that you have said, just the opposite; there is so much to digest;

but I will pray that it becomes clearer in time. You won't mind if I don't worship you yet?"

"No. I wish Christians could see how difficult it was for the Jews when Jesus made His claim. They are about to go through the same thing that you have just gone through. At least you have not said something rude and stormed out; that is quite good enough for now."

He made as if to kneel. "Will you give me a blessing?"

"Just stay a moment, Bill, because you have just said something really important. You will have heard me sing *It's the Sign That Counts* and so it is. The Sacraments as signs are very special; which is why they will enrich people as long as they live on the earth; but signs are not all tied up with the divine. Ringing church bells is a sign which reaches out from the fellowship of Jesus to the whole community. More importantly, our faces are ever-changing, living signs of what is happening inside us. All the time we are giving out signs as indicators of what is happening at our core. So the sign is the outward manifestation of something inward."

"Oh, of course, The Sign'. That song again. I have often wondered about it because I have only heard you sing the chorus."

"There is only a chorus or, rather, a kind of mantra. The idea of a sign is that it is the same every time but different. Ideally you should sing the words to a different tune every time but the tune I sang as a child seems to have stuck. The essence of Baptism is the same for every Christian but it is different for each one. That is true for the Eucharist but even more so because we experience it many times. Above all, it is true for the Church which is a sign of God Our Parent being always with us. We like to sing familiar words to the same familiar tune but in the end, when that works at its best, it ingrains a sense of self rather than of other. A song becomes ever dearer to us and so we never want a different tune. That is when signs become nostalgic rather than living. They talk about past love not present love. Churches have frozen signs and the Church itself is becoming a frozen sign. Even the people who show their faith through the constant sharing of the Eucharist can become so comfortable in its stability, its sureness, that it stops living."

Purple for the way

"If you want to be really subtle you could argue that the best form of music is harmony; so that in the Church all the different ways of singing the tune would end with harmony. The problem with Western music is that it is concerned almost entirely with form; with the working out of an idea; not the organic growth of an idea; with the symphony rather than something even more free-form than jazz; something totally open-ended. The great pieces always come back to where they started; they satisfy the craving for wandering and uncertainty crowned by coming home; but being a follower of Jesus My Brother means that the home is temporary and the going out is the lifelong activity. Prophesy, going forward, has to involve changes of form and also changes of content which cause discord. We can all love where we have been; take comfort from our roots; but because humanity lives in time it must change. And so the Church must change. With God as its constant it needs different ways of saying things and it needs to value the sign which combines elements of God with elements of humanity.

"As soon as we become too comfortable with our sacred signs, including the Cross, we need to make an effort to create new ways of understanding them. One of the 'reasons' why I am here is that Christianity has run out of creative steam. There is plenty of new theology and plenty of report writing and there are so many good people struggling to do God's will but it is really sad that they make such heavy weather of it. Many people say that there are so few Christians because of a catastrophic turning away from God; and others say that there is something wrong with the 'brand' because most people are still in search of the spiritual. It is neither of these things. The real root of the problem is that the incarnation of God—the unity of spirit and flesh; the creative purpose—have been stifled by dualism and formalism.

"There is nothing so opposed to formalism as love. And a love that is dualistic cannot thrive in creatures which are a combination of flesh and spirit. The Churches are obsessed with control and therefore frightened of losing it. If clergy are really servants of the people then the people should choose their servants. On the other hand, obvious hedonism and planetary degradation are leading people to question the goodness of creation. It is another kind of victimhood; another kind of giving in. That is why blessing is such an important sign; the sign of the love of God actually being focused through one child on another child; to show that love is not something we hold onto because there is not enough of it. Blessing is a sign of God's generosity. In blessing, God and humanity act as one. We should all bless."

Bill knelt down and She made the Sign of the Cross in his eye line and put Her hands on his head. "It is not only the clergy who are channels of blessing, from the Bishop to the Priest to the people. Blessing is our way of giving God's strength to one another. It is not our strength, so in a real way we are not giving but channelling, being witnesses that we have faith in this strength which we pass on. We are like a magnifying glass which draws the intensity of the sun into a point that makes fire on earth. You will need this fire, Bill, more than most people. The road you have taken in following me will be hard. Many people who were your close friends will become your enemies. You will suffer humiliation and insult for following me. You will also suffer because it will look to you as if you have caused pain; but faithfulness is more important than anything else. Will you follow me?"

"Yes; with the help of God, I will."

"I bless you
in the name of God Our Parent
Jesus My Brother
My Sister The Spirit
and in my own name as The Sacred Vessel."

Yellow for the promise
purple for the way
red for the sacrifice
and white for the new day.

Editor's Note: Father Bill Midway became a close follower of Perpetua and witnessed Her terrible death. Interview given in May 2007 to www. church&state.net.

Five

The lady in purple smiles wide as the sky
with the set of her head and the gleam in her eye
with a smile that is equal to strangers and friends:
with a smile that you know never ends.

    O lady in purple you shimmer and shine
    like a bowl filled with fruit and a glass filled with wine
    like the banner that waves with the hope of release
    like the heavenly princess of peace.

The lady in purple laughs long as a stream
with a touch of the earth and the touch of a dream
with a laugh that will carry the sharpest of bends:
with a laugh that you know never ends.

The lady in purple loves full as her heart
with a depth that is clear from the moment you start
with a love so intense that expands and extends:
with a love that you know never ends.

The lady in purple dances smiles, tears and love
With a movement divine caught from Heaven above
In a dance that embraces, forgives and amends:
In a dance that you know never ends.

The lady in purple smiles wide as the sky
with the set of her head and the gleam in her eye
with a smile that is equal to strangers and friends:
with a smile that you know never ends

The Lady in Purple!

They thought it would never end. As they came away from the Excelsior Gardens happening, they could hardly believe what had happened. Of course they believed in Perpetua in a vague sort of way; but they had not been able to imagine this. It was a small Channel; but there would be pictures on the evening news. They were a bit alien in Excelsior Gardens; but they had gained some new followers. Andy had collected thousands of pounds. Dexter suggested that they should go back to Grunge Park to celebrate; but Perpetua said she thought it would be better to go somewhere else. "We are wearing just a little thin where we come from. It would be good to take the message somewhere else."

They decided to go to Paradise Common, a small estate behind Paradise Lodge, the old people's home. It had stubby little blocks of flats, warden bungalows and a few semi detached houses; everything looked overgrown and about to fall down. It was all a bit sorry for itself.

They had obviously been tailed from Excelsior by Olly and Rory who came round the corner almost dragging Father O'Helly.

"Good afternoon Father. I hope you are exercising due care over your unpredictable nephew and his mercurial friend."

"Oliver tells me that you have been blaspheming."

"Well, at least he learned something during his brief stay at theological college."

"He says you claim to be a special person sent by God."

"Would you not make that claim for yourself?"

"He said it was more than a general claim."

"It sounds a bit muddled. I wish he was prepared to speak for himself as he was there. Even better, I wish you had been there to hear me but; there will be many other opportunities, Father."

"If you are something special, why don't you give us a sign."

"Shame on you Father. You must have read accounts of that kind of nonsense in the Gospels thousands of times. It sounds as if you want some scientific proof."

Olly and Rory started arguing, so Father O'Helly managed to slip away.

You could hear it before you could see it. There was a tapping and scratching on the pavement and the wall, then a blind old man came creeping round the corner; cautious; creeping.

"Come and meet Perpetua," said Trina.

"Who is she?"

"She is the Sacred Vessel of God. She has come to bring the good news to the poor."

"Well she's found one of the right people."

"What is your name?" asked Perpetua.

"Fidel."

"A nice name."

"So what is this good news you are going to bring? Is it the same good news that Jesus brought?"

"Yes."

"He cured people."

"Do you want to be cured?"

"Yes; but not very badly. If I had been pushy it would have happened already. I could have been pushy and founded my own business and paid to go private; but I have never been interested in that. I could have been pushy and queue jumped; as rich people do; but I am not interested in that. I believe that you have to put your faith in doctors and bureaucrats to do the right thing rather than fighting a guerrilla war with officials. This, of course, is idealistic."

"There is nothing wrong with that."

"I am prepared to wait because it is important to learn how to wait."

"You recalled Jesus. Do you have faith?"

"I say my prayers but I try not to ask for anything. I have faith in a laboured way."

"Do you have faith in me?"

"I don't know."

"Do you have faith in me?"

"In the way that I have faith in God?"

"Yes."

"You are asking for something very difficult. How were the Jews supposed to know that Jesus came from God just because he said so? How can I just take your word for it? I suppose that it depends upon what you do and not what you say."

"You have come quite a long way already."

> *O lady in purple you shimmer and shine*
> *O lady in purple in purple*
> *You shimmer and shine.*

"Fidel. You have arrived at the front of my cataract queue."

"Purple, yellow, red, white purple. The colours! I had forgotten the brightness of the colours!"

> *O lady in purple*
> *you shimmer and shine.*

He almost ran away but was stopped by Dexter who said, rather gruffly "Aren't you going to thank Perpetua?" "Thanking is sharing."

The lady in purple laughs long as a stream
with a touch of the earth and the touch of a dream
with a laugh that will carry the sharpest of bends
with a laugh that you know never ends

Fidel's sharing, however, was short-lived as he had not gone for more than a minute before he came back round the corner being pushed by Father O'Helly.

"He says you have cured him of his blindness. It's a trick."

"I have cured him."

"How can I believe that?"

"Ask Fidel."

"You said you would not do something like this just because somebody asked."

"Fidel did not ask; that is precisely why I cured him."

"It's the work of the devil."

"O Father, you know quite enough about the devil; do not look at me like that; I mean in a professional way. The devil does not go around doing good without a motive."

"Your motive is to drag people away from Mother Church."

"I hardly think that curing the people I meet will make any difference. As long as good, hard-working people like you are within the Church, what have you to fear from people like me?"

"I don't understand."

"Neither do I. But Father, 'understand' is such a strange word coming from you. Believe. Believe!

"At its simplest, I helped Fidel; and you cannot really know my reasons. I say that I called on the power of God Our Parent because I wanted to give a man of faith a little support and joy."

As Father O'Helly became more animated he let go of Fidel; and as they talked Perpetua slowly, slowly turned on the spot, with O'Helly tracking Her so that he could talk right into Her face until he had his back to Fidel; who promptly ran off. Olly and Rory had also had enough. The miracle, as they thought of it, was a bit of fun but they doubted there would be anything else of interest.

The lady in purple loves full as her heart

with a depth that is clear from the moment you start
with a love so intense that expands and extends
with a love that you know never ends.

You could hear it before you could see it. There was a bumping and scraping like somebody pushing a barrow and then Fidel came round the corner so fast that he almost pitched an old lady out of her wheelchair.

"Fidel, there is no need to hurry; I will wait; take your time. What is your name?"

"Cara."

"That is a nice name. Do you want me to cure you.?"

"Of course I do; but if you can't or don't I will manage."

"Do you believe that I can cure you?"

"Of course I do. Fidel is a good man. Every day when it is fine he takes me out to break up the loneliness; but when it's not fine he sits in with me. I can look after myself but it's the loneliness; it means you can't give to people the way you want to. For me, loneliness is not giving."

"I like that. You will have to look round for somebody who wants a wheelchair, then."

She bent down and took Cara's hand and, almost without her noticing, she got to her feet.

"Fidel and me can now do what we have wanted to do for a long time; to found a day club."

"I think we should say a prayer of thanks," said Fidel.

"All right," said Perpetua "but let us keep it short. I think God would prefer us to dance."

O lady in purple you shimmer and shine
like a bowl filled with fruit and a glass filled with wine
like the banner that waves with the hope of release
like the heavenly princess of peace.

They thought it would never end. People came out of their houses helping the disabled and the sick. Everyone who needed to be cured was cured and everybody else was given a blessing. Some people pretended they needed a cure; just for a laugh; to test Her out; but Perpetua just pretended to tell them off and then gave them a blessing. Some people thought that this was a good occasion for a party and began bringing out food and pots of tea; putting them on the half dozen picnic tables in the middle of the scruffy little Common.

Then something strange happened. Things began to appear on the table that could not possibly have been brought out. Some people said that Andy had been to buy special things; others said it was another miracle. Perpetua said "Each of you take a piece of food in one hand and a drink in the other. I offer these to God Our Parent and, in the power My Sister The Spirit, I proclaim that these gifts have become the very substance of Jesus My Brother; eat and drink now, reverently, and receive God within you."

> *The lady in purple dances smiles, tears and love*
> *With a movement divine caught from Heaven above*
> *In a dance that embraces, forgives and amends*
> *In a dance that you know never ends.*

Perpetua began the dancing; slow at first then faster. Fidel and Cara followed and then others joined in. Some people said it was even better than the end of the war.

> *O lady in purple in purple*
> *You shimmer and shine*

As the sun went down the sky turned purple like something in modern art. It could have been natural; but it went on too long for that. The music was heavenly. It could not possibly have been produced by the few instruments that people were playing. There was amazing freedom and energy because so many people were celebrating their cures; telling each other what had happened to them. When the dancing had reached a high level of energy, Perpetua slipped away, saying that she had some thankyous of her own to make.

The next morning Fidel and Cara set up their day club.

"What do you want it to do?" asked Perpetua.

"We want it to help people to share. To share each other and to share what we have with people outside."

"The first point is very important. Communities are about working with and loving difference. Traditionally communities were made up of all kinds of people but now we have 'communities of interest' and 'communities of practice'; but they are not really communities at all; they exclude difference and celebrate; if that is the word; sameness. There is no creativity, no risk, no oddity, no friction, no challenge, no fusion. And how will you decide who should receive your giving?"

"We don't like the idea of deciding. We wish it could just happen."

"That is an excellent starting point."

"But we realise that you can't just go up to the top of a skyscraper and throw money into the street; and hope that the right people get it. So you have to start somewhere."

"The first thing that is important is not to give money instead of giving yourself; as a kind of buying yourself out of responsibility. Give to those around; those you can reach; make them part of an extending community. Today we here so much about community but that is because our social values and public policies are deeply against the formation of community. We are a society based on competition and consumerism and we keep on talking about community. So, good; giving your heart and your time to people who are difficult or different is even more important than the money.

"I suppose the best starting point for deciding who should receive is to think of the people you do not like. Giving should be for the receiver not for the giver. Here is an example. People give to the organisation that provides blind people with dogs. They care about the blind people a little; but what they really like are the lovely honey coloured dogs. They do not like giving to ex-offenders who need to be helped not to re-offend because they are unpopular. So a good starting place for people with that choice is to give to the organisation for ex-offenders."

"We think that is a brilliant idea."

The lady in purple smiles wide as the sky
with the set of her head and the gleam in her eye
with a smile that is equal to strangers and friends:
with a smile that you know never ends

As She was coming out of the flats, Perpetua was almost knocked down by a kid rushing along the street.

"Sorry," She said "I thought you would slow down."

He obviously hadn't heard. She walked past him but then turned round and faced him on the pavement so that he had to stop.

"You were so busy talking into your phone that you almost knocked me over."

"Sorry."

"What does that mean? Do you mean that you are sorry that you almost knocked me over; or sorry that I am now keeping you from your mobile phone?"

"What?"

"What is your name?"

"Rick."

"Rick, could you concentrate for a few moments."

"Why?"

"Because I am talking to you."

"Who are you?"

"Perpetua. That is a little better. A question at last. I am many things: first of all, I am a human being, I am your sister; secondly, I am part of the place where you live, I am part of your community; thirdly, I am the person you almost knocked over."

"Sorry. I was doing something else."

"What were you doing?"

"It's obvious; I was talking to somebody."

"So the person you were talking to was more important than the person in your street?"

"My girl."

"An interesting concept 'my girl'; but we will not worry about that for now. What is her name?"

"Violet."

"Violet will be there even if you do not talk so much to her; and I am here.

"I see you have a media player in your belt. I suppose you listen to that when you are not on the phone."

"Yes."

"One way or another the phone or the player or your hurry means that you do not have time for the real people around you."

"They're boring."

"How would you know? Am I boring?"

"Sorry."

"How do you think you will ever have a proper relationship with Violet if you are not connected with a large number of other people? Do you think that Violet, no matter how beautiful, charming, gifted and sensitive, will be able to stand in for all the other people around you? Is Violet the world? Is that not a rather unreasonable set of demands you intend to make of her?"

"What? I've got to go."

"Send her a message that you have to stay."

"Why?"

"Because you need to meet some friends in your community."

She took his arm and steered him into the flats.

"Cara and Fidel. This is Rick. He needs your help."

"He can have what he needs."

"He does not need your money; in fact I think he will contribute to many of your good causes; but if you do not help him he will fall out with the girl he loves."

"We can't have that," said Cara.

"How do you know?"

"Because I have told you. You are asking too much of this girl; and perhaps she is asking the same too much of you. You might want to think about what you are trying to give to each other instead of asking so much."

"I don't ask. She's got anorexia."

"I do not suppose that you do make direct demands on her; but you expect her to behave in a certain way; to be with you 24 hours of the day, in your bed, by your side, on the phone. She cannot live up to what you expect. She loves you but it is so hard to please you entirely from her own resources when she is as cut off as you are from other resources. The situation becomes impossible for her. Why not ask Violet to come over here?"

"I've seen girls like that," said Cara "and the answer is to help them to meet all kinds of different people. All they see in life and the media are people that look like them; they stop seeing other kinds of people; they just filter them out. They need to re-learn that there are nice fat people as well as rather unpleasant thin people."

After Perpetua had said hello to Violet she left them to it. Fidel and Cara were trying to decide on a project that the new day club could work on. They chose the nearby prison for practical work and decided on a poor country for fund raising. Rick knew all about oil countries. Violet had been a volunteer in an Indian slum. Fidel had fought in Vietnam before escaping to England. Cara had been born in Jamaica and had spent her time, and many holidays afterwards, learning about different peoples. Rick knew about financial management. Violet knew about making posters. Fidel wrote short sentences. Cara put warmth and humour into Fidel's drafts. Rick talked about water shortages. Violet talked about seeds. Fidel wrote a logical proposal. Cara made the proposal compelling. Rick didn't know that Violet knew about seeds and Violet didn't know that Rick knew about water. There had been a series of horrible bomb scares in London which, everybody said, had something to do with Islamists; so they wanted, as a matter of principle, to give the money to an Islamic organisation instead of a Christian church. They disliked the idea of sending something in a package; so they wanted to support a well digger in Yemen. Already they had too many good causes. Rick knew how to weight and score so that priorities could be ranked.

Rick got his work/life balance almost right. Violet started to eat properly. The two 'outsiders' and the resident group never found it easy to get on; but they worked at it and saw the benefit. Rick was too pushy. Violet was too fussy. Fidel was too military. Cara was too soppy. Most members of the day club were too vague. They said they would do something but hardly ever delivered on time. Rick pushed. Violet worried. Fidel pulled. Cara soothed.

The two couples were married by Bill Midway at a joint ceremony. It had become the day club's third project; and the one they enjoyed most. Rick looked after money. Violet looked after presentation. Fidel was responsible for groom matters and, as Violet's mother was not interested, Cara looked after the feminine side. There were too many cars; too many Violet-clad bridesmaids supervised by Perpetua in a stunning purple outfit; too many flowers; too many photographers; too many guests; and too much food. The only thing that was lacking were presents. The four had agreed that instead of presents contributions should be made to the Islamic well digger in a 'terrorist' infested part of Yemen.

As She sat minutely observing the extended families meeting; not each other but themselves; somebody asked whether Perpetua would change some water into wine.

"It will not run out," She said "with Fidel in charge; but I think I can make a more substantial change."

She went to the top table where Violet's mother and father were separated by Fidel's brother and Cara's sister.

"Iris," She said "why are you separated from your husband?"

"If it's any of your business, he doesn't love me."

"How do you know?"

"I just do."

"Have you asked him?"

"Of course not. If he says he does he will be lying."

"How do you know?"

"What difference does it make?"

"Parents who will not speak to each other are launching their daughter's marriage on a sea of discord. How do you suppose she will be better off if she sees you as an example of marriage?"

"She knows what we're like. Anyway, she has always taken her father's side."

Perpetua went round the back of the top table.

"I am sorry to see you so far away from Iris. It is not good for Violet. In any case Iris knows that you love her; and you know that believing her when she says she does not love you is an excuse for being passive; for walking away."

"I suppose."

"Well, Jason, it's time to set out on your journey again by going round the table and setting a good example to your lovely daughter."

Trina could not remember a photo shoot being so transformed as when Jason, without a word, lifted Iris out of her chair and placed her gently on his knee because when Violet saw what had happened her smile was unbelievable.

"After that," Perpetua said "the water and wine thing is a bit trivial."

The day club faltered when they left for their honeymoons but Perpetua dropped in; Andy offered some financial know-how; and Kylie liked going there. On this earth nobody lives happily ever after; but there was enough fuel in all sorts of tanks for a long journey. Of course it did not all end happily ever after; or, anyway, not yet.

Part of being poor is being ignored. The story of the Paradise Common cures and the party that followed became part of the daily conversation of the Commoners but the media were not interested. They are only interested in marginalised people when they cause trouble; not demonstrations, like, but real, real trouble. The poor are full of unkept secrets. There is something about this in the Ethnographic module of media studies.

> *The lady in purple dances smiles, tears and love*
> *With a movement divine caught from Heaven above*
> *In a dance that embraces, forgives and amends*
> *In a dance that you know never ends.*
> *O lady in purple you shimmer and shine*
> *like a bowl filled with fruit and a glass filled with wine*
> *like the banner that waves with the hope of release*
> *like the heavenly princess of peace.*
> *Like the heavenly princess of peace.*

Six

When the party's over
and your friends have gone
when your girl friend throws you out
and you're all alone
when the cupboard's empty
and the telly breaks
when you see the mess you're in
and are trapped in mistakes:
When the music shatters
and the window smears
when a prospect flares ahead
and then disappears
when the silence presses
and your heart beat pounds
when your eyes glaze over and over
and you can't see the ground:
After all there is love
After everything has gone
After all there is love
It just goes on and on.
When love breaks and enters
all the windows clear
light knifes its way through deepest darkness
and you see hopes appear;
Love is more than a second chance
More than being let back in
more than a fire beckoning
love is the place you begin:
After all there is love
After everything has gone
After all there is love
It just goes on and on.
Love is building castles
that rise and never fall
love is giving everything
to find you still have it all:
After all there is love
After everything has gone

After all there is love
It just goes on and on.

When the party's over
and your friends have gone
when your girl friend throws you out
and you're all alone
when the cupboard's empty
and the telly breaks
when you see the mess you're in
and are trapped in mistakes:

One afternoon when they were at Stumpy Knoll Perpetua asked

"Who do people say that I am?"

"You can see the coverage," said Trina "the press clippings and news items and the coverage on our own god4u network. Some people say you are a social reformer; some even say that you are an anarchist. In the Christian churches they say you are a negative force and some magazines say you are some kind of white witch."

"But who do you say that I am?"

"I believe that You are what You say that You are; God's Sacred Vessel."

"Are you having some kind of identity crisis?" asked Dexter.

"No. I just want to know how the mission that we are undertaking together is progressing."

"I'm sorry," said Dexter "I should not have asked that question? I find it difficult."

"Of course you do. I have never said it is easy."

"When I was a kid we learned to say our prayers and recite the Ten Commandments and we went to Sunday School; but I think it was to give mum an hour's break on a Sunday morning. She needed it. It makes it difficult to say what Trina has said when my grasp of basic religion is so shaky. When I'm with You, it's easy; I can say that You are a special messenger or a special part of God. I can even say that You are God; just by being with You and listening to You; but when we're apart I find it really difficult to capture that; it seems to trickle or drift away."

"I know. Remember Peter's difficulty. Humanity is equipped to recognise God Our parent; but it gets shoved into a cupboard by the frenetic way we live. We find it difficult to recognise each other let alone God; so when I say that I am a special Child of God, people find it difficult to see."

They were still having this discussion when they were approached by a small group of people carrying banners: "Justice for all" and "Justice Now!"

"We thought You were interested in social justice," one of them said, aggressively. Immediately Dexter reverted to type; he got all mean, like, and looked as if he was going to hit the man at the front of the group.

"It's all right, Dexter. Those who are not against us are with us; we just have to work out what we have in common with them. Hello, you are Lefty, I think?"

"Yes."

"A handy name. I think I have seen you selling the Proletarian in the Hypo car park."

"Yes."

"That cannot be much fun."

"No."

"How can we help you?"

"You could stop all that mumbo jumbo about God and fight for social justice."

"Jesus My Brother stood up for the poor."

"Yes, I know all that stuff about bringing good news to the poor; but when He died they were no better off than before; they were still the victims of oppression."

"Tell me something about this justice you want."

"You can see that we are poor and we want proper housing and jobs and when we are in jobs we want a fair wage."

"Do you want justice for all as some kind of collateral benefit that happens to arise because you have got justice for yourselves? If you had justice for yourselves how much would you be concerned about justice for others? I say that the place to start is not with an abstract idea of justice for all. The place to start certainly is not the idea of justice for yourselves which might just benefit other people but might not. The place to start is by being just in our own lives. We must be just to each other; no matter how little we can give. Justice is born of sacrifice."

"We have no choice; we are always making sacrifices."

"The only kind of sacrifice that is genuine is one where we make the choice. When we are forced to do something that hurts us it is not a sacrifice at all; it is a hardship."

When the music shatters
and the window smears
when a prospect flares ahead
and then disappears

"Hardship; sacrifice. This is playing with words. It does not matter who gets justice first; it's indivisible. Until everybody has justice nobody has justice."

"That is a wonderful theory to be advanced by people who are not in touch with God Our Parent; but that kind of indivisible justice is only available in the Kingdom of God."

"Opium."

"A strange word in contemporary circumstances."

"This is rich people justifying poverty by saying that the poor can look forward to what You call Heaven."

"Let us start at the beginning. The Kingdom is now. People do not have to wait for death before having a profound experience of the love of God Our parent.

"You say that you want equality; although you make a rather poor start by calling for justice for yourselves first. Perhaps I am being a little harsh but that is how it sounds. It is not possible to have equality without freedom."

"Right wing claptrap."

"I admit, Lefty, that it sounds right wing; but justice is what we grant to each other in freedom. The freedom comes from the way we are created so that we can love freely. Strictly speaking justice is not for us to grant or withdraw as it is God's justice; but God has created us to choose to be just or unjust; to love or not to love. That is the essence of what we are. We proclaim that justice for other people because we are all equally children of God Our Parent. The two ideas are like two parts of a sentence; but the order has to be this way: freedom proclaims that we are all equal under God Our Parent as children; from that freedom we recognise the merit of justice; but the core of being human is to be free."

"We're finished, then."

"We are just starting. To be free and not to proclaim justice is to choose the wrong course; to deny love."

"So will you come on our demo."

"That depends on why you are demonstrating and what for. Just to wave a banner and shout slogans is not enough; although it helps to dissipate your understandable frustration. Let us meet later and see how we can work something out."

> *when the silence presses*
> *and your heart beat pounds*
> *when your eyes glaze over and over*
> *and you can't see the ground:*

Some of the core group were involved in a fierce dispute when Perpetua went away with Lefty. (No taped record; technology!).

"It's all right for Perpetua to talk all spiritual but we won't change anybody's mind unless we have something concrete to offer."

"You can see it from Lefty's point of view even if he is a bit rough and slightly selfish; he wants something now."

"If Perpetua wanted to do something She could make everybody equal right now; like that."

After all there is love
After everything has gone
After all there is love
It just goes on and on.

"I can guess what you are saying," She said "so let me tell you a story.

"On the planet Janus there was a state of terrible injustice and dissent. There was violence and despair."

"Worse than here? Worse than America?" I asked.

"Worse than you can imagine. So there arose a creature on Janus who saw that things needed to change. Everybody called the creature 'Our Good Leader'. They were happy to give up their freedom so that they could be happy and secure. The violence decreased and inequalities were diminished. After a while people grew comfortable with the new situation and after a few generations no creature could remember a time when it had not been this way. There was no real understanding of freedom any more. They re-named their planet Optima and celebrated its virtues; but after a while they forgot how to celebrate. They forgot how to make a difference between days of celebration and days when they did not celebrate. There was no room for giving and no room for being good. There were no causes requiring sacrifice. Optima's spirit died. The creatures were not like humanity any more; we would think of them as something like angels."

When love breaks and enters
all the windows clear
light knifes its way through deepest darkness
and you see hopes appear

"That is the kind of world that Lefty was talking about; and it is the kind of world you were thinking about when I came in. It is superficially attractive; but it is not enough. Think for a moment about how many rich people you know who have nice houses and safe jobs. It would be foolish to deny that there is not a correlation between poverty and crime; but what people do not understand is that it is not physical poverty that leads to discontent and crime; it is spiritual poverty. To use one of Lefty's favourite words it is a lack of solidarity. To use my word it is an absence of love. Let us see if I am right."

After all there is love
After everything has gone
After all there is love
It just goes on and on.

People from the margins of society were reluctant to go inside the Civic Centre with its huge shiny but somehow forbidding glass door; but Lefty and Perpetua persuaded about thirty to come in. They asked the Manager if they could bring in some refreshments; and he said that this was not allowed; but he supposed that tea and coffee and biscuits was not really food; so Bob and Kylie brought in some cartons of Hypo instant drinks and biscuits.

"What do you want?" asked Perpetua.

"Some people say we just want houses and hand-outs," said a woman holding a baby "but it's obviously not true. Look what happens when we are put into brand new blocks of flats and given hand-outs; we behave no better than when we were in the old ones with lower benefits; sometimes worse."

"It isn't the houses," said another. "It's the way they do it. We're the fourth richest country in the world and the rich people could give us everything we needed to become respectable; but it's not respectability we want from them it's respect. They complain about taxes and they complain about the 'nanny state' and they tell us to pull ourselves up by our own boot straps when we have no boots. They don't see us as people; they pass us in the street as if we were invisible; but of course they don't want to pass us in the street so they separate themselves more and more from us until they can pretend that we're not there."

"We aren't there," said a scruffy looking man. "As far as they are concerned. That is the root of the problem. It doesn't matter what they give us in their mean spirited way; they can give us everything we want but it won't be enough."

"Politicians keep talking about the 'Respect Agenda' which means we are supposed to respect the people who despise us."

"That is entirely correct," replied Perpetua "and I recognise how difficult that is; but we must respect people; I would use the word 'love' whether they respect and love us or not. All the same I agree that this is very one-sided. They have less excuse than us; although I do not want us to take advantage of that excuse. We must deny ourselves the opportunity; we must make sacrifices to reach those who despise us."

As people do at these things, they split into groups with flip charts. As he went round the room Lefty got more and more uncomfortable. Thinking of what happens in that building he looked like a candidate counting votes knowing he was going to lose an election. Perpetua sat in a corner talking to people who came to talk to Her. You see the charts were not full of words like houses and wages; they all boiled down to three things:

- Respect
- Sacrifice
- Love.

"Well, Perpetua, I'm a fair man. You've won hands down. I'll think about it."

"Not quite; watch!"

Love is building castles
that rise and never fall
love is giving everything
to find you still have it all:

"Just watch," She said. The people were still in their groups. Kylie came in with a huge Hypo box of children's purple building blocks. Other boxes followed. People began to build, cautiously. You could hear comments like

"If you put that there, the whole lot will crash!"

"Their tower is higher than ours."

"Look how quick they are."

and

"We're winning!"

"You see," said Perpetua "how it starts."

Then something strange happened.

It didn't matter how high bricks were piled, no matter how thin the towers or narrow the bases, no matter how crazy the construction, nothing fell over. After a while people could see that there was no need to compete; everything was just cool.

"Isn't this like Optima?" asked Trina.

"No. Optima is a permanent state of being, this is just an interlude, a way of telling people that they can work together and build, that they can learn about the Kingdom where there is no competition, to put earthly competition into perspective. It's the sign that counts. This is a sign of love. Love is about building together."

After all there is love
After everything has gone
After all there is love
It just goes on and on.

when the silence presses
and your heart beat pounds
when your eyes glaze over and over
and you can't see the ground:

As the sun set in another of those modern arty sort of purple skies, they walked to The Stump Tavern. Perpetua sat with a man who looked very distressed.

"I wish you would perform a real miracle," he said "instead of playing with bricks."

"What kind of miracle? What do you want?"

"My wife is dying of cancer. I don't know what to do. Part of me wants to be with her; part of me can't stand being with her; part of me wants to love her; part of me wants to get drunk; part of me wants her to live; part of me just wants it to be over."

"Do you believe that I can cure her?"

"It isn't like it was in the time of Jesus. I know what I am supposed to say; I am a sophisticated postmodern person; so it's easy for me to say I have faith."

"It does not matter what you say; it is what you believe. I do not have to know that. Anything I do is through the power of God Our Parent. I am only the Sacred Vessel; I try to draw down the loving power of our Parent to bring peace to all God's children. I think that when you get home you will find that your wife has taken a turn for the better."

When love breaks and enters
all the windows clear
light knifes its way through deepest darkness
and you see hopes appear:

She look straight into his eyes.

"You can never tell with cancer. God be with you."

As he went out, trying not to to hurry, an anxious looking man walked in.

"You should not be here," he said to Perpetua. "You have been invited to preach at our Chapel on Sunday; highly irregular; but it will not be possible if you are seen in here."

"You must be Pastor Drone. I am sorry that you do not approve of The Stump."

"It's the people."

"How can you be a pastor if you do not like people?"

"I do like people."

"I wonder whether you only want to be a pastor to the people you like. But how can that be a way out? You have a dwindling congregation and a leaking roof which must be a worry for you. Why not consider reaching out to the the congregation of the whole world and abandoning the roof?"

"Look over there at those sinners."

"Pastor, I am sorry, I do not think you heard what I have just said. They are children of God Our Parent."

"They are shameless, openly flouting the Word of God."

"Ah, Pastor, openly, that is an interesting idea. I presume you accept that we all fall short but some of us are better at keeping our 'sinfulness' secret. We also have to remember, Pastor, that for every prostitute there is a pimp and a stream of clients. What do you think of their sins? Just because you only see these women it is wrong to conclude that they are the only 'sinners'. Like Jesus My Brother, I came to be a pastor to sinners just as He said that the sick needed physicians."

"There are Government services for these people. They should use them."

"How would the sinners have fared if Jesus had abandoned them and left them to the Pharisees?"

"It is not like that now. People have so many opportunities and benefits. It is my job; and the people in my Chapel agree with me; to maintain a high standard of morality in our society."

"But, Pastor, it has to be a morality based on love not judgment."

"Well, that is a liberal point of view. I am sorry that we extended an invitation but it is too late now."

"Stay for a drink, Pastor."

"The work of the devil."

"If that is the worst the devil can do I am not worried; but the devil is turning your head away."

He had a small sherry, drinking it fast and slow at the same time, looking and not looking at the people.

"When you have finished your drink we will go and talk to those ladies."

He stopped drinking.

"That will only delay the moment," said Perpetua. "Come on."

She dragged Pastor Drone over to a table by the door where two women were sitting.

"Good evening ladies. How is trade?"

"Not good."

"What are your names?"

"Real or trade?"

"Whatever you prefer."

319

"I'm Stella and she's Lucia."

"Very nice."

"Better than Anne and Mary."

"Those, too, are nice in their different ways."

"Are you some kind of social worker trying to get us off the streets?"

"No. I want to listen to you; and my friend here also wants to listen."

"He doesn't look as if he does."

"Never mind; help him to overcome his discomfort."

"He doesn't need to be uncomfortable. We know all there is to know about men. You don't suppose we're proud of what we're doing, do you? And as for him, I'm what he calls a 'common prostitute' because his organist is a fraud. He used to be a fast bloke. He made promises to me; got me pregnant and then threw me out; changed his name and his outside appearance; and now he goes nice and respectable to play the organ. If I were you I would tell your Chapel women to watch out!"

"What about you?"

"My boy friend said he loved me but he got me on heroin and then I discovered he was a dealer and a pimp. I think I might have been able to kick the habit but I was so depressed by what he did that I just sank deeper and deeper. I can't get out and I'm tied to a man who lied to me, made me an addict and now forces me to have sex with customers and with him."

"What are we to do, Pastor? I think that if the people of the Chapel will not reach out to these people they will have to come in. Will you come and listen to me on Sunday evening?"

"Why not? An hour won't make a difference."

She did not preach at the Chapel; She told a story:

"Once upon a time there was a good man who was full of love for all people. He was deeply loved by his congregation. The Chapel was a place of peace. One day as the Pastor was preaching he noticed a woman wearing a sleeveless top. He had a quiet word with her so as not to cause embarrassment. She never came again. He had a similar word with a man who had come to church straight from his allotment in gardening clothes. He never came again. And as time went by the congregation dwindled. The fewer there were the fewer of them seemed to fit. The roof began to leak. In the end there was no congregation and the Pastor moved away with a heavy heart. The windows of the Chapel were boarded up. Squatters; beggars and addicts; moved in. They had a home but it was not a spiritual home. They looked in lucid moments at the books and wondered what they were all about. They kept seeing the name Jesus and wondered what it meant."

When She had finished Pastor Drone thanked Perpetua and asked Her to lead the congregation in a prayer. Slow; nervous; he walked down the aisle and stood between Stella and Lucia dressed in purple.

Love is building castles
that rise and never fall
love is giving everything
to find you still have it all:
After all there is love
After everything has gone
After all there is love
It just goes on and on.

Seven

Gather round,
all the outcasts of the nations
join the throng
of all the souls that thirst for life
sing a song
for the road that lies before you
tell the world
that the freedom bell has rung:
There's only one road to freedom
There's only one song for the joy of life
There's only one love that sets us free:
the only road to freedom is heaven.
Gone at last
the oppression of the mighty
sunk to nothing
all the highness of the great
smashed to dust
all the towers of the tyrants
brought to us
all the tribute they have lost:
And when you're on the road
carry for the children
and when you see their load
carry it all
until they grow when you
hand over easy
and still be prepared to
lift them when they fall:
Love the journey
with all the gifts we have been given
love the struggle
to make them count for everyone
love the struggle
to bring back the stony-hearted
love the freedom
of the road we're travelling on:
There's only one road to freedom
There's only one song for the joy of life

There's only one love that sets us free:
the only road to freedom is the road to heaven.

Gather round,
all the outcasts of the nations
join the throng
of all the souls that thirst for life

"Who is in your life?" She asked a man on a crumbling bench.

"Nobody much now. They left one by one. There's nobody now."

"What is your name?"

"Max."

"Would you like a cup of tea, Max?"

"Thanks."

"Shall we go over there to the Paradise Cafe?"

"No. I don't go in there anymore."

"Why?"

"They threw me out. I'm banned."

"Come with me.

"Two cups of tea, please."

"We don't mind you but he can't come in."

"Why not?"

"He upsets the customers."

"We can ask them. Hello, do any of you mind this man sitting with me?"

There was an embarrassed shuffling but nobody said anything.

"These customers don't seem to mind."

"Well I mind."

"But that is very different from your customers minding."

"Look; it's my place and I don't want him in here. And who are you to come round interfering? Jesus Christ?"

"A good question. What did he do to upset you or your customers?"

"He was rude and I don't like that."

"You are being rude and I don't like that either but we have to learn to love all kinds of people who we think are being rude. If you do not change your attitude you will have no customers at all."

"I'll take that risk."

She looked round at the people. They began to get up.

"No," she said "do not disturb yourselves. You have made the point. This man is a good man. He just needs to think a little about what it means to own a community centre; to keep an open door. Are you going to serve us?"

"All right; but he better behave himself."

"Ask him. By the way, his name is Max."

"Will you behave yourself, Max?"

"Of course. I am sorry that I upset you and your customers that time. I was under a great deal of stress. Have you ever been under stress?"

"Yes, of course."

"What did you do?"

"I got drunk."

"So did I but I got drunk and came in here because I had nowhere else to go. I suppose you got drunk at home?"

"Yes."

They went into a corner. People looked at them for a few minutes but then got bored and turned back to their own concerns.

"Do you want to tell me about yourself Max?"

"It isn't very difficult. I was a banker. I was wealthy. I had many people who said they were my friends. I had a beautiful wife. My bank was taken over. I was thrown out. I had spent over my income as most people do. I went bankrupt. My wife left me. I lost my home. I began to drink. In the end I was in a filthy little flat. I'm lucky in a way; I'm still there now; but without vodka I can't stand it. I compare it with the big house. I sometimes prefer the street."

"Do you really not have any friends now?"

"I suppose Brod is a friend. He hangs on to me because I'm a failed banker and he thinks my luck will change. But I suppose he's a friend. He's the only person I can talk to or, rather, he talks to me."

"What about Jesus My Brother?"

"I used to say my prayers to a kind of fairytale Jesus but He faded out as I got into my teens."

"This is so sad Max. I hear this all the time. People work at their lessons and their skills and their friendships but seem to think their friendship with Jesus will just work and grow automatically; and then it disintegrates."

"It's all so distant."

"But if Jesus walks towards you and you keep on walking away from Him what can you expect?"

"But I haven't walked anywhere."

"Doing nothing is a decision. It is in reality a walking away even if indifference feels like standing still. Better to shout at your friend than turn your back."

"What can I do?"

"The first thing is to recognise that Jesus as part of the Godhead is not a theory. God Our Parent is not an abstract idea. Who would choose to love and worship a theory? It is the love of theories that has brought the world to where it is now. You were a banker. You know about theories. You never loved economic theories. You used them. That is what happens now with God. People use Godhead as a theory to suit their own ends. It is in competition with other theories; it is unscrupulously used to advance selfish ends. When people say that God 'wants' this or that they are putting themselves above God."

"What must I do."

"You are very lucky. For two thousand years Christians have been trying to know God through the life of Jesus My Brother but it has become ever more difficult for people to understand what He said and did. Theology, science, selfishness, the simple passage of time, have all made things more difficult. It would not have been so difficult if people had tried to maintain a relationship with God Our Parent, Jesus My Brother and My Sister the Spirit but people have put philosophy above trying to grow their relationships with the Godhead in its different aspects. As I say; you are lucky because God Our Parent has sent Me to renew the idea of the personal relationship between God's children as created and their creator. In a way; in talking this way; we are turning the idea of relationship into another theory. Let us go outside and see the world that God created."

sing a song
for the road that lies before you
tell the world
that the freedom bell has rung:

They came to a girl with a baby in a beat up old pram.

"How are you, Marta?"

"I am very nice, Perpetwa; but no money."

"I have brought a friend. He will help you."

"He has money?"

"No; but he will help you manage better. He knows about how to be clever with money."

"I clever; not enough money."

"Of course I will help you," said Max "but what has that to do with what you said earlier about a relationship with God? Anybody can be a financial adviser. There's the Citizen Viability Directorate."

"Yes but in serving the children of God Our Parent you are serving God and being a witness to Jesus My Brother."

"But that means that everybody who does good is supposed to be in a relationship with God."

"You are getting there Max. But do you not think that it is nicer and easier to work within the love of God rather than working in parallel with that love?"

They passed an old man struggling with a large bag of fertiliser. "Going to your allotment, Gordon?"

"Yes."

"Max will carry that for you; and he might undertake a small session of digging; under strict supervision; needless to say. You see Max you have the pleasure of digging away your hangover and Gordon has the pleasure of supervising you. You can both be irritated with each other and then you will learn how to become friends."

"And Jesus?"

"Think of Him while you are digging and being supervised. If you dig in His name you will be blessed. I will see you later Max; and Gordon; be gentle."

> *Gone at last*
> *the oppression of the mighty*
> *sunk to nothing*
> *all the highness of the great*

She joined Dexter, Trina and the others. She told them about Max, Marta and Gordon.

"I want you all to go out into the community and do what I have done. Be gentle and constructive. Talk about your relationship with God Our Parent. If people want to talk about theology do not get into tangles. We are not cut out for that kind of thing. There are plenty of good clergy who can handle these matters."

"But they won't know about You?" said Jim.

"They do not need to know about me. I am preaching The Word of God; helping people to understand that the Kingdom is here. When people hear and see me it might help. By all means tell them what I have said to you but always get back to the essential love of God for all humanity and its purpose of loving God."

"But we are so weak when we are not with you," protested Dexter.

"You will have the strength of the Godhead but remember that a spark of love destroys a den of hate. Be gentle with the mighty and they will fall."

They divided the surrounding area between them and went out in twos and threes to give strength to each other but Dexter got above himself and thought he could manage on his own. Without strong support he found it difficult to control his aggression. He got angry when people said he was a fraud because he could not perform miracle cures. As usual when Perpetua rescued him from his own foolishness he went through a period of deep sadness. Nobody struggled more than him towards understanding God; nobody tried harder to pray; nobody was so up front about admitting when they were wrong.

> *smashed to dust*

all the towers of the tyrants
brought to us
all the tribute they have lost

Mostly the followers came back amazed. They had expected to meet materialist hostility but they were told over and over again how empty people felt. They wanted a spiritual life but the only things on offer seemed to be the grim churches; lifestyle and therapy gurus; or nothing. Some people said they wanted clear answers but most said they needed constructive dialogue. No matter how economically and socially comfortable they were they only seemed to talk to themselves and people like them. Instead of trust there was suspicion and fear; instead of conversation and debate there was confrontation; instead of partnership there was competition.

What upset them most was the deprivation of children.

"Let us go and look," She said.

There's only one road to freedom
There's only one song for the joy of life
There's only one love that sets us free:
the only road to freedom is the road to heaven.

They drove through the night when the roads were empty to get the best value out of the bus. Perpetua was wakened by a shout:

"The brakes have gone!"

They all started shouting. Perpetua looked ahead for a moment and said

"Calm down. There is nothing to worry about. Bob; press gently."

He pressed; the bus slowed. They were relieved and confused. Bob said

"The brakes weren't working; honest."

"They are now. Peace. Peace. Have you learned nothing from the things that I have said and done? Am I just a girly preacher or is God working through me? Have you forgotten the way I have fed the hungry? Do you think that God Our Parent would let me die in a car crash in the middle of the night on a motorway? Look; the sky is purple coming on to dawn. Let us stop and pray."

And when you're on the road
carry for the children
and when you see their load
carry it all

They thought Grunge Park was bad enough but they had never seen anything like Borton before; except for Jo and Beth who had been sent there.

Grunge Park was shabby but it was feisty; Grunge Park was mashed up but Borton was a wreck; Grunge Park had crime but Borton was past it. There was nothing worth burning; nothing worth stealing; nothing worth breaking; nothing worth mending. Most of the houses had been designated unfit for human habitation years ago but there was no new housing.

Media Studies research module Abstract: every scheme for building new houses had been blocked by middle class campaigns. The alternative was to provide temporary housing and completely rebuild the estate but middle class people resisted any attempt to settle the estate people among them. A small group of Councillors who had fought for the people on the estate were thrown out at the last election.

Perpetua knocked on door after door but hardly anybody bothered to come. At last she found a mother with a little girl. They were encouraged by the biscuits She had brought and the mother said she would make a few calls on her pay-as-you-go.

"What do I tell them?"

"Tell them it is a party for adults and children."

"We don't have them."

"Try; just once."

The mother; reluctant; made the calls.

They came slowly; looking like they was trying to hide behind each other.

"Bob will take you for a ride," She told the children. "We all have Child Subjection Clearance. Then we will have a party."

They looked bewildered but Bob was so friendly that they went.

"Now," said Perpetua "we have some peace. Tell me about you.:

The mothers hardly even looked at one another.

"I am going to cry," said Perpetua "unless I can help you find something inside yourselves."

"There is nothing," said one; Libby. "We are the end of the world. God knows what will happen to our poor, half starved, listless, hopeless children. Dads gone, teenagers gone; money never came. Too poor for drugs; too helpless to steal. Telly and chips."

She cry.

When She recover Herself She said

"I know you have so many people who come and preach at you about your lives."

"Not even that; they've given up."

"I have not given up. You are all God's children and you are loved more than the richest people in the land."

"It doesn't feel like it."

"Everybody asks the same question 'How can God love me if I am poor and the other person is rich? God must love the rich person more than the poor person.' This is really difficult and the people who say it is easy are wrong."

until they grow when you
hand over easy
and still be prepared to
lift them when they fall

"We are all children of God but we are not all the same. Because we are human and different and imperfect some prosper and others do not; but that is a sign of our humanity not of whether God loves us or not. God loves most those who suffer from earthly oppression because they most need love."

"We need more than that! What did You come to do?"

"I came to do three things: to listen; to tell us that God loves us; and to remind us that there are things we can do together."

"Like what?"

"Well Libby; you are very brave and articulate. Teach our sisters to be brave and articulate with you. All of us must dredge deep to find out what we can give to each other."

"We have so little," said Mo.

"Watch how when you share a little it will grow. I will come again tomorrow after the children have gone to school. We will go out to the country with the little ones."

The bus came back and smiling children got out. There had been plenty of things to eat and drink on the bus and they had driven round a small wildlife park. There was plenty left for the mothers who were almost frightened by the liveliness of the children.

Next day the mothers and those too young for school (and a few who were not) went into the country. Perpetua was surprised that so few had ever been even though it was only a few miles away. They walked through fields and had lunch at a country pub before they came back to the school gates.

"It's a bit pathetic," said Brian.

"You have missed the point. We are here to bring hope; to help people to work together. When we go back they will remember us and over time they will come to see Jesus through what we do. Giving them everything they want and then going away would be trivial."

After a week of constant visits and long discussions in which the women talked more and Perpetua talked less the atmosphere was completely different. They had set up a discussion group; found out what skills they had between them; and had learned the Our Father. Digging up a childhood memory a mother suggested they should organise a nativity play. This pleased everyone because it would mean dressing up. Where would they perform it?

"We hate the so-called 'Community Centre" said Libby "because it isn't ours. There were so many rules at first; and then cuts; and then vandals; and then nothing."

Love the journey
with all the gifts we have been given
love the struggle
to make them count for everyone

On the last day of her visit Perpetua took Libby with her to a nearby church where she had been asked to preach. She was met at the door by a small welcoming party who didn't seem to like the look of Libby.

"She's with me," said Perpetua "so it is all or nothing; I am afraid. I thought that the Church of England was open to all not a gathered church of the faithful. In any case what do you know about Libby's faithfulness?"

It was the angriest that anybody had ever seen her

"I have just been on the nearby estate and seen poverty that should be impossible in our rich country. I have obviously seen financial poverty but this is coupled with poverty of expectation and ambition. There are Children of God Our Parent living less than a mile from here who do not feel that they are part of society. They have been abandoned by the public authorities; by voluntary organisations; by churches and worst of all by you. Usually when I talk about problems I say what 'we' need to do because that is a polite way of speaking but on this occasion you are responsible.

"Our country is so rich that Champagne is part of our General Retail Analysis Basket. We spend three times as much on Champagne alone as would be needed to eliminate officially defined child poverty. What are you doing filling these people with despair by your indifference and then complaining when some of them turn to crime as an expression of their frustration? The people I have met like Libby are so worn down they are even past addiction and crime; they live in the middle of nowhere."

love the struggle
to bring back the stony-hearted
love the freedom
of the road we're travelling on

Before she left Perpetua went to the local Hypo and asked to talk to the Manager Mr Hide. He wasn't pleased to see her.

"I've heard about You from Annie Price and some of Your people have infiltrated my store."

"We will not argue about that at the moment. I propose that when people come to your tills with luxury goods they are asked whether they would like to make a contribution to reduce child poverty."

"We have to be very careful about supporting charities. If we give to one the others will object."

"But children?"

"It's difficult. We've just finished a big appeal for the donkey sanctuary; it went very well indeed; so people might have compassion fatigue."

"Compassion fatigue!"

"I am sorry; I can't help you."

She stood outside the main door and said to people coming in" "Good news for the poor; give to children; good news for the poor."

The on-screen arrays at check-outs had changed from their usual configuration and the blue/grey background was now a vivid purple and when people came to check out every cash register asked the question automatically repeated by the staff; lots were Perpetua's people; whether they wanted to make a contribution to abolishing child poverty. It would be rung on the till and shown on their bill. At the same time when poor people got through check-out they found a discount marked on their bill. The operation went so smoothly that it was more than two hours before anything happened; the check-out staff worked like automatons; the generous thought this was a novel way of giving; and the poor dared not go back to check although Perpetua found that some poor people had donated and got a discount.

> *There's only one road to freedom*
> *There's only one song for the joy of life*
> *There's only one love that sets us free:*
> *the only road to freedom is the road to heaven.*

The major alert came when Corporate Centre began to detect a strange pattern of small movements payments and discounts that did not link with stock; but the transactions kept cancelling themselves out and having no effect on the overall ledger. When Mr. Hide came out of his office at last he was very angry.

"I suppose it's you with your do-gooding that has messed up our systems."

"Mr. Hide; I think it would take more than a little good intention to effect the changes you have finally detected. Do not worry. Everything will balance; but just see how easy it is to help. There are many generous people waiting to be asked; and a clever little programme can always analyse the purchasing patterns of the poor. But" She said turning to her followers "this simple sign from God Our Parent is not the end but the beginning. You have seen that the poor need solidarity as well as money. In the end we cannot buy ourselves out of the responsibility for our sisters and brothers. Mr. Hide; talk to my friends and see if you cannot organise a little scheme to link your organisation with the Borton Estate. They need you; you are a good and honest man."

He looked shocked but nodded slowly.

"And by the way God Our Parent will look after the donkeys."

Gather round
all the outcasts of the nations
Gone at last
the oppression of the mighty
Love the journey
The only road to freedom is the road to heaven
is the road to heaven

Eight

When the night is fearful
and the words are sharp
when you know it's over
and there's nothing but dark;
when they're all against you
and the insults fly
when you're all for turning your back
so they don't see you cry:
Everywhere you go
everything you do
everything you say and think
There's only one you.
When the anger's over
and you're all alone
when the days get longer and longer
and nothing feels like home;
when the footstep frightens
and all voices jar
when being alone is the best you can do
and you forget who you are:
No matter how loud the hostile crowd
no matter the pain to make the gain
no matter how rare the simple prayer
no matter how long love will keep you strong.
Love is not a question
but an answering light
even if you don't find what you look for
the question makes you bright;
love is always giving
and taking without pride
love is always the space made for others
not the small space inside:
Everywhere you go
everything you do
everything you say and think
There's only one you.

When the night is fearful
and the words are sharp
when you know it's over
and there's nothing but dark;

This is the most difficult thing I have ever done. Living it has been difficult, writing it has been worse; but I know it has to be done, that there is no alternative, that there is no turning back.

The first time I ever saw Perpetua, she did not see me. I was in the crowd when she performed what I can only think of as a waterless baptism. There was a cross made of fragments of glass and other rubbish and it was bathed in intense yellow light. We met on and off after that but I found her freelance, somewhat cavalier, approach to Christianity highly irritating; but she was always cheerful and polite and seemed to do more good than harm. Then she took most of my congregation, saying that the Christian churches, including the Roman Catholic Church, were too introverted. I grudgingly agreed with the analysis but her action hurt me deeply. I had less and less to live for.

I knew right from the beginning that she knew my secret and that it was safe. My poor congregation were not worldly wise enough to see what she saw. Right at the beginning when she insisted on buying me a drink in the local pub, she followed my eyes which could not conceal what was happening. Then there was the strange incident with the—shall we say—adult magazines. She somehow knew what I was carrying but when I got home they had been replaced by worship materials in respect of the Blessed Virgin Mary.

when they're all against you
and the insults fly
when you're all for turning your back
so they don't see you cry

Shortly after that she persuaded me to spend a day with Her. It wasn't the routine, inculturated antipathy which made it difficult to accept; I knew we were going to have some sort of catharsis.

We went in my lovely old Volkswagen Beetle out into the countryside. She knew I liked walking. "I was going to choose your favourite walk, Father," she said, in her light but deliberatively formal, half-Caribbean prose "but as both of us know what we must talk about may be painful, I don't want to spoil your favourite place by inhabiting it with such memories, so I thought it would be best to go somewhere new and not altogether remarkable to which you might not want to pay another visit.

"Tell me about yourself. It is very difficult to get a picture of you from day-to-day gossip and apart from what you would expect, COBBLE says nothing."

I told her I was born in Liverpool of a strict Roman Catholic family which seemed to be fighting a rearguard action against Vatican II. We hated the "trivial" and "immoral" world of Bill Shankley and the Beatles but, worst of all, we thought Pope John XXIII was a traitor. All through my childhood we bemoaned the lost age of the Latin Mass and Solemn Benediction. I was therefore brought up in a house divided between veneration and resentment. What I took from this was a deep love of the traditions of the Church but an element of sadness has always been there. I was lucky to get into Theological College and was ordained in the early '80s when I thought that Roman Catholicism was in terminal decline. I did not feel resentful that I was to dedicate my life to a lost cause; I very strongly felt that Jesus Christ would stand by me if I was brave enough.

"I know," she said. "I can always see the suffering and the bravery in your face."

I told her a little about parish life but there was not so much to tell. I had been in line for a place in a private school for boys but a sharp-eyed member of the care staff had noticed something. Nothing was ever said, let alone written down, and I was 'asked' if I would like a difficult parish. Once, out of the blue, I received an anonymous letter saying: "You're in the right place; the Irish dislike blacks more than queers." She winced.

Everywhere you go
everything you do
everything you say and think
There's only one you.

I thought she was going to ask another question but she just looked kindly at me and walked on in silence for a while. "So brave," she said. "What sacrifices we all have to make when we distort our lives."

I told her I had not intended to do anything with the boys. "I know," she said. "You have far too much self-control for that. I can see that it almost strangles you sometimes."

The problem, I told her, was that the whole tenor of my life and mind, bound up with Holy Mother Church, was as far away as it ever could be from this other feeling. But the more I tried to use the force of my will to shut my feelings in, the more stressful it became. I had begun to exceed the one tot of whiskey I allowed myself of a Sunday evening after Vespers.

She said nothing for a while. "I know," she said at last. "I know."

I hate the word "gay". It's a silly word which used to describe innocent village merriment; and I hate the word "Homosexual" because, being Greek, it

336

sounds like a medical condition. And I hate "Same sex relationship" because it has the word sex in it and I don't even like "Partnership" because it sounds too legal. I like the word "Couple" because that's what my parishioners call themselves. Of course they all pretend to me that they're married, to save my blushes but, whether they are married or not, they still use the word "couple"; it's a word that speaks both about two people being separate and about the physical act of coupling. I like that. Some people say that the Church is against sex but that is not true; it simply believes that when Jesus said that marriage was for life, he meant it. There is some doubt about what He might have thought of sex before marriage in our own time, though there is no doubt what He, as a human being, thought about that during His own time. The problem for the Church of Rome is that it won't make compromises; it still holds to what Jesus said, on sex at least. One wishes it had been as faithful over worldly goods.

Where was I? I was telling Perpetua about why I hated these words.

"But it is what is in your heart that counts, Father, not the words you use."

I wanted to hit back and say that I was a trained Confessor and knew all about that. I was suddenly very angry that we were talking about me in this way.

"You have cause to be angry, Joseph," she said. "The Priest and the Joseph in you have been at war and they are both used to it. In a very strange way, bringing peace between them will not happen until you have been through the anger, anger most of all about what you will think of as wasted years; but they are not. You have been a good Priest; and still are a good and faithful Priest; and whatever you do I know you will stay faithful to Jesus My Brother."

I ignored this last designation which always annoyed me. Who was she to claim any special relationship with Jesus who is brother to us all? Then I wondered about what I had seen of her and had to admit that, special sister or no, she was surely a remarkable young woman.

> When the anger's over
> and you're all alone
> when the days get longer and longer
> and nothing feels like home;
> when the footstep frightens
> and all voices jar
> when being alone is the best you can do
> and you forget who you are

We went to a nice pub and although it was early November we sat outside in our thick clothes, in the pale sun. I supposed I would have to make a choice between my feelings and my vocation.

"Someone as well trained as you, Father, should not make such a simple mistake as that. You should not choose; you should integrate the different parts of yourself; others, sadly, will choose for you. They will tell you that you have to choose; they will make you choose, under duress, and you know that that is no choice at all. They will proclaim the primacy of conscience in Vatican documents and deny it to you. They will say that your conscience cannot be properly informed. They will forget how foolish they were about Galileo and Darwin. For an institution that is 2000 years old, its grasp of history is strangely weak."

> *No matter how loud the hostile crowd*
> *no matter the pain to make the gain*
> *no matter how rare the simple prayer*
> *no matter how long love will keep you strong.*

I knew she was right but she was going faster than I was prepared to go. I knew that there would be a long inner struggle but I did not know the outcome. In the long silences she kept looking round. "I do not know anything about the countryside," she said. "I visit it as a curiosity, the way some people go to the zoo. I do not understand nature but I wonder who does? Who can tell what God Our Parent meant? I doubt, however, that people like you were deliberately created to be unhappy. Individual people have all kinds of crosses to bear, some that they choose, some that they do not choose. But we are not made to be what we are not. If we are born blind, for whatever purpose of God Our Parent, we are not expected to behave as if we can see. If we are created so that we are attracted to people of the same sex, why should we try to be what we are not?"

I told her that I had tried to discuss it once with my Spiritual Director but it was a disaster. "You know the teaching of the Church, Joseph," he said "and you also know that this fad of yours is a dangerous piece of self-indulgence. Let's face it, we know your mother was a tyrant and we know that your four sisters bullied you even though they pretended to adore you. As the youngest of five you did not have an easy life. This tendency you say you have results from the way you were treated by your mother and sisters; you just have an antipathy to women; but it doesn't mean that you have an attraction to men. Thank God this tendency can be reversed. We all have urges of some sort from time to time. Say your prayers and, if you must, look at *Playboy* now and again, but for God's sake be discreet."

She laughed. "Did you look at *Playboy*?" "No," I said; by the time I had worked out how to buy such magazines without detection I didn't think it worth wasting the opportunity to buy what I really wanted; so he did me a favour. She looked grim. "Yes, Joseph, but remember how these magazines are made. It is better for you to fall in love, to have an honest relationship which you can celebrate, than it is to have a vicarious relationship based on the exploitation of boys and young men. I daresay some of them are willing enough but, even if they are, it is a sorry business."

I blushed.

"There is not that much to say about it," she said. "I am always surprised that people find so much to say about it. They are so zealous on behalf of God Our Parent but they turn that commitment and that longing for a sharing in the mystery into moral sound bites."

I said that people needed a moral compass, something to help them deal with the difficult issues in life. "But," she said "do you not see that these sound bites only solve the very simple problems such as: people who have enough should not steal, people who are safe should not kill, people who are unmoved by others should not commit adultery. When it gets difficult and the sound bites are applied it causes all kinds of confusion. That is when it is important to have a muscular conscience and by that I mean a mechanism which is subjected to rigourous training. A fatty conscience is no more use than a puny conscience. No matter what situation people find themselves in, they can always exercise conscience. Sometimes they are wrong but we can only be wrong if we hear what our conscience says and do something different. If we try really hard to listen to our conscience, and if we always exercise a strong preference against what we personally want until such time as we genuinely see that what our conscience dictates and what we want are the same thing, then we will have fulfilled our obligation to God Our Parent. Most Christians believe this but then they play a game saying that a conscience is not well-informed unless some factor over-rides all others.

"That is like, to continue our athletic metaphor, insisting that the way the muscle behaves should be dictated by a drug. It is very difficult to make connections but I somehow feel that the connection between the moral drugs we take that are supposed to save us from ourselves are somehow related to the drugs on the street that are somehow supposed to save us from something. All drugs of this kind, that we go on pumping in to make things easy, are somehow the same. I know this argument would be shot down by doctors and psychologists and, I suppose, theologians, but we need to think about it."

The afternoon was drawing on and although She never pushed me, I was getting tired. I could feel that active muscle of my conscience fighting against all the 'drugs' that had been pumped into it since before I could remember. Of course she knew this. "That is quite enough for today," she said; but then I said something I did not mean to say. I asked why she had not formed any attachments. To an extent, I said, she was like me; she could make all kinds of pronouncements but she had no direct experience.

"That is not so," she said, "on either count. First, I have had many experiences of longing, of wanting to be physically involved with people; and I know you have too. Just because people stay celibate it does not mean that they do not understand the pull of physical love. If they stay celibate they know something of joy and pain but not the joy and pain of the journey. That can help sometimes. The problem with celibate priests is that they try to solve these problems on their own, thinking their moral compass is enough, not understanding the biology and psychology, the social and economic pressures. On the second count, I see no reason why you should not form a physical attachment. Celibate clergy are a strange anomaly. For myself, however, I know that I cannot commit myself because that will involve another who will have to go through intense pain before very long. I was sent here to undertake my mission and then be killed by those I came to save. This is inevitable because only the murder of the Saviour points up the unfathomable depth God has for God's children, created imperfect to choose between not loving and loving. They can only see the starkness and the promise in the ultimate deed.

"Now that really is enough," she said. "I do not like to think about it. I accept that it is inevitable. Let us talk about other things."

What she really liked talking about was the development of small groups where trust could be built and where people could work through their problems together. She said that the current structure of Christianity was so artificial that its decline was inevitable. If people came to church and simply went through a ritual, each in a dialogue with the Priest, and were then sent out to love God and their neighbour, they were being asked the impossible because they were not being taught how to love God and their neighbour while they were in church; they were always being told what they should do but never how. They heard all these stories about fishermen and seed being planted and the obstacles of the Law and Temple worship and it made no sense. And it made less sense to non-churchgoers. "Just ask a person in Grunge Park who is of average intelligence, but who has not been to church, to pick up a Bible and see what sense they can make of it. True, there are people like you to help them make sense of it; but the essence of a church of equality as opposed to a church of hierarchy is that the real effort should be in doing what we ought to do not in working out what these books tell us we ought to do."

I asked, no longer horrified, if that meant she renounced the Bible. "No," she said, "but there is a point in history, as there is with Shakespeare, when the Bible stops being a common source of inspiration and becomes the object of scholarship; and at that point hierarchy kicks in; and it is not long before the honest pursuit of scholarship turns into the exercise of power. That is one of the things that happened with the Jewish tradition, so Jesus My Brother added a contemporary layer of the understanding of God and I hope and believe that people will write the equivalent of Gospels about me so that that will form another contemporary layer. It is like geology; the later does not invalidate the earlier which is the foundation; and, as I have said before, there may be other layers to come when Planet Earth is very different. Just think how little we know of what it will be like even fifty years from now."

> *Love is not a question*
> *but an answering light*
> *even if you don't find what you look for*
> *the quest makes you bright;*
> *love is always giving*
> *and taking without pride*
> *love is always the space made for others*
> *not the small space inside:*
> *Everywhere you go*
> *everything you do*
> *everything you say and think*
> *There's only one you.*

In the weeks after our long talk I sometimes thought it had not happened as I said the routine things and went to the routine meetings; and as habit was such a strong force in me I could take great comfort in the Eucharist as if the talk had never happened. But at other times it cut deep. It made me look at boys in general and one in particular in a quite different light, with the vague, distant prospect of possibility. Then I would go through the struggle and it usually ended up with the whiskey bottle. When I went through these dark periods I thought of going back to talk to her again but I never did. I saw her often enough, sometimes in almost comical situations like the time I led a kind of demonstration against her when she was holding a big service in the Civic Centre. We were accusing her of taking people away from Christian (well, no, Catholic) churches but she did not argue, she laughed, not at us but, in the end, with us. She turned our rather grumpy little manifestation into something joyful.

> *love is always giving*
> *and taking without pride*
> *love is always the space made for others*
> *not the small space inside*

I never forgot what she said about her future and I prayed for her every day but what happened yesterday finished me off. It is, honestly, the first time in my life I have tasted alcohol on Good Friday. Her last hour was on television as if she was just another episode in the endless opera that is not soap but is filth.

That is why you found me, stupefied, on the floor when you came back last night for whatever reason. You never come unless you want something. I suppose it was money; and I have precious little of what I was given by the family to try to look after you.

Oliver, I am writing this today, in the strange blank time between the Death of Jesus and His Glorious Resurrection, to tell you that her death has forced me to a decision which you will not like but which cannot be avoided. I am in love. If he will have me, I will not flinch but will go to my Bishop and tell him. Of course I should go to my Bishop if the boy will not have me because of my feelings; but I'm not brave enough for that. When I have told the Bishop it will be up to him what to do; but I doubt you will want to have anything to do with me. You are so contradictory, with your income from making pornographic movies and your disgust with same sex relationships. What I feel is genuine and I will suffer greatly; what you film is fake and will bring you riches I cannot imagine.

Please keep this confidential until the news breaks, which it almost certainly will. I want to tell my Bishop in my own way. Try to be gentle if we meet; and God Bless you if we do not—your Uncle Joe.

BLOG ENTRY POSTED 18:37:22 07/04/07

Confidentiality Be Damned! I am posting this as a lesson to all pervert priests.

COMMENT POSTED 19:23:34 07/04/07
Olly, you bastard!—Rory

*Everywhere you go
everything you do
everything you say and think
There's only one you.*

Nine

Prepare to crown the Infant King:
Though we wear purple at His Court
The time of reckoning is short,
His royal star is beckoning:
Prepare to crown the Infant King.
Prepare to meet the Prince of Peace
And pray that Bethlehem may see
The fruits of his nativity,
That zeal for earthly power might cease:
Prepare to meet the Prince of Peace.
Prepare to greet our Little Lord:
Emmanuel for all our days,
The joyful centre for our praise
Of life renewed and hope restored:
Prepare to meet our Little Lord.
Prepare to love our Blessed child
Whose humble birth was made complete
When He washed His disciples' feet
Who suffered Him to be reviled:
Prepare to love our Blessed Child.
Prepare to tread the Pilgrim Way
From Jordan's Bank to Galilee,
From Bethlehem to Calvary,
From Advent until Easter Day:
Prepare to tread the Pilgrim Way.

Blood. Deep, red blood. It would get in your eyes and in your hair; it would seep like water into every crevice and stay there; glistening; sticky. She saw it. I saw it. I wonder who else saw it. Whoever they were they behaved as if it wasn't there. You would see Her putting Her hand through Her hair with a worried expression; you would see Her wiping Her eyes like weary; you would see Her wiping Her hands like compulsive; it was like Lady Macbeth except She was the victim. She could see it coming.

Strange that it started at Christmas; the red time; the Father Christmas time; the robin time; the holly time; the promise of blood in the strange old Carols.

> *For Eden's tree Calvary's cross;*
> *For what man knew Our Lord knew pain:*
> *The tree of life, the tree of death*
> *He gathered what the world had sown.*
> *For honeyed apples bitter gall*
> *For what man gorged Our Lord took none:*
> *The food of life, the food of death*
> *He offered what the world had strewn.*
> *For comely Eve a virgin pure*
> *For what man ravished Christ was born:*
> *The seed of life, the seed of death*
> *She cherished what the world would scorn.*
> *For Satan's serpent Yahweh's lamb*
> *For what man flattered He was torn:*
> *The source of life, the death of death;*
> *He conquered what the world had hewn.*

When everybody had left the Midnight Service and Her followers had finished clearing up She said She needed to be alone but She went out into the darkness to talk to those who were left alone on that Christmas night. She had put food and drink into a sack on her shoulder like a Father Christmas; and She handed it out to anybody who wanted it and left gifts beside the heads of the sleeping. She said she was taking Communion to all those who had not come in. When She thought nobody was looking

She cry.

They all gathered in the early afternoon to celebrate Christmas. It was a typical mixture: some people wanted to be there and some did not; some wanted to be there but not with some of the others who were; some forced themselves to make polite conversation and others pretended to be very jolly; some found genuine peace in the day but others remembered happier Christmases and were sad. Bob brought his mother who lived alone and loved company; Dexter brought his mother but she spent almost the whole time saying she would be better off in her own home. Trina brought her sister who showed off her great learning; and Jim brought his sister who was as gentle and simple as he was. Except when she was serving the meal Perpetua never stopped moving from person to person or group to group seeing that they were as all right as they could be. She didn't tell anybody to cheer up or cheer down; She just took people as they were.

When She sat them all down Dexter refused to sit.

"I can't have You serving while I sit down."

"I want you to see that your teacher and leader must also be your servant."

"I know the theory but..."

"It is not a theory, it is a way of living. I will serve you now so that you can remember that I was your servant when it is time for you to serve me. That time will come."

There was a turkey but only a small one because She said they had to enjoy food from many lands and traditions. Christmas was for the whole world not just for Christians and Christians themselves lived in many different cultures. "This is not the time for another sermon; you will be pleased to hear," She said. "I know I am rather too fond of preaching; but today Jesus My Brother speaks for Himself. Here's to the Baby!"

After the meal She said they must watch her Christmas special. Brian found the god4u channel and there she was; but who was it? There was a picture of Her in a kimono sitting on the floor with Japanese children. She was a black woman in a Soweto slum. She was an Indian princess standing outside a temple giving food to the beggars. She was standing on a snowy mountainside. She was wading ashore to a palm fringed beach with a cross in Her hand. She smiled in yellow; She walked along a road in purple; she knelt on a rock in red and she glowed white coming out of a cloud.

"You never said You had been all over the world," said Dexter.

"I have and I have not," She said. "All the world is mine; and all the world will be yours. I know the world and I want the world to know me. Wherever there is poverty; I am there. Wherever there is suffering; I am there. Wherever there is hopelessness; I am hope. Wherever there is death; I am life. Have you not understood yet? Do you think I was sent by God only to save a few people in England? I have to be in a place and England is the place I am in but I am here for the whole world. I have shown you the extent of your mission; the mission I have begun but which you must complete. Dexter; who do you think that I am?"

"Perpetua; I have already said that you are the Saviour of the world; God's

Sacred Vessel. How often must I say it?"

"It does not matter how often you say it. What matters is that you mean it."

"I mean it," he said almost shouting; and crying.

"There! there!" She said. "I only ask you so that you will continue to ask yourself. One minute while I am talking it is easy; the next minute when I am out of the room it is difficult. You have said so yourself. But I need you. I need you more than anybody else to hang on. There will be terrible times ahead; and this is not the day to think about them too hard although there is always joy in sorrow and sorrow in joy; but for all your problems you are a leader and as I said when we were talking about serving I need a leader to carry on where I will have to leave off."

> *Virgin of the Raj*
> *Geisha full of Grace*
> *Bearer of Our Lord*
> *For all God's human race:*
> *Mother of the sick*
> *Sister of the poor*
> *Sheds a lonely tear*
> *Outside the stable door.*
> *Exile in the dust*
> *Wanderer in the heat*
> *Home at Calvary*
> *To see His last defeat:*
> *Servant of the dead,*
> *Waitress at the board*
> *In the upper room*
> *Heard of the risen Lord.*

"I need you too; Jim," She said "for all the simple joy you bring. Play us one of your very own tunes."

> *Thy starlit throne a manger bed*
> *One star alone a heavenly thread:*
> *Angelic praise soft cattle lowing*
> *Their quiet ways the prophets bowing.*
> *Eternal might an infant's sleep,*
> *The darkest night nearest to deep,*
> *Yahweh's disdain a baby crying*
> *His mother's pain a saviour dying.*

The crowded inn an empty cave
Adam's first sin a vanquished grave:
The weak whose cries hailed His descending
Shall with Him rise, world without ending.

People were strangely quietened by the music; even Dexter's mother seemed content to be there. After a selection of Jim's music they sang traditional Carols and meant them.

"It does not matter whether there was snow or a star or a stable," She said. "What matters is that He was there; He came down to earth to be a human being; and I am doing the same thing for the same reason. It is not that He failed but that it is so difficult for humanity to believe that God became human. People in churches talk about it as if it was easy. They say their doctrines like the multiplication table but it is not like that. It is the most difficult thing that humanity ever has to grapple with; why it is here and why it is difficult and why God Our Parent knows it is difficult and is prepared to share the Godhead with everyone."

Then they all gathered round the tree. It was like no tree you had ever seen before full of Buddhas and Krishnas and strange objects. "Still," She said "I have put Jesus My Brother under the tree in His crib and there is the customary angel at the top; between Him and the Angel hangs all the world."

An angel tall and bright
From heaven did appear
In all his power and might
He filled a maid with fear:
O angel so bright,
O maiden so pure
A soul full of light
A servant so sure.
"Fear not, O gentle maid,
God wills a Saviour Son
If you will give Him shade
Within your virgin womb."
"I am the Lord's" she said
"May His sweet will be done.
His servant, yet a maid
I shall bring forth His son."
Then was Her calm restored
That spot so bright grew dim,
She felt her little Lord

And knelt to worship Him.

After the singing was over they went into action. Perpetua had arranged for the god4u channel to advertise a Christmas tension help-line; mostly they answered calls and listened patiently but on a couple of occasions Perpetua went out. Her first call was to Kish mother.

"You saved his life once," she said "and I thought that would keep him out of fights and make him safe; but the same thing has happened again. I tried not to call but in the end I could not bear it."

"Did you tell anybody what happened last time he was hurt."

"No. I just said that The Lord had seen fit to save him; I didn't mention what you did."

"That was true enough. Thank You. Your obedience to my request for silence is rewarded just as your faith was before. They say that lightning does not strike twice but in this case it does. He will be all right. Let us hope he learns this time because he will not have a third chance. I will not always be with you in the flesh."

"What should I do?"

"It is Christmas Day so no time for sermons; but remember what Christmas Day was like and rejoice. My Auntie Mary had a lovely baby and you have got your son back again; so be happy."

> What treasure can we offer to our king
> Who, seeming weak, is Lord of everything?
> No Tarshish hold
> of Ophir gold
> Could ever please, for all its glittering.
> What worship can we offer to Our Lord
> Who gave Himself as the Incarnate Word?
> No reverence
> Of frankincense
> Could ever praise, for all its sweet accord.
> What sorrow can we offer for this cor'se
> Who gave Himself for us without remorse?
> No bitterness
> Of Myrrh's caress
> Could ever mourn, for all its sad resource.

Next she called on Max who was almost at breaking point trying to get through Christmas Day without vodka.

"Well done; Max," She said. "I know what we will do. I know how you hate this flat so let us leave it and call upon Marta to see how the baby is doing. It is a day for babies."

When they arrived at Marta's; a tiny flat; shabby but spotless; she offered them a drink.

"Not much but nice," she said.

Max would have refused but Perpetua said:

"It's safe here to have a little; and it will show you that you can enjoy a little instead of being miserable after a lot."

"I know," said Marta. "Underneath; very nice. I care for him Perpetwa."

"I know," She said; and left them.

> *Smokey and faltering I shine*
> *Upon a babe so newly born,*
> *And with new light my powers decline*
> *As He awakes on His first dawn.*
> *Shiny and glistening the star*
> *New born shines over Bethlehem,*
> *But I am luckier by far*
> *Because I shine so near to him.*
> *O faltering lantern, beam so low,*
> *Shining upon that sleeping face:*
> *Who came for us that we might know*
> *In flesh the God of endless space.*

Gordon could hardly manage the pain of his dying wife. It was her pain and his pain; and the pain of knowing it would be their last Christmas together which stopped them enjoying it; thinking of next year rather than now. Gordon got rid of the pain by going to his allotment but that was unthinkable on Christmas Day. She said:

"You never told me."

"I never mention it out of doors."

"Now I understand better why you are sometimes grumpy. You have so much to bear."

"Not as much as her."

"Who is making league tables?"

"Anyway that's not the main reason I rang."

"No."

"I've heard about you. They say you can; well; they say you can do miracles."

"Do they?"

"That Brod who trails behind Max says he saw you do a miracle."

"He says all kinds of things."

"Yes but he said so and I want to believe him."

"Want to believe him?"

"Well yes. It's difficult to handle stories of miracles but I want to believe him because if he's telling the truth you could do a miracle for me."

"Even if he was not telling the truth I might be able to do a miracle; as you call it; for you. What God Our Father can do through me does not depend on what others say about it. Is your wife awake?"

"She will be waking about now."

"What is her name?"

"Emma."

"Emma; how are you? I know it must sound like a silly question."

"I'm not too bad; he makes a fuss like men do; it isn't as bad as he says it is."

"I am not sure it is possible to make that kind of comparison. Anyway let us not go there. How is the pain?"

"I can bear it."

"Emma! I was not asking about you but about the pain. You have made bearing it what you are instead of only part of you. In a strange way the pain has conquered you because you are so concerned that it should not."

"All right."

"How is the pain?"

"Not as bad as it was a minute ago. In fact I feel a bit hungry."

"That is always a good sign," said Gordon. "I like it when she's hungry,; it shows she is in less pain; no matter what she says about it."

"What is your favourite?"

"She likes mints."

"No she doesn't; you just think she does and she's always been too considerate to tell you otherwise. Just because she accepted one of your mints on her first date it doesn't mean she really likes mints."

"I never knew that; but at least she's showing a lot of spirit. She must be feeling a bit better."

"How is the pain?" asked Perpetua for a third time.

"You won't believe this but it's completely gone; for now."

"I believe it," She said.

On Her way out She said to Gordon

"I hope you have got plenty in."

"I got everything for Christmas just in case she would be fit for a bit of something."

"If I were you I would make a big dinner."

A dancing snow flake calms a bleating lamb
A star shine cheers a weary king
A berry stores the blood unshed
In the beginning.
An angel sets alight the secret sky
A chorus makes the whole world sing
A mother hums a lullaby
In the beginning.
The snow melts and the star declines
The blood bursts in the gloom
An angel bears a golden cup
On the darkest afternoon:
A lamb starts awake in a golden haze
An angel greets the risen king
A mother feels her womb ablaze
In the beginning.

Her last call; late at night; was to Father O'Helly. His dull little Presbytery was in darkness but She knew he was there. When he let Her in it was clear that he had been drinking heavily.

"I don't know whether to let You in," he said. "It was bad enough as it was but today you stole my congregation. Why did you lead them out of my lovely little church?"

"I am sorry Father; but your own lonely state makes it seem obvious. I led your congregation into the street and into the houses of other people many of them non believers; that is where they and you should be. What kind of birthday is it for Jesus My Brother that finds you drinking alone? It is not the drinking it is the alone that hurts me."

"It hurts me too; but you took them."

"Joseph; even if I had not taken them; if they had just stayed in your church for Mass; looking inwards; you would still be alone tonight. Was there not one who would ask you to their table or come and sit with you? So so much loneliness Joseph. Pour us both a little one to celebrate the birth of Jesus My Brother. Considering how you feel that is good of you. Take it slowly and enjoy it. That is what worries me so much. There are people all over the country drinking wine and whiskey and it is not a source of enjoyment but an escape from something. We do not need to go into what you are escaping from; we have been through all of that. Just take a last little one; then say a prayer to My Auntie Mary as it is her big day too; and then sleep."

She kiss him and left.

My soul lives in the greatness of the Lord
And rejoices in the Grace of my salvation
For He has rescued me from servitude
To be His servant queen for every nation.
All peoples for all time will call me blest
Not for myself but folded in His fame
Which unites heaven and earth in one dimension
To celebrate and glorify His name.
His strength and goodness compass all who love Him
Beyond the ancient strictures of the Law;
His mercy heals all earthly degradation
To liberate the sinful and the poor.
All earthly powers will crumble at his coming
And justice will prevail in every land;
The hungry will be fed, the weak will flourish,
The prostrate will receive the strength to stand.
The promise given to His chosen people
Extends to all the people on the earth
And I will serve them through my intercession
Because He made me fit to give Him birth.

Ten

What do you want of my heart
Do you want its beat or the blood run cold?
Do you want the thrill of my defeat
or to love me gently when I'm old?
What do you want of my heart
do you want the pain in my frightened eyes
do you want the power of sole command
or the joy past fear and compromise?
What do you want of my heart
now the blood is ebbing from my face
do you want the final fatal stab
or the liberty of common space?
What do you want of my heart
When the music stops and the dancing ends
do you want to be left alone with a crown
or live in love among good friends?
Answer no questions my love
for we both know now it is too late
I am dying for our common good
that the world will learn to love not hate.

What do you want of my heart?

On Ash Wednesday Perpetua said She was going to fast during Lent; nothing excessive; nothing that would damage Her mission; but keep eating and drinking to a minimum. It began to affect Her sleep and She found Herself watching television in the middle of the night. It was as if Her power to affect the media had been turned on its head because She kept being tempted by what She saw. The same themes went round and round a core which was all about power.

Night after night She saw pictures of Herself making speeches at celebrity events; walking into No 10; addressing the United Nations; shaking hands with Nelson Mandela. Every time She turn on a chat show She was there; every time She watch the news She was there; every time She saw people in danger She was there; every time there was a natural disaster She was there.

The worst thing was starving children. When She was at her weakest after a hard day with very little to eat or drink there would be starving children.

"I could go there and fix it!" She thought but then; sadly

"No. I am only here on behalf of God Our Parent; I am only a channel; a vessel into which God's goodness and the world's wickedness are poured and mixed. If I am to go I will go but My Sister the Spirit tells me I must stay here and complete my mission."

It got so bad that She began to pray to be freed to visit far-off places but the answer was always the same. At last She thought

"Jesus My Brother did not fast and watch television; he fasted and prayed."

So She refused to watch television and She prayed but as She got stronger She prayed less and watched more and this brought on a new set of anxieties. Instead of being tempted to eat more She was being tempted to eat less. Every time She switch on the television there was somebody on a chat show eating less than her; somebody on a movie being braver than her; somebody on a religious show holier than her. She found herself enmeshed in a holier-than-thou competition.

"It is the wrong reason," She said and abandoned television for praying. But again as She grew stronger She pray less and watch more. This time it was transformation: every time she watch a chat show there was a criminal who said She change his life; every time She watch the news there was a politician who said She change his policy; every time She watch a documentary there was a clip of some pundit explaining how She tip the balance. Night after night She was turning the world into a better place. There were no more criminals; no more starving babies; no more natural disasters.

She was horrified. She had almost gone over the edge wanting to make a world that was not Hers to make; wanting a world that would have all the love squeezed out of it by a kind of angelic Utopia. She; of all people; the believer in the freedom to choose to love; dreaming of being all powerful in a perfect world. She thought of getting rid of the television but She thought of Max.

"I must learn to handle a little properly instead of going for all or nothing."

What do you want of my heart?

Then it got worse. The people She had refused to help began to hit back. The starving babies pointed at Her and said She had condemned them to death. The mother of a murdered son said She had refused to reform the murderer; politicians said She had refused to intervene in crises. Whatever She watched it was full of people blaming Her for the shocking state of the world.

By now even though it was as bad as it could be She was ready. She watched television in moderate amounts to check that She was under control and She prayed regularly. What was most important was that She got her balance back

"It is; after all; the same old dichotomy; power and love."

At that time She could talk about nothing else

"If you really want to understand a situation," She said "look below the surface and see if the people involved are exercising power or love. Usually when they say it is love it is power. They say they are doing things for our own good; out of love for us. The difficulty is that power is visible; you see it being exercised; but the best kind of love is invisible; it is in a way the lack of something being exercised. Even in personal relationships the love is the quiet thing that provides space for otherness; the noisy love that fills the music shop and the knicker shop and the chocolate shop is the love of 'I want'; power masquerading as love."

"Talk about something else," said Trina. "You're too 'on message'."

"I know; I have to become more balanced but it is difficult to be balanced about love."

"But by being unbalanced about it you are shouting love instead of letting it flow."

"True."

"Wow! I didn't think you could be wrong."

"I hope as God Our Parent's Sacred Vessel that I will do no wrong but I can be wrong; I was about to say 'I am only human'."

She laughed for the first time in days.

"The other thing," said Trina "is that you are getting your fasting wrong; it has become too important; it is beginning to be an end not a means; it's throwing you right off balance."

"I know. It is better to eat more and praise God than it is to eat less and concentrate on eating less. Lent is supposed to be a time of renewal; getting ready for the Resurrection; and fasting is only a small part of getting ready."

Half way through Lent when Perpetua had quietened her demons they went on a tour of witness carrying a Cross into town centres and telling people about Easter.

As the days went by it got worse. The red; the blood.

First it happened at sunrise and sunset but as the days went by the gap narrowed until it was always red. I wonder nobody else saw it but Her and Jim; and me. She kept putting Her hands through Her hair; she kept rubbing Her eyes; She had that worried look; like Lady Macbeth only She was the victim.

She saw it coming.

Before the road trip She had got rid of Her house and most of the little She owned and during the journey She had steadily given her things away until She only had a few clothes. At first they thought She was scaling down and would make a new start at Easter when Her 'Lenten Blues' ('reds') went away but She just smiled a bit sad

"I have had this bag since I went on my first school trip," She said giving it to a girl who didn't look all that pleased.

"It looks like it," said the girl. "I wanted one of those that looks like a lap-top bag but more fashionable; but my mum says we can't afford it. Do you expect me to be grateful?"

"No of course not. We do not show our gratitude by making an exchange; my old bag for your gratitude; we make an onward commitment. I give you my old bag; you give something you have to somebody else so that it goes on going on."

"Cool. When I've got something I don't want I'll hand it on so the going goes on."

"Not quite. I am sorry to lose the bag but I have to. It is giving what we care for but somebody needs more than we do. You know what I mean; stop pretending you do not."

Perpetua smiled and the girl smiled.

> *What do you want of my heart*
> *Do you want its beat or the blood run cold?*
> *Do you want the thrill of my defeat*
> *or to love me gently when I'm old?*

One day as she was passing a scruffy second-hand shop she saw a woman in the doorway.

"I remember you," She said. "Earlier today I gave you an old coat."

"You don't want it back do you because he's got it."

"Let us go in."

"I needed the money you see; so I brought it in here. We're desperate; nothing to eat."

"I give unconditionally. I suppose I might expect you to keep warm and you could have asked me for money though I realise how difficult that is."

They went inside.

"The ten Pounds tag is a bit steep."

"Nice coat."

"Yes; I know. How much did you give her for it?"

"Fiver."

"So you have doubled your money."

"That's the idea. Trade is trade."

"In this case trade is dishonesty. You have done nothing but put a label on the coat and doubled its price."

"As I said; trade is trade; but it isn't yours any more so keep your nose out."

"Give her three Pounds; 25% profit is quite enough."

"No."

He opened the till to deposit the five Pounds.

"Robbery!" he screamed. "The till's empty. How did you do that? You two are some criminal double act. I'm going to call the police."

"I do not think I would do that if I were you; your sort of people are usually short of necessary paperwork. What is the last time you paid any tax for example?"

"None of your business; but what's that got to do with it?"

"I suppose your character might be under some scrutiny if you appeared for the prosecution in a legal action. Juries don't like people who; shall we say; pretend to be helpless victims when they are quite sharp really."

"Well; where's my money?"

"Promise to give this poor lady another three Pounds."

"Done."

"Close the till. Now open it."

"Blimey."

"Three Pounds. Now; or something worse will happen."

"That gave me a fright. What kind of person are you?"

"A friend of the poor."

"All that for three Pounds?"

"It is a lot to her even if it is very little to you. Now; what else can you do for us."

"Tell you what; sign of goodwill; here's another two Pounds for the coat so you get ten and I sell it at ten. Not good for trade. Too much of that and I'd go bust; but goodwill; goodwill."

"Yes," said Perpetua "we are going."

On the Wednesday before Palm Sunday they were heading South when Jim noticed that Perpetua was missing.

"She must have got out at the last stop. I could swear I saw her get in," said Kylie who usually did the counting out and the counting in.

"We will go off at the next intersection and go back to the service station," said Bob when he heard what had happened.

"I swear I saw her get in," said Kylie.

The sun was setting and I saw this red again and like before it got deeper and deeper. I said nothing but nobody else seemed to notice except perhaps Jim who had some special gifts but didn't mention it. We were on a long stretch of empty road but Bob suddenly put his brakes on.

"Christ!" he shouted.

"No; Perpetua," came a voice seemingly out of nowhere.

"I know," said Bob. "I saw you walk in front of the bus."

"Sorry Bob," She said. "Can somebody let me in."

Bob slowed down; Kylie opened the door and Perpetua kind of floated in.

"What was all that about?" said Trina "except for a demonstration of your divine powers?"

"It was not a piece of magic," She said. "I just want you to be aware that when I have gone you will sometimes see me like this; not quite what I was before. There. Let us settle down and pray for calm."

Nobody said anything; they were all too frightened of what they had seen and what She had said.

> *What do you want of my heart*
> *do you want the pain in my frightened eyes*
> *do you want the power of sole command*
> *or the joy past fear and compromise?*

On the Friday evening when the advance party had gone to set up the event for Palm Sunday in Royal Park She gathered her closest followers together in the back room of the Down and Out.

"It all really started here," She said. "If you do not count Hypo; so this seems like a good place to come clean."

Silence.

"As you know; I came here on a mission. My mission was to be God Our Parent's Sacred Vessel here on earth; to carry some of the Godhead within me (it is indivisible but we will not bother to go into that) and also to carry within me; to soak up; to absorb; the sinfulness and yes the sadness I see around me. I came to bring people back towards God Our Parent just as Jesus My Brother had done. My poor Brother suffered so and My Sister the Spirit worked with all Her might but over time God's children have slipped away into contempt and even apathy. I had to come not because human history in some way offends God Our Parent; God is not affected by human behaviour in that way; but God's purpose was that the created should choose to love. Over time as we all know things have become unbalanced; just as they did in the time of Jesus. God Our Parent chose the Jewish people because in spite of their apparent unfaithfulness they were serious about God even though this became rather constricted. I was sent here rather than anywhere else because I needed to be with the poor as we all have been but I also needed to be able to communicate with a wide variety of people. Just as the Jewish people got constricted so have the Christians of the rich countries. This seemed like a good starting point.

"All this you know but I think you also know deep in your hearts that it cannot go on. You know the story of Jesus My Brother. Nothing so grandly significant will happen to me but I know now; in my soul; that I will soon be killed. I do not know how but it is inevitable."

What do you want of my heart
now the blood is ebbing from my face
do you want the final fatal stab
or the liberty of common space?

"We can stop it," shouted Dexter. "If you knew where it was coming from; you might," She said "but I doubt it. It might surprise you to know given my behaviour that I do not actually want to die; yet. I really would like to go on a little while; I love being with God's children for all their little shortcomings; but even though that is what I would like I recognise that I will have to face it when it comes and not back off."

"Why?" asked Trina. "I have thought about it so much but I don't see why."

"Because there are three simple truths behind the life of Jesus My Brother which I need to re-live in my own way so that people can be re-connected with them: first, He was born a human as I was born; secondly, He died to show humanity that killing Him would not kill His love; thirdly, He rose from the dead to under-write the promise of universal salvation. I tell you that even if you do not really know what that means I will rise and be with you but not be with you.

"hAnd will we go where you have gone?" asked Brian.

"If you try to follow in my footsteps and freely love God and all that is created one day you will be enfolded into the Godhead. From the Godhead we all came and into the Godhead we will all be enfolded."

"What about sinners?"

"Nobody is completely evil. Nobody that has ever been has not been a child of God and a sinner; except Jesus and my Auntie Mary. People will always choose not to love; choose to do evil things; but they are still God's children."

"So," said Heather a bit petulant "if we all get there what's the point of choosing to love; of being good?"

"Because that is what we were made for. It is rather like asking why a flower opens in the Summer. That is what it was made for. This is what we were made for. We were made to be good; made to love freely; not to get some kind of reward for good behaviour. The joy of loving is that we are then doing what it is in our nature to do. Contrary to popular materialist prejudice people are happiest when they are loving because they are behaving naturally. What we are tempted to do by (people say 'The Devil') our free will is to behave unnaturally by pretending that we are not creatures of God but are totally self-determined. That is the difference between love and power; love is the essence of God's world; power is the essence of a world without God."

"So," said Jo also a bit sour "are you saying that it doesn't matter what people do; mass murderers for instance; they will end up in the same state as good people?"

"Yes; enfolded back into the Godhead from where they came."

"I am sorry; I don't really see the point."

"The point is that love is not competitive. You cannot construct a league table which shows who has loved more than somebody else. Only God knows how we deal with the situation we have been given and God is not saying."

"So are you saying that the Christian churches have got it wrong?" asked Wayne. "And if they've got it wrong about this could they be wrong about; er; being gay?"

"I am glad you got that out at last," She said; smiling. "It has been a long time; but the answer to your basic question is yes; yes and yes again. That is one of the reasons I am here; and notice how badly my message has gone down with many Christians. You can see the divide between the official Church and what Jesus taught because they cannot come to grips with what I teach which is exactly what Jesus taught. It is not a failure to understand but a failure to carry out. All human institutions are flawed because that is the nature of being human; but the Church needs such a huge change of direction and I am puzzled about how I can say things again without simply repeating myself. If Jesus had wanted to establish a new kind of moral law he would have been some sort of politician with a legal background; or a High Priest. If God our Parent had wanted a world of good order and strict justice with proportionate punishments for those who do wrong I am sure that could have been arranged. It did not appeal to God to create that kind of earth with those kinds of attributes.

"The Christian church started out all right but it soon merged with the legal and political systems and became obsessed with making laws and judging people. No wonder most people have turned away; it makes me sad that they cannot endure the difficulty for the sake of Jesus but I can see their point. They read the Gospels which are full of unconditional love and then they are subjected to a barrage of rules about good conduct. People will not readily submit to that kind of authority; nor should they. At least when we get bad politicians we have voted for them; but the Christian church has become an arrogant and unaccountable imposition and bless them it is only for the love of Jesus that so many people have the Grace to stay with it."

"So what must we do?" asked Andy. "Should we get rid of the churches and give the money to the poor?"

"A good question from our financial man," said Perpetua. "Not entirely. Churches are very special places that can and often do bring people to God Our Parent but they should be places of gathering for celebration. The vast majority of the time we spend being good Christians should be spent in the worship of life; of every day. You do not need a church for a Eucharist. You do not even need a priest for a Eucharist. The Eucharist is being abused as a focus of clerical power. Those who truly believe that they are bringing Jesus My Brother into their presence in the gifts God Our Parent made by calling on My Sister the Spirit to aid them are doing what Jesus commanded. He did not ask anybody who came for His help whether they had a certificate; he simply insisted that they had faith. Even that sadly warped great pillar of the church Saint Paul knew that the central requirement for following Jesus was to have faith in what He said. It is a pity that such a mighty person as Paul should have been warped. That is where it began to go wrong. Although he is always talking about love he introduced a note of harshness and wrote lists of sins; he denied The Law but he could never truly escape from it. That is humanity; beautifully flawed."

> *What do you want of my heart*
> *When the music stops and the dancing ends*
> *do you want to be left alone with a crown*
> *or live in love among good friends?*

"Sorry. I rather went off the point there Andy. I believe that hiding inside churches is not good for people. I do not think it brings most of them closer to God. But I say again that churches are places of celebration. They are better off with crying and dancing than with the Creed.

"Well then; let us dance."

After all that sadness and theology it started a bit slowly but Jim got the guitarist out of the main bar and there was a slow elegant bitter/sweet sort of dance.

She dance so nice.

Answer no questions my love
for we both know now it is too late
I am dying for our common good
that the world will learn to love not hate.

Eleven

Stop looking for your brother
He's everyone you see
stop looking for the nice one
and see him in me
stop looking for an angel
who behaves the way you do
and stop looking for the idol
who says she will be true:
The grass is always greenest
at the place you see it grow
and the flavour is the keenest
in the thing you're eating now
and the friendship is the surest
when there's nothing in return
and the love is brightest in the hearts
of those who look as if
they cannot burn.
Stop looking for the sister
who is solid, swift and sure,
and stop looking for the alter ego
living in your core
stop looking for the signpost
to which you can relate
and stop looking for the wise man
who will open up the gate:
There's a brother in the beggar
and a sister in the weak
The angel is a mirage
and the idol is a freak
And the shadow you are looking past
is what you need to see
for the shadow that is nearest to you now
is me:

The grass is always greenest
at the place you see it grow
and the flavour is the keenest
in the thing you're eating now
and the friendship is the surest
when there's nothing in return
and the love is brightest in the hearts
of those who look as if
they cannot burn.

"I didn't like to ask in front of the others," said Dexter "because they might panic; but if I am the leader as you say I have to ask; what is to become of us when you have gone?"

"It is all right. I know you are frightened. You should be frightened. What is love if not overcoming fear; fear of rejection; fear of getting it wrong; fear that we will not be good enough; fear that it will not turn out as we planned which it never will because you cannot plan love that way. You are right to be frightened and perhaps it is best that I talk to you and you talk to the others in a way that you think is right. After all; it will not be long before you are doing all the talking."

"I have never been very good at talking."

"The world puts too high a value on people who are good at talking rather than people who have something to say. We know where you began; we go back a long way although I was frightened of you when I first saw you as a teenager."

"Yes; I suppose I was frightening. The only thing I wanted was to be respected by everybody else; to be the leader. I read all this stuff about kids needing role models and leadership and joining gangs to get respect because there is no other way. It's a lie of course; we both know there is another way; if the wealthy society we live in wanted to change our world by giving us respect and a respectful share rather than giving us handouts and sneers it could do it. So the answer is that I looked for the only kind of respect I thought I could get. I see now that I did terrible things and that people did not respect me at all; they were just frightened; but it felt like respect. And another thing. I can't blame bad parenting. I had a good mum and dad and they stayed together for more than thirty years until he died young in an accident when he was told to disobey basic safety instructions or he wouldn't be paid. And then because he had flouted the safety instructions mum got nothing. The easy way out would be to say that I have been fighting back but that would not be true."

"I never thought you would be leader."

"Nobody did; but I had set my sights on it and I thought about nothing else. I was not the cleverest person who wanted to be leader and I was far from being the most violent; but I wanted to be leader so I disciplined myself. I didn't drink; I didn't take drugs; I prepared everything carefully; I didn't make any mistakes."

"Why then did it take so long?"

"I went into periods of self doubt which I suppose some people would call depression. I stopped believing in myself and while I was in that state other people would make up the ground I had gained."

"Then?"

"Then I had a long spurt without self doubt and took my chance. I had the power base of the Hypo stock room; I could get stuff for people who needed it. You always need the tacit support of a lot of people to survive without getting into trouble. It doesn't matter how much active support you have from close followers operations based on violence fall to pieces without the tacit support of a lot of people.

"As I said; I had the Hypo base which meant that a bottle of rum here, a blanket there; a television with a slightly damaged case. Hypo knew the game as well as I did. Little by little; never too much; stay within the 'permitted' margin and keep the labour force content and it's all right."

"Annie Price?"

"No. She changed all that as soon as she came. She said that the workers would not thrive where they didn't respect the people who let them break the rules. It happened just before you came; that is one reason why I was glad to quit."

"You have a very strange way of paying a compliment."

"Sorry; of course I wanted to follow you when you asked but I was thinking of getting out of Hypo."

"And what about getting out of the gang?"

"It was easy. I got out when you called me and look! Nobody asked me back; nobody said they were sad I was leaving; nobody did anything; they just started fighting over the next leader. I could have covered Grunge Park with blankets and televisions and drowned it in rum and it would have made no difference. After all; they didn't respect me; they were just frightened when I was tough and grudging when I brought stuff. There was no respect; no gratitude; nothing."

"And now?"

"I know I often fall down. I shoot my mouth off and regret it; but you know I'm not a fool. You know I will be faithful to you."

"I know you will try and sometimes fail but I know that you have the resilience to come back when you have failed and that is the most important thing of all."

"And what should I tell them?"

"Tell them that it will all come clear when the terrible events are over. Tell them it is not possible to paint a complete picture now but I promise that I will not leave you stranded. I will always be with you; as will My Sister The Spirit."

"And what must we do?"

"You must do what I said earlier. Help people to love one another and to love God Our Parent for their being and their freedom to love. You have a great advantage because after the experience of the televisions and blankets you know what love is not. You will not be fooled."

> *Stop looking for your brother*
> *He's everyone you see*
> *stop looking for the nice one*
> *and see him in me*

"Some people will try to trap you. Do not try to be clever with your answers; bad theology is worse than no theology at all; and there is quite enough bad theology without you adding to it. You can rely on Bill Midway. There are some who will betray me but Bill will fill a gap and become one of you."

"What about the divine power bit? You remember when I got carried away and tried to heal that poor lady and upset her and you?"

"I remember. You were so busy concentrating on the lady and your determination to fix her that you forgot to call on God Our Parent where all power lies. Be careful. To call on the divine power is a very serious matter and to call on it frivolously is the truer meaning of the word 'blasphemy'. I am sure that God Our Parent does not really 'mind' when all kinds of unthinking people say: "My God' in the street but God definitely 'minds' when powerful people invoke his name to exercise control and oppression.

"You are the leader. I could make some kind of formal announcement but we all know and it is better that your authority grows in spite of setbacks through your own spirit. Lastly; never be jealous. Some people need a little more gentleness than you; do not begrudge it them. Which reminds me; I really must talk to Jim as he will be upset when things become difficult."

"I know. I try to look after Jim but it doesn't really work."

"I know; but Bill needs somebody to look after and keep him company."

> *stop looking for an angel*
> *who behaves the way you do*
> *and stop looking for the idol*
> *who says she will be true:*

"Now Jim; you are not going to like what I have to say but you are not to be frightened and above all you are not to blame yourself which you too often do; you have done nothing wrong."

"I know; I trust you; but ever since I can remember people have treated me as if I had done something wrong; as if I was guilty of choosing to have Downs Syndrome just to make life difficult for everybody else; as if it didn't make life difficult for me."

"That is terrible."

"I don't know why and how I got this syndrome but I have learned to accept it particularly with help from you. You have never made me feel embarrassed or a nuisance."

"We are all God's children and I know this must sound like a platitude to somebody who has so much to put up with as you have; but God has a purpose for each of us; and the human race would not work as it does if we were all the same. You just have to believe that God has a purpose for you and that you are to go on loving in just the way you always do."

"But; O Perpetua; I do so want a girl friend who I can cuddle. They all look through me; I don't know whether I am a piece of glass or a piece of dirt."

"O Jim!"

"They told me when I was ten that I wouldn't live past twenty and they told me when I was fifteen that I wouldn't live past twenty-five; but I am still here. They used to say I should not try to develop affections of that sort because I would die and it would all be over too soon. I often wonder if what I was told is the truth; that it would not last and that I would soon die; whether some kind girl would still love me. I get so lonely. I am not very bright. I see these lovely girls smiling at men; and I just want one of them to smile at me."

> *Stop looking for the sister*
> *who is solid, swift and sure,*
> *and stop looking for the alter ego*
> *living in your core*

"I know it is difficult for you to accept that individual personal relationships are not the only joy in life. I have chosen not to develop any relationship because I have known that I would not live past twenty; no; wait; I will explain in a moment; but I have found a full life in other ways. You have music and I know but nobody else does that you have special powers of seeing things."

"Yes; I have the music but people always typecast disabled people. I heard a woman say to a blind girl once: 'You are so lucky to be blind because it makes you so gifted musically; and you can always smell the flowers.'"

"I know Jim; there are a lot of insensitive people about but try to remember the pleasure which you give to people when you play. I am not fobbing you off. For you a genuine attraction is more difficult but its authenticity is if anything more important.

"Now about what I have just said; do not be alarmed. I will soon be going away but I will come back in a different way. You know this because you have the power of seeing. You will see more of my glory than anyone else. You will see my rendezvous with Jesus on the Cross and you will see me rise from death to a new life."

"How?"

"You stick to Bill Midway. He needs somebody to help him. He is so lonely. You would be doing him a service by staying close by him; and he will; I promise he will; bring you among people who will treat you as a full rounded human being. He might even introduce you to a nice girl. I make no promises but I am extremely hopeful."

"I trust you."

"I know. In the next few days when things become alarming stick to Bill."

"I will."

After he went out

She cry.

stop looking for the signpost
to which you can relate
and stop looking for the wise man
who will open up the gate:

Next it was Wayne's turn.

"I am glad you finally brought yourself to use the word 'gay' yesterday in front of Dexter."

"It was difficult. He is really homophobic."

"He is not; and do not use that foolish word unless you are properly explicit. People find it difficult to deal with difference. They find it difficult to deal with Jim who has much more to put up with than you do. People find it difficult to deal with people not of their own race or tribe. Now that people can please themselves much more about where they live and who they meet they are losing the ability to cope with difference as part of living in a community; of exercising the faculty of love."

"All right then; but he gives me funny looks."

"Dexter is having to learn like everybody else that following God Our Parent is not an easy business. I know he will try; but you have not been over keen on spending so much time with a black man; have you?"

"No; true. I have to admit it."

"The first thing is to get things into proportion and dispense with the self pity. What is wrong with your life?"

"People make fun of me because I'm gay."

"That is a bit like black people saying people make fun of them because they are black; sometimes it is true; but sometimes they hide behind this knowing that people make fun of them because of other factors. People should not make fun of anybody; but face yourself Wayne before you start on other people. Tell me about how you see yourself?"

"I know. I am vain. I like to wear nice things and I like people to notice me. And I love talking; really clever talking; to impress people; but part of the dressing and talking is to make up for the fact that I feel lonely and isolated. It isn't so much people making fun of me really; it's that nobody takes me seriously. It's like if you're gay you can't be anything else; they can't see past the gayness."

"But Wayne a lot of the time nor can you."

"True."

"If you can see past it other people will see past it. What you are going through is no different from what heterosexual people go through. There is a point in their lives when they cannot see past their need for a relationship; and once in the relationship they can get so caught up in it that they cannot see the whole of themselves any more but just the bit that is in the relationship (you can take that literally as well as metaphorically). You are still at the first stage. Stop seeing the whole world as a potential trap or at the same time as a potential source of pleasure. Take the idea of a relationship seriously.

"I know somebody who is deeply in love with you but you are so busy worrying about yourself that you have not noticed."

"Who?"

"He will tell you when you have got yourself ready. It will not be easy for him and this will teach you that there are people in much greater difficulty than you will ever be; and you will have to help him because in committing himself to you he will be abandoning most of what he has ever known. He will take a huge plunge into the unknown for you and you will need to respond with more sympathy than you have ever summoned before. I know you can do that."

"Who is it?"

"Honestly Wayne; what a foolish question. Do you not want to hear the words from the man's own lips instead of through a girly messenger like me. This is not light fiction where gossip spreads; this is serious love."

"I am sorry."

"Go and get ready. This will be a difficult few days for us all."

There's a brother in the beggar

and a sister in the weak
The angel is a mirage
and the idol is a freak

"Oh dear," said Perpetua when Trina came in with the latest report on the Palm Sunday preparations. "Whoever got the strange idea that God our Parent is a man? How are all the others?"

"Bob is a bit upset about losing the bus but he will get over that; and the rest have plenty to do. The only problems are Heather and Jo who seem to have dropped out; they are showing no interest at all in Sunday."

"And what about you?"

"If we can't predict the crisis that is coming or; even better; prevent it; we might as well just get on with things."

"Yes. You have not asked about your future; afterwards."

"Just once or twice I have resented Dexter's leadership. After all Kylie and i have kept a lot of things going. But I see why it has to be Dexter and I will do all I can to help."

"And why does it have to be Dexter?"

"Because he always says sorry and he won't quit. He finds the word 'love' really embarrassing. I am not sure I have ever heard him use it full on the way you use it; but it is there for all to see."

"Remember Moses. You will have to do some speaking for him particularly when he gets into ecclesiastical tangles as he surely will. Anyway; I believe that you will very soon want to spend more time on your private life."

"Oh! Miles. Nothing serious."

"Everything about Miles is serious. That is where you can help him change. Miles is a good man just as old Father Joe is a good man. They stick at it. They make mistakes but they stick at it. What I can't stand are the ones who call the committees and make the rules and sign the papers and then say they are doing it in the Name of Jesus My Brother or say that they have been told to do this or that by My Sister the Spirit."

And the shadow you are looking past
is what you need to see
for the shadow that is nearest to you now
is me:
The grass is always greenest
at the place you see it grow
and the flavour is the keenest
in the thing you're eating now
and the friendship is the surest

when there's nothing in return
and the love is brightest in the hearts
of those who look as if
they cannot burn.

On the day before Palm Sunday they said goodbye to the bus and went through the final preparations. Then Perpetua took Dexter Trina Andy and Kylie to a private place to show them Her glory (and somehow Jim slipped in and then out without being asked). They saw Perpetua with an array of prophets and martyrs and with Jesus Her Brother.

"This is not a God spectacular show," She said. "You just need to be sure of the promises I have made. It will not make sense for a while but I truly am a part of the Godhead and now you have more than my word for it."

Out of the red light came white.

She came into central London on an open-topped bus and appeared for all the world like a queen about to be crowned; not killed. Of course everybody was interested in the spectacle rather than what it meant. I could see red and white pulsing, as if some kind of issue was in the balance; but it was mostly a white day with lots of Her special signs. I had never seen Her smile like that before; it was out of this world. She took London by storm: the people in the park; the people crowding the streets; the sick people that she cure; the party afterwards. It was the biggest thing London had ever seen.

And it all came to nothing. Within a week She was dead and nobody; no power in the land; had been able to save Her.

Blood. Red blood. She saw it coming and if She could stop it She wasn't going to.

The grass is always greenest
at the place you see it grow
and the flavour is the keenest
in the thing you're eating now
and the friendship is the surest
when there's nothing in return
and the love is brightest in the hearts
of those who look as if
they cannot burn.

Twelve

I thought that love was something
that lovers gave and took
of bravery and sacrifice
all written in a book
of courtly love and heroes
who kept their love from harm
and came from dark and danger
into the light and warm
Then I thought that love was virtue
standing up for what is right
being firm against all evil
always ready for the fight
when the battle was all over
and the victory was won
you would hold me in your loving arms
for the bravery I'd shown
Then I thought that love was loving truth
with the certainty of right
that our safety lay in judgment
shunning darkness seeking light
if we held onto each other
and rejected all the wrong
we would always be united
in the lyrics and the song
But I know there is no answer
and no gift that is enough
and no truth and right to save us
from the tangled and the tough
and the only thing I give you
to show my love is space
to be the supreme mistress
of your time and space.

I thought that love was something
that lovers gave and took
of bravery and sacrifice
all written in a book
of courtly love and heroes
who kept their love from harm
and came from dark and danger
into the light and warm

I am a sinner. I have been changed by Perpetua but in this I have not changed. I am a sinner. It can never change. I am a sinner. I need to get that straight immediately because some people too easily draw the conclusion that if you stop thinking like an Evangelical and start thinking more like a liberal you automatically stop thinking that you are a sinner. Some people may think like that. I do not. I am a sinner.

I first saw Perpetua at Her weird graduation ceremony when She made a cross out of all kinds of rubbish. I could see the significance of it—how that word resonates differently now—but it reminded me of the kind of mumbo-jumbo, as I thought of it, that Catholics go in for. I still dislike it, make no mistake, but I have come to see that we have all become too bound up in what we like and dislike in our approach to God.

Then she came to my youth club. I say "my" without any sense of pride. I hated every minute of it but I knew from the time I first left Excelsior Gardens and wandered into Grunge Park that the Lord's work was waiting for me there. I could have gone from learning at Bible Class to being a junior teacher there but it did not seem right. I saw vice and degradation and it was my personal mission, from God, to bring the light. I thought then that the degradation was a direct result of the vice. I am not so sure now; I have come to think that it might be the other way round, that the vice springs from the degradation; but I am not yet competent enough, or maybe the word is committed, to see it that way.

Looking at it now, that first time might be seen as a new wind of the Spirit blowing through that place but at the time I could only see it as a takeover. It looked like some form of witchcraft, the tricks with the light and the strange invocations. Even though I hated the place, it was mine, and I did not want it subverted. The kids might sneer at me and make my life difficult but my feeling that I was doing the right thing and that She was subverting it was powerful.

I see now that what I was doing was a kind of penance for my sin. It is really hard to admit it, particularly to you who are so good and pure, that I was doing penance for my obsession with women. I told myself that buying soft porn magazines was a better way of dealing with my inner lust than trying to impose it on real women. I told myself that it was some kind of vicarious working out of my obsession that would harm nobody. I did not see then that it involved buying a product which was produced through exploitation. Perpetua showed me that without ever saying anything; She never said anything.

That was what began to change me. My approach was to preach, to set a list of moral imperatives against what people actually did, to see the gap and describe that as sin. If I put my own weakness aside—and how easy that was most of the time—I could make comparisons between the ideal and the real and then draw conclusions which allowed, permitted, me to judge other human beings.

Judgment came easy. I inherited it from my parents and community. From the earliest time I can remember I was judged and found wanting. I was lectured, punished and given penitential exercises. I ploughed my way through Deuteronomy and Leviticus, I read stories of God's vengeance with a kind of pornographic relish. My father beat me and I did not complain. My mother hectored me as she consoled me for the beatings and I did not complain. I see now that it was love gone wrong but then it seemed just; they had to be cruel to be kind. Now I see that you have to be kind to be kind; but how could I understand kindness when I had never met it? For me, for us, you could, you must, have love which is above kindness.

Of course, you will recognise immediately, the change came about when She discovered my wickedness when She saw me in the newsagent's. My automatic reaction when I was found out was to find some way of seeking forgiveness through penitence. You will rightly say that if I had not been found out I would have gone on in the same way. Although the theory in my upbringing was that we sinned in our hearts, the truth was that the environment was so punitive that I was trapped in a closed world of game playing. The reality was not what was in my heart but in what other people saw. Once She saw what was in my heart my reaction was to try and put it right, to play the game, to wipe the slate clean. I saw that the game was only a game but I had been playing it for so long that it was difficult to escape. The game was cruel but it was easy in its way; the rules were easy, the boundaries were defined, you knew where you were.

Perpetua introduced me to a life where you never knew where you were. I had to stop playing the game but for a long time this just made me feel insecure and vulnerable. I once saw Her sitting enjoying herself with a boy who was obviously a dealer. I was confused. She kept reminding me that Jesus had spent time with "publicans and sinners" but I had always tried to brush that under the carpet; after all, I thought, Jesus was really trying to get to know these people so that He could put them back on the straight and narrow way. And, indeed, He was, but She showed me that this was not achieved through telling people what to do but through helping them to look into themselves.

The biggest problem I had at this time was coming to grips with her idea that we were created to choose the good, that our humanity was deliberately flawed so that we might choose. I had always been taught to believe that we were flawed as the result of 'The Fall', that this was a terrible state in which to be and that it had only been put right by the death of Jesus, that He had paid the price of our sin and put things right in an act of what I might now think of as supernatural accountancy. I can see that is a very odd way to look at the death of Jesus but at the time it looked logical; it was part of the game. Humanity had been playing this game and was losing badly and Jesus had come and loaded the dice. The game went on but now we had the advantage over the Devil because of what Jesus had done. No matter what we did, no matter how we fell short, we all knew that Jesus had loaded the dice and it would all come right and, in the meantime, when we came face to face with others who were falling short, all we had to tell them was that they did not understand the rules of the game because they had not learned of the dice that Jesus had thrown to put things right.

> *Then I thought that love was virtue*
> *standing up for what is right*
> *being firm against all evil*
> *always ready for the fight*
> *when the battle was all over*
> *and the victory was won*
> *you would hold me in your loving arms*
> *for the bravery I'd shown*

I went on with the youth club even though I was no longer so sure that I was doing any good; but after a while that was not so difficult as I thought it would be. Not knowing that I was doing good was my own kind of new penance for all the time I had been certain that I was. I did not have the tools She had to come to terms with the people around me but at least I began to learn about doubt. It was a hard lesson. As you can imagine from what I have said, doubt was not an element in my early life. Doubt was always dismissed as wilful sinfulness.

In a paradox that I only recognise now, doubt was thought of as pride. If you doubted the rules as they were set down you were putting yourself above the game. How could you play a game if you questioned the rules? I did not know then what I came to learn later from Perpetua that this game reduced God to something anthropocentric, that we were turning God into one of us, chief of us all but still one of us. I had lived so long in the game, in the shadow of the great rule maker, that the idea that God is above our kind of language and that our language is just a metaphor, an approximation to try to approach God, came as a shock. I remember the day when Perpetua came into the empty club when I was reading the account in Genesis of the 'burning bush'. "What do you think," She said in her slow, deliberate way, "of a God who deliberately hardens His heart in order to make Pharaoh vacillate when He could just let the people go?" I said that God needed to show His power to Pharaoh. "That would be true," She said, "if God was 'He'. A God who was manifested to human beings in the metaphor of a woman would have taken a different approach." She showed me that our idea of God was absolutely bound up with our idea of God as male.

I began to think about her idea of God Our Parent and realised that I was in great need of a God who in some ways represented the mother I never had. My mother was so frightened of God and my father, who was a tiny version of that God, that I had never known the kind of God that modelled the kind of love that I had missed in my mother. By coincidence, I went to see Father O'Helly to talk about my worries. He was the opposite from me but I had nowhere else to go. In a strange way I thought we were the same even though some of his rules were different from the ones I had been brought up with. He had just finished celebrating a special Mass for the Virgin Mary and I immediately saw something I had never seen when I all too easily dismissed the Catholic obsession with Mary. O'Helly and his kind, no doubt brought up in similar conditions to mine, was looking for his mother in God and, not finding her there, had instead fixed on Mary as his mother, the nearest thing he could find. All the lonely people.

She must have known, of course she knew, that I was struggling because She was unfailingly kind even when I was terse and sometimes bitter. I began to see in Her the virtues She so often preached of Jesus Her Brother and after a time I think we were both confident enough in each other that She was able to advise me not to spend so much time reading the Bible without causing a shocked and destructive division between us. She said that I should spend more time looking carefully at the world I lived in to see if I could see God in it. She asked—no more than that—whether the Bible reading was some kind of escape from the real world in which I was supposed to carry out my mission. No matter how different we were, and no matter how easily She saw through my surface righteousness to my inner sinfulness, She never called my mission into doubt. She sometimes made fun of me in a gentle, kind sort of way but she never doubted me; I know that now, looking back, although I thought sometimes that She did.

I began to walk around Grunge Park, particularly at night. I saw all the evils I imagined I would see and I tried to do what She did but I could never get alongside the people. I supposed that it was because I was white and middle class but I came to see that it was because I found it hard to see God in the faces of people. For a while I thought I would not see God anywhere. I had stopped playing the game, I had stopped escaping into the Bible and I was stranded here, amidst all this wickedness and degradation and I could not see God.

Then I thought that love was loving truth
with the certainty of right
that our safety lay in judgment
shunning darkness seeking light
if we held onto each other
and rejected all the wrong
we would always be united
in the lyrics and the song

Then I saw you; adored you. God forgive me if that is some kind of idolatry, which at one time I would have thought it to be but do not think so now. Of course there is no doubt that what I saw was not simply a good human being with God in your face, it was also a human being that I wanted to love; and, yes, I wanted you to love me but the starting point, I swear, if I may, was the person you were, working alongside Her. I saw you working tirelessly without complaint; I saw your tiredness which others—apart from Perpetua—seemed not to see. And I thought: "I am seeing something of her that others do not see" and I thought: "What Perpetua said is working inside me. I am seeing people as they really are and I am seeing God in what they really are." And, like Her, you never judged, you never made fun of me, you never sent me away. I was occasionally—God forgive me—frightened that you might know of my terrible sinfulness; but of course I realised that Perpetua would never say anything.

Then I saw something else. I saw that beneath your quietness and your dedication there was another layer which you never showed. I discovered that you were very clever, that you read difficult books, that you understood theology and philosophy, that you might have been a great teacher in your own right; and of this you said nothing. I even wondered for a short while why you were not the leader instead of Dexter but then I knew—and this was the biggest breakthrough of all—that leadership does not depend on human knowledge. I knew that you would accept what was given unto you. I knew that you had found deep contentment through working with Perpetua. I saw that you were fulfilled in your work and your quietness.

Of course we both know what happened during that dreadful Good Friday but I want to set something else down now for both of us, in case we ever come to forget it or, as is so easy, re-write history when circumstances change. We both knew that Perpetua was in terrible danger although we did not know what it was. You came to see me, crying, in a terrible state, on Good Friday afternoon when you had left her in Bill Midway's church after the Service. I asked why you had not stayed with her, as one of her key helpers, and you said: "I wanted to stay but Perpetua told me that my place was with you. She said that at this time of crisis we needed each other and that we should explore our commitment to each other. She said that such exploration should not be delayed." I remember you saying: "Perpetua says that what must befall Her must befall Her and the rest of humanity must go on trying to love instead of holding its breath, waiting for something to happen." I want to record this because there will be many, I have no doubt, who will ask why you, of all people, you who are so wise, were not there when She walked into the trap and was brutally raped, injected and murdered. There is part of me that regrets that we were not there as good companions should be but I have to recognise that Perpetua saw Her death as inevitable.

Nonetheless, it may be that you will need to face up to your absence, no matter how She sanctioned it. We have already talked about your feeling of guilt, that you think you abandoned Her and then rushed back when it was too late. I keep going back to the conundrum that the Disciples abandoned Jesus but in some way they were meant to, that they had no choice. If they really were acting in such a way as to fulfill the Scriptures I can only say I find it difficult to understand. But perhaps their very denial, which was meant, was to strengthen them for their mission, a presence within them that never let them stop doing what the Spirit prompted them to do. Set against this, I should not worry that you are condemned because we both know that you behaved with integrity under the loving care of Perpetua; but I still cannot help it. I still care more than I should no matter how little that is.

It was then that I truly understood Perpetua. When She went to Her death, having sent you to me, I understood what it truly means to lay down your life for your friends. I knew, as certainly as I have ever known anything, that She was laying down Her life for the kind of love which we wanted to show to—or maybe it's allow to—each other. She was not laying down Her life for an abstract love but for the hard love that we are determined to forge together no matter what difficulties we face. She was laying down Her life in a way I will never understand, as once I thought I did in the case of Jesus, for the whole of humanity but also for each individual. She was laying down Her life for you and me.

For this reason I was not shocked when She appeared to us all on that wonderful Easter morning; and I was not even shocked when She appeared in person when we were at the market looking for a tea pot. I was not surprised because I was ready. I had undergone a transformation. The last vestiges of the game had been swept away. The last thing to go was the doctrinal baggage I had held onto for so long. I saw that the Trinity was a useful idea as long as it lasted but it could not be the end of everything. I saw that the game was over; that we have to go out into the wide world and risk ourselves for God Our Parent, for the love which Jesus showed and for the love which we saw face to face in Perpetua.

> *But I know there is no answer*
> *and no gift that is enough*
> *and no truth and right to save us*
> *from the tangled and the tough*
> *and the only thing I give you*
> *to show my love is space*
> *to be the supreme mistress*
> *of your time and space.*

I am writing this now, on the eve of our marriage, so that you who are wise may know me better perhaps than I know myself but also to show you how hard I am trying to know myself. Perhaps lovers should only talk and touch and never need to write but it is my weakness that I have not got that power of speech. As you are so reticent in your own way I know you will understand this reticence in me.

I need not say that I love you but there is one last thought which at least carries through from my beginning until now. For all my weaknesses I never thought that what good I did came from me, but rather came from God, and so now I know that whatever good there is in us comes from God whose glory we have seen in the life, death and Resurrection of Perpetua.

I grew up amongst people who said that they were sinners but that they were saved. I can truly say now, as we prepare to live our lives together, that I am still a sinner and always will be because I will not always choose to love; but I will try; and in trying, I know that I am saved.

All my love, by gift of the Godhead through Perpetua, to you—Miles.

> *and the only thing I give you*
> *to show my love is space*
> *to be the supreme mistress*
> *of your time and space.*

Letter published on www.fortress.net after Miles was killed, the first Martyr for Perpetua, in June 2007, two weeks after the marriage.

Thirteen

When we arrived, about 20 of us, for what would be our last meal together, She was warm and calm like the lover who promises but will not hurry. She was wearing a beautiful red outfit with white trim, silver and red jewels, like a bride waiting for Her husband. Nobody ever combined such joy and sorrow in such flawless charm. We, by comparison, looked bedraggled, confused and untidy.

"Come in," She said "and take comfort here." (It's only my memory; it had been such a confusing day that I forgot the recorder.)

She sat us down and gathered our shoes and, putting a pinafore on, knelt down and cleaned each pair as if it were being prepared for a wedding or a dance. Dexter, of course, protested and Trina blushed but said nothing. She put our shoes back on as if She were a mother with a child who could do it for herself but who chooses the shared joy of the mother helping and the child being helped. It was all done in a sad, light silence; no panic; no hurry; no outbreak of emotion.

When She had finished cleaning our shoes She took two bottles of Champagne and poured them into a large crystal jug; clear and uncut; with a red band at its rim. She held the jug in front of Her and said

"Look, look at the bubbles of life breaking in the liquid. Look at the delicacy of the bubbles and their strength as they break through the liquid to the surface and then die. Look at the way the light passes through the glass and the liquid. I offer this wine to God Our Parent in the power of My Sister the Spirit as a sign of the sacred union between the blood of Jesus My Brother and Me as the mediators between God and all people. In the name of God Our Parent' Jesus My Brother; My Sister the Spirit; and their Sacred Vessel I pray that through the drinking of this blessed wine all those who love God shall be one; on earth and then in the glory of God when they are enfolded back into their Creator; creatures no longer but again flames of the living fire; currents of the living water; beams of the eternal light. This is the Third Covenant for the Third Millennium."

There was a pulsating white and red light so bright that Jim and I had to close our eyes.

"This is the vibrant essence of God Our Parent, made alive in the blood of Jesus My Brother and brought to us in the Spirit; remember who made you, remember by this blood who rescued you, remember in the clarity of this glass that I brought you hope; and when it is shattered remember me still."

She poured the wine into an amazing variety of glasses

"Take this wine and drink it for after the blessing I have brought upon it, it has become one with God Creator Brother and Sister. This crystal container is a symbol of My mission which contains the love of God, the blood of My Brother and the power of the Spirit.

"Never again remember Our Parent with gold and jewels but with glass through which you can see the meagre beauty of your offering. Remember me."

We drank a calm and sublime toast; our eyes fixed on the jug which stood before Her.

Then She took bread and looking up to Heaven She said

"Dearly beloved God; Parent of all; we each and all offer You this bread through Me that we all may be united in Your presence here with us now. Send down My Sister so that by Her power this bread may be the very essence of the Godhead present in the body of Jesus My Brother Presided over by the Father and empowered by the Spirit; Parent' Brother; Sister; and held in Me as the Sacred Vessel of hope."

Again there was pulsating white and red light.

"Through this offering may all sin be forgiven; may all choices not to love be counted for nothing so that all may begin afresh to revel in their love for You."

She broke the bread; dipped it in oil and salt; and gave it to them saying: "This is the very God who made you, sent Jesus to rescue you, sends The Spirit to strengthen you, and has sent Me to bring new hope of everlasting life, of being enfolded back into the Creator from whom you came. Teach all your followers to bless wine and break bread as I have done so that all may invoke the very presence of Their true parent. Make sure that never again is that sacred power of bringing God among you reserved to a special class of people, to those who are men, to those who have read difficult books. Promise me now that you will preach a Gospel of universal empowerment that all those who have been created as God's children can invoke the true presence through their free choice to spend time in the company of God. Teach all to believe that they have the power to draw near to their creator here on earth before they are enfolded back into the very being of God Our Parent when they have fulfilled their role, loving the free and free to love."

We began to eat dinner. She had found dishes from all over the world; like the meal at Christmas; and although each of us had been asked to choose a favourite all the food was passed around so that each might eat something of each dish. She encouraged without pushing; she seemed to be everywhere without ever rushing. She seemed to be part here and part not here; as if She was already conscious of Her return to God Our Parent.

"There is only the ordeal between me and reunion now," She said "and then I will have to leave you for a while; as you know; before I return. I was sent to bear witness to God in the world and to regenerate the worship of Jesus My Brother and My mission in the power of the Spirit is almost accomplished."

When She left the room we began to argue about our places at the table and to say what places we would occupy in Heaven

"I might be a long way from her now," said Brian "but when we meet again in Heaven I will be right up there."

"Heaven," She said coming in quietly with an atlas under her arm "is not a hierarchy. There are no tables and banquets and other human-like things there. The whole point about being enfolded back into the Creator is that you will relinquish your flawed creatureliness and return from where you came as part of the very substance of the one true and loving God.

"Here are the dishes of many lands; here is a map. Instead of choosing your hypothetical places at a mythical table choose where you might take my message. When I have gone there will only be you to start with to carry on the mission."

Heather and Jo made as if to slip away but She caught them and spoke quietly with them in the hall where the others could not hear

"I do not know exactly what you are planning to do but I know what it will mean. I am sorry for you that it has come to this. For Me there is no choice; I must take what is given to Me; but I will pray for you."

When She returned we were quarrelling over the map. "I am going to America," said Dexter "because that is the biggest place."

"Is there not enough territory to go round?" She asked almost exasperated. "My poor sisters and brothers; you cannot help competing. I pray that you may compete for the glory of God and not for your own glory.

"Look how big the world is and how few you are. You will need courage patience and a willingness to engage others whom you do not yet know. You will be insulted and beaten; you will be brutally attacked with word and weapon; you will be shunned as irrelevant and shunned as if you were fatally diseased; you will be lifted up on high as good people and then smashed to the ground so that your reputations are nothing; you will be idolised and trivialised; but however you are treated your end will be the same. You will all suffer and die for My sake and for the sake of Jesus My Brother and God Our Parent. But I will send you My Sister the Spirit."

When we had finished She again left the room and again we started quarrelling; this time about what powers She had given us. Again She came in quietly

"Oh children; remember; they are not your powers; nor even mine. All come from God our Parent who has made everything. Do not seek power or it will be the wrong kind; it will be the earthly power that makes love more difficult. In the end there is love and power and the one (if love can be said to have an enemy) is the enemy of the other. Always remember; love is opening space for others freely to love; power is closing down space; making it more difficult for people freely to love.

"Power is tight; love is loose. Power is closed; love is open. Power is hard; love is soft. Power breaks down barriers and invades; love finds its way into the tiniest places. Never overlook the tiny places where love has found a place. They are the precious gardens of God Our Parent where the flower of love may briefly bloom; die; and then bloom again. Power is like a forced vegetable a thing of nature that has been perverted by earthly lust. Love is the flower that grows as it will; that gives pleasure; that is itself; that calls for nothing; asks for nothing; serves for nothing. Its beauty is in itself and all may see it; but to own that beauty is to destroy it. People will struggle for power; as you poor children are tempted to struggle for power; but there is no struggle for love; it belongs to no-one; it is the gift of God Our Parent; it is ours to enjoy in unlimited bliss but to try to capture it is to banish it."

We looked puzzled.

"Do you not realise after all this time that you will be wonderful large lively people in love; and in all other things you will be almost invisible; nothing? Do you not yet realise what I have told you all along that your stature will be measured in the space you make not in the things you take? Do you not realise what I have told you all along that you love God to the extent you have chosen to love all the children of God? Sometimes my sweet brothers and sisters I think that there is no way in human language simple enough to tell you about God and the love of Our Parent for all children. Sometimes I fear that I can hardly prepare you for what you will suffer for the sake of love. Poor children! Smile now and drink more wine because the day of my terrible suffering is not far away."

"We will defend you," said Dexter.

"Dear children. I do not blame you. I hardly dare tell you; but you will run away. I was meant for a lonely death but I hardly know how to tell you."

They look sad.

She cry.

Then She smile and said

"But that will come when it comes. Until then we will enjoy our evening together. Jim I have a new song for you. After all these years of humming a chorus I have finally found the words I want. Let me sing it and you catch up with me

It's the sign that counts
the glass we see through and shatter
the bread we offer and break

the gifts we offer and take
the ash we gather and scatter:
It's the sign that counts
it's the sacred sign
it's the joining hands
and the broken line
it's the space we dance in
but we never own
it's the love we fashion
in word and bone.
It's the sign that counts
the dance of passion and danger
the working and weaving of fragments
the sound of laughter and laments
the fire of warmth and anger:
it's the sign that counts
the kiss bestowed on a lover
the sex unwanting and open
The child born of emotion
the smile that says it's forever:
It's the sign that counts
the melody that bends its line
the bridge that crosses a river
whatever brings us together
it's the sign.

It was all white.
All the red had gone.
She laugh.
We dance.

"Do you not see now how the divine and human connect? What Christians call Sacraments which they received from Jesus My Brother are only special instances or connections that have been distorted through the use of power; particularly male power. All creation is divine. All creation is a sign. They will call it 'sacramental' but that is both to make too much and too little of it. If it is 'sacramental' they own it; but they cannot own everything. In fact they cannot own anything. They just think they can.

"What we have to create for all people are signs that give divine significance to human lives; that show the promise of what is to come so that we can enjoy it now. God Our Parent did not create children to live in some kind of ante room; temporary exiles waiting to go back; creation allows freedom to enjoy the prospect of God before being enfolded. Once enfolded there is perfect freedom but the taste of human freedom is so sweet. Likewise to be enfolded in total love is the end of all our being but to taste the possibility of total love is the sweet fruit of humanity.

"All this lovely sweet fruit and so often we choose the bitter. All this sweet fruit and we look coldly upon it and let it go rotten. So much fruit my children for you all to gather. How I wish that I could have stayed longer to gather it with you. For although I am the Sacred Vessel I am as human as you and so love to see that fruit before me; before you; before everyone.

She smile; sad.

"It is too late now. You will have to say what I have not been able to say. You will ask 'How can the world be so sweet when Perpetua has gone?' and the Spirit will say 'Because She pointed Her finger and nobody followed where it pointed until She died and then it became clear.' So sad that humanity has to be driven to extremes before it recognises the simple. People say 'you only miss something when it is gone'. Love never goes but so many people miss it; perhaps love only grows when it seems to be under threat. I have sometimes wondered what would have happened if Jesus My Brother had died quietly in the shade of a tree; and I think that His life; His teaching; His very incarnation would have been quickly forgotten. People needed to see Him absorb the world's wickedness; it was not good enough for Him to say that He would. People need to look at the Cross and see their own deed and compare it with His love; then they recognised Him.

"So it is with me. The world will only see My Godhead when My body has been transformed. It is a necessary sadness; a necessary suffering.

"Lovely rich earth with such sweet fruit and so many poor people starved of love who can hardly imagine it let alone see it. Take the fruit of love and freedom and carry it all over the earth that it may bear seeds and grow lovely trees. The more you scatter the more there will be; this is my promise. You will never want for fruit; you will always even when your hearts fail know deep down that as you lift your eyes back up towards the world away from your inward fears there will be fruit.

"You are looking tired. It has been a long day; part of a long week. We have done well. We have prepared the way. Whatever happens do not forget tonight. Do not forget to celebrate love and freedom in God Our Parent. Let us have a final verse and chorus

> *It's the sign that counts*
> *the melody that bends its line*
> *the bridge that crosses a river*
> *whatever brings us together*

it's the sign:
It's the sign that counts
it's the sacred sign
it's the joining hands
and the broken line
it's the space we dance in
but we never own
it's the love we fashion
in word and bone.

She said goodbye to each one of us as if She would never see us again but Dexter Trina and Andy stayed behind.

As we left I could see the light going red.

The others did not stay long. They helped to clear up and then she asked them to pray. They dozed; their minds wandered; it had all been too much. After a while she tried no more. She did not want them to leave but She knew they must.

They left.

She cry.

She prayed alone for the strength to go through with what She must face but like earlier in Lent she was tempted. She saw what good She could do if She stayed alive; if She waited a while before returning from where She came.

"Just one more year," She thought. "This time has been so short; not even nine months and everything so fragile.

"I must go back to God Our Parent. I must trust My Sister the Spirit; I must keep always in my mind the life and death of Jesus My Brother; all three which are part of me must give me strength now."

She took a Crucifix from the mantelpiece and held it at face level; arms length; in Her hands.

She dance.

Round and round the room in the red light with the Cross in Her hands.

She laid the Cross on the table where She had sat at dinner and put some bits and pieces around it; flowers, an unused spoon, a red ribbon; remembering that night when She had begun Her mission. Now that She had survived the temptation of wanting Her mission to go on the memories were sharper and more precious.

"To be human," She thought "is to live in a permanent state of Schadenfreude but to be divine is to know the word that makes them one."

She sat in the chair and looked straight at the Cross.

"There is really nothing more to say. I offer myself tonight knowing that My time has come. It was only a tiny wobble. I am firm. Thank You for putting

Me here to do Your will. I am ready."

The red light went out.

Jim knocked softly at the door.

"I thought you might like some music to help you sleep; you look so tired."

"That is so kind of you."

"What should I play?"

"Perhaps just one last chorus of our new song. I will sleep in the chair."

It's the sign that counts.

He played it in a series of magical variations; like Goldberg for a prince; until She was asleep. Then he left quietly and made his sad way to Father Bill's.

Fourteen

I am She

After witnessing in the streets to the death of Jesus Her Brother She stayed at the back of the church for the Liturgy of the Cross. When it came to the Veneration She could hardly walk but She gathered all Her strength and fell at His feet in a gesture of unembarrassed abandon. All who saw Her were moved to tears. In Her adoration they saw the meaning of the Cross. As the Gospel was read She focused on every incident crossing each off as it came saying to Herself

"I am She."

In his sermon Bill Midway said

"Today we recall the bitter passion of Our Lord Jesus Christ but it should not be a recalling as of a thing of old; something that has passed; a memory of a bygone age when Jesus suffered among us. For He is here now; suffering with us now. He suffers in the slums where the people live whom we abandon and He suffers equally among the rich who have abandoned Him. There were many including His friends who abandoned Him in His hour of greatest need but there were even more who were not there because they did not know or care what was happening. During the past few months we have tried to reach out to the abandoned of both kinds; to the poor and the rich; to bring His Word to harassed and hardened hearts. Some of you have been with me to the house groups with the poor; some of you have braved the insults and worse the indifference of those in prosperous areas. You have sacrificed the shelter of this church for the open and threatening places of the world. But wherever we have felt most abused that is where He has been. We have felt Him among us through the leadership of Our Sister Perpetua. She would not on this His day want His message to be obscured by raising Her up before you but where we have recognised Her we have recognised Him. His mission went largely unrecognised but we must not make the same mistake today. Those who were most committed to following God made the mistake of not seeing The Word fulfilled in Jesus our Messiah but we must not make the same mistake; tying ourselves to an unchanging tradition; locked in a human understanding of God that owes everything to who we are and nothing to the greatness of the mystery. Once the death of Jesus ceases to be a mystery it becomes a tool of the religious oppressors. We are today presented with the same opportunity of witness which those who condemned Jesus failed to take. We must take it. It has cost me much to wrench myself from the comfort of the God I saw to see God renewed again in the promise of hope; to see that our doctrine is always in danger of becoming a prison and not a force for liberation. Again I would not want my own situation to obscure what we are remembering today; but to deny what has changed is to cloud the meaning of Good Friday. We must see God's love anew and we must move from a theoretical framework of religion in which we are comfortable and renew our personal relationship with God. We must move from a necessary recognition to an indispensable love for what God is. Perpetua has taught us that God's love is never-ending; that we will not be abandoned; but in return; although this is not equivalent in any way; we must not abandon God; we must not abandon Jesus on His Cross but be with Him today as He is with us always."

After the service when the tempest was raging outside Perpetua stayed at the foot of the Cross in an island of calm. She lay on the cold stone and prayed and then in a cloud of red light She danced with Her Brother in a last dance of commitment to be with Him.

"I will be with You today mirroring confirming everything You did; and then I will be re-united with You," She said.

She lay down again as if to take one last moment of rest at His feet; and Her mobile phone rang.

While the service was going on and for hours afterwards there was a terrible storm. On the stroke of Three O'Clock a huge tornado tore through the middle of London; tearing away the doors of churches; trashing media offices and shopping malls. The radio and television services went over to emergency procedures and people struggled to reach their homes to evade the storm frightened of what they might find when they got there.

Some said it was a judgment on the country for its greed and indifference to the threat of climate change. Others said it was God's punishment for the wickedness of materialism. But most people simply cursed and said it was one of those freak events that insurers ironically call "Acts of God."

Father Joe sitting bleakly in his Presbytery saw it as some kind of punishment for what he was thinking. He saw Wayne struggling towards him in the pouring rain and then the image turned to darkness. To his horror the image of Wayne and the image of Jesus on the Cross on the opposite wall kept changing into each other. He reached for the whiskey bottle.

Forgiveness is unending

The message said

"help! the hollow".

As She closed the door the lights came on. She walked through the sodden and empty streets; slow and quick at the same time. She noticed the wrecked shop front of Hypo and wondered about Annie Price. Whatever God was saying in the storm She knew that it would be just. She did not know what it meant; and certainly did not connect it with Her own impending death; but She felt its weight as She walked steadily down the slope towards The Hollow.

When She arrived She saw Beth and Jo standing uncomfortably just in front of Roy and some of his gang.

"I came as soon as I could," She said in a level voice.

"That is Her," said Jo to Roy.

"I know. It's hardly necessary for you to say that. Now get lost. You have done what you came to do."

"What did you come to do?" She asked. "These are not good people for you to be with."

"They are our people," said Heather "and when we left them you promised a better life. But nothing has changed. You said you would change the world; but look at it. Look at us."

"I never meant to imply that you would be materially better off."

"All that stuff about good news for the poor," said Jo.

"Cut it out," said Roy. "You have done what you have done."

The two girls flinched at his brutality but then decided that the sooner they left the better. Their only route was past Perpetua and they tried to dart past to avoid Her but She put Her arm out; slowly; so as not to frighten or hurt them.

"Forgiveness is unending," She said as She put Her right hand in turn on each of their heads. "Remember; when things look desperate; as I fear they may; forgiveness is unending."

<u>Love Transcends Power</u>

When they had gone trying not to run She was left facing the gang. Then She was aware of Rory and Olly coming forward.

"What are you doing here?"

"We are appearing for the prosecution," said Rory.

"We charge you with subverting Christianity," said Olly.

Roy looked bored. "We have to go through with this for the sake of his father and my uncle," said Olly.

"Oh go ahead then. It's your party after all," said Roy turning away.

"We put it to you," said Rory trying to look formal "that you have subverted the Christian religion. You have claimed to be part of the Godhead and in doing so you have denied the doctrine of the Blessed Trinity."

She say nothing.

Olly hit her in the face. "What do you say?"

"I ask how you in your lives have paid respect to God Our Parent; Jesus My Brother; and My Sister the Spirit? What I have done is for God and me; what you have done is for God and you."

"So do you claim some special relationship with the Trinity which you describe in your quaint; or is it subversive; language?"

"You have heard me talk many times. I will not deny anything I have said."

"So do you claim to have supernatural powers?"

She say nothing.

"I ask you again; do you claim to have supernatural powers?"

"You know that all power comes from God."

"That is an evasive answer."

She say nothing.

"We further put it to you," said Rory "that you have attempted to over-throw the Christian Church by calling on people to abandon it in favour of 'congregational' house groups."

"I see your brief study at theological college did not include the early church."

He hit Her.

"That's the kind of clever answer I would expect from you. Answer the question."

She say nothing.

Exasperated Rory came very close so that their faces almost touched.

"You have wrecked the life of my uncle. You have told him that his life is worthless."

"Only he and I know what we have said."

"It's plain to see what you have done."

"Nothing is plain to see except to God."

"Another clever answer."

"Get on with it," said Roy with television on his mind. "This is boring."

"We won't be long," said Olly. "Just one more question. Do you deny that you have been trying to overthrow the Christian Church?"

"I was sent to build up the church of God. What happens to structures and hierarchies and power are only incidental. Love transcends power."

"We will show you what love is." said Olly.

<u>I am the Sacred Vessel in which all love and denial of love are contained</u>

She was desecrated. The Sacred Vessel was smashed. She who was the most wonderful person that our world has ever seen; Pardon me Jesus; was laid low and all the wickedness of the world was poured into Her mingling with all Her goodness. And yet I know that it could not overcome Her. She absorbed the wickedness so that we might start again.

The gang formed a circle and started to chant

"It's the thing that counts! It's my thing that counts!"

First the two prosecutors raped Her and then the rest; brutally; joylessly; methodically. Then the prosecutors began to fight over her god4u t-shirt and Roy had to pull them apart.

"Don't be stupid," he said. "Take another bit of her clothing as a souvenir."

Then they all took their drug of preference and with Rory and Olly holding Her down Roy injected her with a cocktail of drugs. As they waited for them to take effect they stood about drinking beer and insulting Her; occasionally giving Her a kick.

There were shadowy figures in doorways and on walkways in the flats but everybody hurried by as if nothing unusual was happening on that degraded piece of land. Occasionally somebody would venture to the edge of the muddy patch but would then go away again frightened; ashamed. They knew better than to interfere. Word had got round that the police were nearby; they would sort it all out; there was nothing else they could do.

Then a horrible noise began to emerge from the knot of people around Her. They were seized by a collective wave of anger and hysteria and began to curse Her.

"Posh bitch who didn't know her place!"

"Preachy little girl always on about sex and drugs; well she's had them now."

"Where are all your friends? That wimp Dexter and all your other mates? Why don't they come to save you?"

"Come to think of it; if you're that special why doesn't the almighty come down and give us a beating?"

She managed to sit up; Her face crumpled with pain.

"I am the Sacred Vessel in which all love and denial of love are contained," She said. "It was meant to be this way. Better to pray that God will save you rather than worrying about me."

Rory kicked Her fiercely in the face and this started an orgy of violence. One pissed on Her; another vomited. They stamped on Her hands; ground glass into Her face and stubbed out cigarettes on Her arms. They went on pounding until Her body was broken and limp; with blood pouring from Her mouth and stomach.

They left Her for dead. They had grown bored with the violence. They needed something else on which to vent their anger. She was not an object of searing hate but a piece of collateral damage; something to provide entertainment and then be cast aside. She was the bringer of light; of so much promise; and yet She was the victim of those She had come to save.

O poor, broken queen. O Queen of Heaven come down and rejected.

<u>The Beauty of Imperfection</u>

She thought She was in heaven. She was bathed in a light and warmth She had not known since Her mission began. She looked down on Herself laid on the ground surrounded by the detritus of Her violation. It reminded Her of that Yellow evening when Her work began.

Jesus said:

"I know how you feel. It was hard for me to leave. I loved them so much. All those people created by Our Parent struggling to love; struggling to create beauty out of the material around them; struggling to love when there were so many barriers."

"Yes," She said. "I loved the beauty of imperfection. I know now why they are so precious to God Our Parent. They are so much more beautiful than angels. What love they offer is so precious emerging from trouble and pain. I love their endless search to understand the mystery that we are. How much more worthy this is than what they think of as the chorus of the angelic choirs. I love the brokenness of their prayers; the sadness of their songs; the incompleteness of their words; the woundedness of their gestures; the hesitation of their actions; the naivite of their signs."

"Even when they denied me I could not help smiling. They thought their imperfections were so serious and they were so sad; and yet I knew; as I know you must have known; how small are their shortcomings in comparison with their striving."

"They loved us more than they will know until they are here, within us. I tried to tell them but they were so hard on themselves and so hard on each other."

"That is what I found hardest to bear. How their imperfection made them hard not soft. They used to come back from fishing tired and dispirited when they had tried so hard."

"They came to worship after a long day at the supermarket stacking shelves and thought that I would be displeased with them when their minds wandered. I found it so hard to convince them how wonderful they were."

"They do not understand the joy of imperfection; the preciousness of the love they offer."

"But Jesus My Brother what have we done wrong?"

"Nothing. It is their joy and their sorrow that they are imperfect. God Our Parent created in them the most wonderful difference from what we are. Without that difference the love we are would simply be contained within itself. God has opened up love into a new domain; into a space where it grows in such variety. I have often thought when I see them how our perfection is paradoxically limiting. In a strange way their love for us is more wonderful than our love for them."

She shifted slightly and the vision fragmented.

"Are you still with me Jesus My Brother?"

"Yes. You are passing back to earth for the last time."

"How glad I am to go once more to see them still struggling."

"I wish I was coming with you."

"I wish they could see it; not in the grand formulations they so piously construct to reach us. I wish they could see it in the journey; in the individual act; in the incomplete but so beautiful prayer."

She shifted again and saw Max shuffling towards Her in the mud.

<u>In Loving one We Love Everyone</u>

"Max," She said struggling to raise Herself on Her elbows. "What are you doing here?"

"I lost heart. I slipped back."

"Yes; but do you not see that slipping back gives you the opportunity to go forward again?"

"It sounds all right but I am ashamed."

"Max; what has happened to Marta and the baby?"

"Never mind that now. What can I do to help You?"

"The best way you can help me is to go back to Marta."

"She said if I slipped back she would not have me."

"She will. You must try again."

"I have lost hope. There is nothing left."

"How can you lose hope when you see Me here in front of you dying to show the value of love? You cannot love the whole world; in loving one; in loving Marta; we love the world."

She stared into the distance. "Poor Dexter," She said. "He will need you. He will be so desolate; and he has tried so hard."

"I don't claim any credit for being here."

"No; but it will be harder for those who were not. Look after them; my poor people. Go back to Marta and love her as I know she loves you."

"Are you sure?"

"Yes. There is nothing more for you to do here."

As he went he was vaguely aware through his tears of people coming the other way.

"Bill," She said "and Jim. You already know that you need each other. You have the solid experience of God's people Bill; and Jim although he will not admit it has seen God's presence."

"Strange lights," said Jim; crying.

"Do not cry Jim. Those strange lights you have seen are God's way of showing you that you will never be alone."

<u>Blessed Are They Who Have Taken Up Their Cross And Followed Me</u>

The pain crumpled her face again. Bill bent down in the mud and put his ear near to Her mouth.

"Blessed are the chosen," She said "but more blessed are those who have taken up their Cross and followed me."

She made the figure of the Cross with Her poor arms across her bleeding chest and with a last effort She said:

"It has begun again. I thank you God Our Parent that it has begun again."

She die.

Figures appeared out of the gloom. They picked Her up gently and carried Her away. After the journey they wrapped Her in some old red choir robes in the vestry of Bill's church. They knelt in prayer and then rose to leave but Bill was so overcome that He did not notice when he left that Jim was not with him. He stayed by Her broken body.

Fifteen

She was God's own Daughter and we killed Her
we ran when they captured Her and killed Her
She had been so kind
She had won our hearts and minds
we thought we left that all behind when we killed Her.
But She rose in a blaze of glory
yes, she rose in a blaze of glory
triumphant star in Her own love story
in a blaze of glory She rose
in a blaze of glory
She rose.

Jim thought he must have dozed off. When he woke he was aware of the now familiar red light over the place where She lay. As he looked intently at the spot the light changed to intense white so that he had to close his eyes; but the light still got through. When he opened them again She was gone. The old red robes were folded neatly in a pile and tied with a white ribbon. He looked for a frightened moment and then he ran faster than he had ever run before. He knew he was carrying the most important news that he would ever carry.

"She's gone," he told Bill who had never really slept. "She's gone!"

"It's all right," said Bill. "Don't be frightened. She will come back. I know now She will come back but we must be prepared to wait. Stay calm; don't be frightened."

"Shall we phone Dexter?"

"No; let things take their course Jim; that's best."

Jim could hardly contain himself as the day wore on. He helped Bill and the ladies prepare the church for Easter; he played his flute; he went for a walk round the overgrown graveyard; when he knew nobody was looking he went to look at the spot where She had been laid. Time dragged. He kept taking his mobile phone out; looking at it; switching it on to check if there were any messages he told himself then putting it away.

"I know," said Bill "it's a strange time between the death of Jesus and when He rises again. It's bad enough when you know what is going to happen but it must have been so much worse for the followers of Jesus; Peter; the other Apostles; the followers and perhaps worst of all His mother Mary. I wonder whether she had any inkling of what would happen. And it must be like that for Dexter and our friends now. I would let you join them if I knew where they all were but there does not seem to be anybody at Bleak Villas so you are better off with me."

For Trina and Miles the roles were reversed. He had this idea that Perpetua would rise again. He kept telling her that he was sure this would happen. She said that of course she must hope for this from what Perpetua said; but her spirits were low. He tried to tell her there was no more she could have done but she could not be convinced.

They went to where Jo and Heather had killed themselves. They asked her if she was prepared to sign for the few bits of property they had left. When she turned on Beth's damaged mobile phone she saw an unread message

4giv infin—p

She must have written it in the minute after they left; before She faced Her mock trial.

Jim hardly slept. When he woke he had the sense of lightness that you get when you wake up on a snowy morning. Everything was bright and still. He could feel the lightness of the air but of course when he went to look outside the window there was no snow. He said nothing when he met Bill for the early service. When it was over he took a quick look at his phone and there was a message from Dexter

SOS All god4u 2 BV

He told Bill. "He would not say that without reason," said Bill. "He is our leader now. I will ask the Curate to take the main Communion. I will explain later; but perhaps I will not need to."

Restlessly waiting in the hall Jim picked up the TT; and She was there. She was there! He showed Bill. "But I knew anyway," he said "after the light on Friday night. I knew."

They were all gathered in the kitchen looking tired and grey. They did not know what to do but Dexter said they were to wait there until they were told what they must do. Then Jim rushed in

"She's alive!" he said, "She's in the paper and I know She's alive because I saw it."

"Slowly," said Bill.

Jim told his story.

Then the television came to life and the room went so bright that even closing your eyes was not enough.

Then She was there. She was there! Jim thought he was going to faint but he held onto Bill.

She was standing as if on a cloud

"I promised that I would never leave you. God Our Parent and Jesus My Brother want you to know that everything they have done has been re-confirmed in Me as Their Vessel. You do not need to do anything drastic. Remember what we learned together. You must now go out and practice what you have learned."

Dexter lay flat on the ground barely raising his face to the screen.

"My God! How could I have doubted you?" he said; quietly.

"It says in the Gospel that there were fifty days between the Resurrection of Jesus My Brother; His return to God Our Parent; and the sending of My Sister the Holy Spirit; but the world does not work like that any more. Be ready at noon today to receive further help for what you have to do."

Dexter said

"Where are you? It looks like the top of a tall building or maybe you have already returned to God Our Parent."

"I am alive but not in the way I was when we were together. I am taking this earthly shape so that we can talk. If you think back to all the things that I have told you it will become clear."

She explained carefully all that had happened and what it would mean for them.

She smile.

Then the screen went back to Her picture.

They wanted to run out into the street but Dexter told them to stay put and wait for what would happen next.

They were so intent on talking about the future that they were jolted when the screen lit up again.

"I have taken the highly unusual step of speaking to you all on every media channel on planet earth in your own language because I want you to know that God Our Parent loves all of you. That love was shown when Jesus My Brother was sent to demonstrate God's love on earth; and it was shown again when I was sent as a witness; as the Vessel of God's fullness. I was killed but I have returned to proclaim God's love afresh to all the world.

"In matters concerning God forget complexity; hierarchy' tidiness; cleverness; and calculation; these are simply human attributes for human situations.

"When you think of the divine love of God for everyone think only of returning God's faith in you expressed in creation with faith in God; God's hope in you expressed in the Resurrection with your hope in God; and return God's love for you expressed in my space through your love of God; and in all three recognise the constancy of My Sister The Spirit."

After a few moments of silence Bill said

"Let us pray."

And they prayed to God Our Parent; Our Brother Jesus; Our Sister the Spirit; and our own special Sacred Vessel. It was not broken; it had somehow miraculously been put together and in memory of its brokenness it was no longer smooth but shining with millions of facets; no longer smooth and uniform but made up of countless facets of light.

We rushed down the street towards the Easter Market shouting

"Alleluia! Perpetua is risen!"

Nobody was more animated than Miles whose obvious love for Trina was totally bound up with this new beginning. Except for Her face I have never seen happier faces.

Father O'Helly still feeling hung over after struggling through Easter and writing to Olly switched on the television to see The Pope's Easter message; and before he could turn the set off when it was over

She was there!

He felt full of new hope and rang Archdeacon Varnish.

"Did you see it?"

"Yes. We are going to have to undertake a little re-thinking to take account of the emerging situation."

"Anglican fuddle!" O'Helly almost shouted. "Come for a walk."

"Yes; I think a little fresh air would do me good."

Before he left the house he threw away all his magazines.

They met at the Easter Market and walked round not saying much. O'Helly had plenty to think about and Varnish was still caught between worry over Rory's exploits and relief that Perpetua had in some strange way come to no harm. Then Dexter and his followers came shouting and dancing between the stalls.

"Yes Archdeacon," said O'Helly not quite able to suppress his customary dry humour "I think a little adjustment will be necessary."

Dexter began to speak and it was amazing how the tourists stopped to listen as if each were hearing him in their own language. Even the Chinese students seemed to understand what was going on. When Father Joe spotted Olly he tried to hide without it being obvious to Varnish but the kid just came right up to him and said

"I'm terribly sorry for what I've done."

"What?"

"The blog."

"What blog?"

"Never mind. If you see it I'm sorry. If you don't see it; well; I'm still sorry but there will be less harm done."

"What harm?"

"I put your letter on my blog and I'm afraid I wasn't very enthusiastic."

"No harm done Oliver. I want to be a witness to Perpetua in my own small way and what happens to me doesn't matter."

"Good luck," said Olly and walked off.

"There's a rumour," said Varnish "that that nephew of yours and my son Rory were in some way involved with what happened to Perpetua."

"I've heard that too; but if She was; er is; the sort of woman; Oh dear; not woman; as She is who She says She is I doubt anything will happen. They know what they did if they did anything."

"Most reassuring," said Varnish. "I must leave now to get ready for Evensong. Nothing like a powerful set of Canticles and an Anthem in a fine building."

"And what She has done; and the rest," said Father Joe.

It was then that he saw Wayne. He tried to hang back but as with Olly the boy; as he thought of him; came straight towards him.

"Don't say anything," said Wayne "not because I don't want you to but because we need time."

"I know; you have your work to do with Dexter."

"When the day's work is over we can talk."

"What are you doing?"

"I'm learning to do some of the jobs Heather and Jo used to do. I need to be in a place where I don't keep opening my mouth trying to sound clever."

"I know the temptation," said Father Joe. "We will be a fine pair keeping each other quiet and then competing in cleverness."

"Baby is heavy," said Marta. "Have you named her yet?" asked Max. "Never got settled really; gypsy baby; Lucy baby. Now she's Perpetwa; not just light but perpetwal light."

"Good."

"Well; if she's heavy we better find a pram."

"Too dear. Even second hand pram too dear."

"I've got a bit left. Let's buy a little pram."

"Only if you promise."

"I know. Friday was the last time and it changed me forever. After I've had a word with Andy about god4u funding we'll go and find a pram."

They were walking past a shabby second-hand stall when Marta saw a little pram.

"So sweet; but how do you say? Scruffy."

"Yes. But we can clean it up."

"Yes. We try. How much this pram?"

The young woman who had been turned away looking intently at something turned round and Perpetua said

"A gift for a new love."

And the pram gleamed with white newness.

Dexter told all the people that they were welcome to come to a special celebration.

"Bring Father Joe," said Dexter to Wayne. "Bring the baby," he said to Marta and Max. "You won't have to stay too long," he said to Miles and Trina.

"As long as you like," said Trina.

"There is so much to celebrate but sometimes the personal takes precedence over the collective; sometimes vice versa; And we can't work without you Bill."

"I'm going to dash round my congregation and say what's happened and then bring them."

It was a deadly deliberate choice. Dexter walked at the head of a procession through the down-trodden streets of Grunge Park straight to the Hollow; the scene of Her death and His denial. Before he reached the spot Dexter knocked on Roy's door.

"Come out. There's no need to hide. We all know what you did. In a way you don't know it was what was meant. I have returned but not to take physical control. I have come to mend broken lives; to bring people back to themselves and to God. Bring all your people out and all the stuff you've got in there."

They brought out their knives bats bits of metal and two guns.

"Put them down there," said Dexter. "Put them where she lay when you had finished with her. Make them into the shape of a Cross. Now do what you think is appropriate."

The crowd went completely silent. As if by some invisible message people began to come out of the houses and I_in the crowd that Dexter had brought.

Roy kneel.

He touched the bottom of the long stem of the Cross where his own knife was laid.

"Sorry My sad Sister," he said. "I have done wrong and I want everybody here to know it."

Dexter shook Roy by the hand and then he said

"We must start; even at the height of our joy and thanksgiving; in the mud; to remind us that we have all done wrong. I do not want my personal sadness to dominate Her most glorious day but to avoid any misunderstanding I want to confirm publicly and openly that I denied Her. I did a much worse wrong than Roy here. I ran away when I was needed. Only Jim and Father Bill were there at the last.

"But what is important is that whatever I have done; flawed though I am she wanted me to lead her mission. We are simple people. We have not come from the universities; we are not high dignitaries of the Church; but She chose us because She wanted people who were most in need of Her. We live in a land of many peoples and many sadnesses and we must take God Our Parent into the lives and hearts of all of them. She has promised us the gift of tongues and we must use these gifts with reverence and care. The tongue can be dangerous. We must take care.

"Before I carry out our promise to remember the Sacred Godhead in the way She asked I just want to say that I am your servant. I will sometimes answer back and sometimes drop the dishes; but I am your servant to the end."

His followers handed round bread; and wine in small plastic cups. He looked up to heaven and I saw again that white light descending upon him; surrounding him.

"In the name of God Our Parent and Jesus Our Brother and in the memory of our Beloved Sister God's Sacred Vessel I call upon Our Sister the Spirit to make these gifts we offer into the very presence of Jesus and Perpetua."

Father Joe could not help wincing.

They ate and drank and danced and talked of the wonderful things that had happened to them since She had come among them. Trina and Miles would not leave before the clearing up was completed. Father Joe tried to slip away but Wayne caught him.

They went to the sad Presbytery which saw real joy for the first time since Father O'Helly had entered it. They both wanted to talk but exercised a kind of reverence. The day had filled them with joy and they were quietly happy in each other.

"It will be difficult," thought O'Helly "but She will see me right."

"I am still uncertain," thought Wayne "but She has given me strength to decide."

When Miles and Trina got home they were exhausted and exhilarated.

"Will you marry me?"

"No Trina. I won't be here long enough."

"What do you mean?"

"I already know that I can't last long with what is going on inside me. Your gentleness will try to moderate me so that I can serve God for many years but it won't work."

"But Miles; I want you so badly. I need us to be one. She told us that you could not separate the spiritual and the physical."

"I know. It was the last barrier to fall. Yes of course we will marry. She would want us to love each other with our whole selves until the time that God Our Parent calls me to be enfolded; to be taken back (or is it forward?) to where I came from. Until then there will only be Her and you; and in a way that She would understand the two are the same thing."

She is God's own Daughter and we love Her
when She rose again we ran to Her forever
She had been so kind
She had won our hearts and minds
We gave all that we could find to show we loved her:
And She came in a blaze of glory
yes, she came in a blaze of glory
the sacred babe in Her own love story
in a blaze of glory She came.
Such a start; such a start
When She gave her sacred heart
such a sense of failure turned to glorious fame
such a gracious space when She came to us in grace
when we promised Her that we would bear the flame.
And She came in a blaze of glory
yes, She came in a blaze of glory
the sacred babe in Her own love story
in a blaze of glory She came.
We live in the brightness of the day
With its sweet and mellow curve
In the gentle light of hope, the space of love,
With the sound of silent prayer and such radiance in the air
when She said She had come back again we knew it.
And She came in a blaze of glory
yes, She came in a blaze of glory
the sacred babe in Her own love story
in a blaze of glory She came.
She is god's own daughter and we love her.

DAMIAN

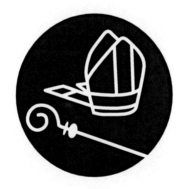

I.

In the beginning, God created the beginning. Where there was nothing, there was something. The Creator, and all the reified manifestations of the Godhead that there will ever be, and their Sister the Spirit, smiled upon time, space and matter: for time, being imperfect, having a beginning and an end, is the framework in which space may exist, but space is impossible without matter, and space is the theatre in which love is shown; for love is the choice freely to clear space for the other, and freedom is the fruit of imperfection which is space, time and matter.

And the creatures—created freely to love or not to love God Our Parent, the undivided unity of spirit and flesh—were given language and called themselves humanity.

And the Creator caused such a light to blaze that the earth looked perfectly beautiful, but there was no night, so the Creator caused a hint of night to interrupt the day as the heavenly symbol of the difference between loving and not loving, between the perfection of God and the imperfection of humanity, the choice for which humanity was created.

And in choosing between loving and not loving, humanity learned the power of fire and water, the power of the fatling and the barn, of the knife and the brick, all of which made it more difficult to choose to love; and difference became not a celebration of choice but alien, and instead of striving for choice humanity strove for uniformity. And the nights grew longer and the days grew shorter.

And one language became many. Some say that God created different languages to re-inject difference where power to impose uniformity waxed strong; but others say that fear of power drove people apart so that separate languages evolved. And the nights grew longer and the days grew shorter.

And over time, technology strengthened uniformity and empires emerged based on brick and grain. Empires rose and fell. And the nights grew longer and the days grew shorter.

And God chose a people to rescue humanity from itself and they listened and then did not listen, and they looked and then did not look. And they were faithful and unfaithful; exiled and reconciled; and those who had been chosen to undertake the rescue foundered and were in need of rescue. And the nights grew longer and the days grew shorter.

And God caused a mighty fire to burn on Mount Horeb so that the night was red bright, and the people saw each other in the red light and knew that they had failed, and they swore an oath at the foot of the mountain that they would never forget that God had made time and space and choice. But the nights grew longer and the days grew shorter.

And they listened and did not listen; and they looked and did not look; and they re-discovered the power of the fatling and the barn, the knife and the brick; and they would have a king; and God was angry, but they had chosen as they were free to choose. They were chosen but were free not to be chosen and they were swept into oblivion and the sun rose no more, so they lived in eternal night, a world of sickly moon and guttering fire. A man called Nehemiah lit a great fire, and it flared and died.

And God so loved the world that a Son was caused to be made of human flesh so that the abstraction of God which had driven the chosen people to despair should be made manifest among them. Jesus was born of Mary and Joseph in Bethlehem and, being both human and of the Godhead, His Sister the Spirit was always with Him. Some say that there was a great star to signify the birth, but others say that His mother was the morning star which shone before the new sunrise of the Lord. And the nights grew shorter and the days grew longer.

And Jesus, Son of God Our Parent, truly God and truly man, was doomed to death because His perfection was beyond the tolerance of the chosen people, but they were only the incident which represented the whole history of wrong choices which humanity had made and will make, all the indifferences of all time, all the choices not to love of every place and time. In His death He reconfirmed that no matter how much pain God suffered, pain borne in His humanity so that humanity might understand the pain, the freedom to choose would abide so that we, in our indifference and failure to love, crucified Him and crucify Him still, and when He cried out from the Cross, the darkness descended in the day but the critical point had been reached and was passed; and when they had buried Him they thought that night would descend as it had done before, but He came to us in a blaze of marvelous light and He said that because we were created to choose, and that to choose freely meant that we were made imperfect, we should not be punished for being what God had made; and He whose flesh broke into history as the star shone bright, broke again into history in another flesh, and He told the world that His own conquest of death should be to us a promise that we will all be enfolded back into the Creator from whom we had come; that God is creator and kenosis; and that kenosis is the only true love. And the nights grew shorter and the days grew longer.

And the Cross of love's freedom travelled through swamp and sand, through storm and shipwreck, to senator and slave; and the tale of old Abraham was told on Celtic mountains and the deeds of humble fishermen reached lakes that froze in Winter; and the nobility of reason and the necessity of worship, the probing and the prayer, became fused in a culture of adoration; but the Cross of Christ conquered the imperial eagle and a hint of night broke the blaze of the eternal day.

And in spite of the shadow of darkness that never completely vanished, a high point of affirmation was reached, a point where freedom to love was recognised as humanity's purpose; and the Angelic Doctor and Dante ruled the earth. And the days were long and the nights were short.

But the love of difference in the other was disfigured by love of difference in the self, and the ego escaped from the knife and the brick into the prayer and the book. And the nights grew longer and the days grew shorter.

And God Our Parent was no longer a person but a dispute and an explanation, a caricature and an insult; and then a class of object that made sense of the world. But the microscope and the telescope, the fossil and the geological fault, the turtle and the finch, the pigeon and the barnacle, the falling apple and the splitting atom, made more sense than the class of objects or object known as god; and so what had been a person and then an explanation became a curiosity. And the nights grew longer and the days grew shorter.

And the power of uniformity and the hatred of difference massacred millions in the mud and gas of war and in the brick and gas of extermination camps. Every time a catastrophe took place the people said, this will never happen again; but it happened again and again, all over the earth. The barbarity and slaughter were so great that the language was fractured, some say forever, so that talking of ourselves as children of God became almost impossible; and the sense of the gift of the earth became dulled. And day ceased.

And the sickly moon sinks over the horizon and the fires' dull glow is all that is left. There is fighting still in the trenches and fighting in the queues of idle labourers where a vineyard once flourished. The vines have been smashed by shells, the vines have been poisoned by gas, the vines have been uprooted and earth levelled for the gas chambers and the gulag.

And now? And now we live in a permanent state of darkness with a sickly moon our only memory of sunlight, of the sacred light once seen. It is so dark that we have lit our own savage fires, the fires of the forest, the flares of the plant, the dull glow of the death camp. Dante turned upside down; with Nietzsche as our guide we have descended from Heaven into hell.

We have built palaces of glass and planes of gleaming steel to take us to beaches where the sand is white and have deluded ourselves into thinking this is Heaven but it is a vain dream. We are running, we are running away, but there is nowhere to go.

There was a time when the people of Leipzig heard the music of Bach before that critical moment when the cantata became a concert, when worship gave way to philosophy, when the personal became the abstract, when the narrative became a theory. Now we listen to Bach through the filter of Schoenberg's strange shadow. How the philosophy has failed! We have climbed the mountain of Kant and Hegel to sit on the sad summit with Mahler in our ears, watching the fires in the plain. There are moments when we think that the mist has cleared, when the trumpet sounds and the dance of joy will break through, when the way to God seems open as if we could hear Bach for the first time; and then the sadness seeps in and it seems more like art than worship. And we cling to the moment like one who wakes up and tries to remember a dream, but Mahler creeps back, mordant and sarcastic, looking for a time to which there is no way back. Where there was a world there is now only the self, the sad self at the centre. And then the music rises from its grave and the rattle of the kettle drum is momentarily silenced and we look towards Heaven; but it is the sad Heaven we have made with hands. Our Saviour has no hands but ours and we have used them to build our own vision of heaven. How have we lost Heaven, why is there only this?

Our minds know glory in the pages, even amid the tawdriness of Florentine bickering it blazes; we hear it in the Leipzig dance of the trumpet but our hearts are so sad and sick that we would have a Requiem if there were one sad enough. For all that was bright makes us sad at what we have lost.

Or so it seemed.

And then God Our Parent broke again into the history of earth and sent Perpetua among us, a sacred vessel to contain all our false choices and failures to love in Her divine kenosis. She came in the night in the form of a young woman. She came in a blaze of glory that lit the lowering skies. She gathered the people together to make a cross of all the fragments of their shattered lives: the glass and the guns, the knives and the nails. And she knelt before the Cross of Jesus Her Brother, knelt in the brokenness of lives lived in the dark, and she prayed for the world, and the sky lit up as if it were day with a yellow light that had never been seen before, beyond the capture of the camera and the skill of the painter.

It started with a few but as the cross was made and the word got round, the crowd swelled to hundreds of people. It was as if everyone was under a strange influence because the rival gangs mixed without scowling, and the gangs and the people mixed without threatening on the one side or cowering on the other. She told them to bring out the old folk and the sick so that they might be comforted. People who never came out of their houses after dark came out to join in the celebration.

Perpetua said: "What did you come out to see? Some sort of sign or miracle, I suppose. Well, what you have is a sacramental occasion where the broken objects that you have brought—the glass and the fragments of wood and stone—represent your broken lives which can be put together into one whole, communal object, the Cross. And the nails and the knives and the guns which you have laid around the cross represent repentance and forgiveness.

"You are beyond self-help: it does not matter how many special schemes are introduced; it does not matter what new initiatives there are; it does not matter how much money is poured in here. There will be gun amnesties and dealer amnesties and mentoring programmes and role models and all the other paraphernalia of social engineering, but you are past all that. Only repentance can save you, only turning back to God Our Parent in thankfulness for the gift of your lives can put anything into perspective. Come to me in remembrance of Jesus My Brother and you will be healed. Your humanity, that fusion of flesh and spirit, will be set free, you will regain confidence and self-esteem in your renewed relationship with God."

"But," said one of the crowd, "we know you. You went to the local school and weren't all that bright, I seem to remember. Where did you get all this fancy talk? You never got an 'A' level and you're spouting like a professor." "I am sorry it sounds that way but God is not easy. You have to persist. You have spent too much of your lives wanting things to be easy; and when they prove difficult you have given up and turned away. I never did well at school but God Our Parent has always been with me and I have read and prayed regularly at the beginning and end of every day. I do not say this to boast but just to let you know that what I say comes from God and that I have done my part, only a small part, to earn the right to speak in the name of the Creator."

"But," said somebody else, "you didn't go to church." "I think that was partly a mistake," Perpetua replied. "I have found my search very lonely, particularly since I came to believe that I am God's Sacred Vessel. I needed support from sisters and brothers in Jesus but I had not built up that companionship. On the other hand, most of what you know about church is not from personal experience. You have a vague idea about church being boring and hierarchical which makes you hostile to it. It is easy to be hostile when you are ignorant; that is what our parents suffered when they came to this country from distant lands. Racism was the child of ignorance. There are many faults in the established Christian churches but they are not the faults of which they are mostly accused by people who know nothing about it. Words that you make no effort to understand are going to be boring; in structures where most people expect to get something for nothing there is bound to be hierarchy. Equality can only exist where everyone plays their part, where giving is unconditional."

And someone else said: "Yes, I remember you from school but there is obviously something different about you or this crowd would not be here. Who are you now and why have you come?" And she said: "Because the world has forgotten how to remember Jesus My Brother; because the language has gone and the feeling has gone and the sympathy has gone, and the words of the Creed have killed the conversation between God Our Parent and humanity, and we have seen how your hearts are sad, how the light has failed, how you live on the dark side of the earth; and just as Jesus My Brother absorbed all the sin of the world forever in his own body, so I come to do the self same act, to absorb all sin, the self-same act but at a different earthly time."

And a Priest said: "You are denying the integrity of the Passion and death of Jesus as the full and final sacrifice." "I am not," she said, "for it was indeed full but not final. The Godhead could do nothing that was not 'full' but nothing with the Godhead is final. Why cannot the Godhead undertake the self-same action at different points in human time? There is one act only but it might take place at times innumerable. Do you presume to know the 'mind' of God Our Parent? Who are you or, indeed, the Church, to say that one manifestation of the divine sacrifice is enough? Language grows thin, memory fades, empathy leeches away. The story of Jesus My Brother has become a story, like a fairytale, as the story of Moses came to be for the contemporaries of Jesus. Freedom becomes eroded and freedom must be renewed; love grows tired and must be revived. Imperfection must be a pilgrimage and not a prison. God Our Parent so loves the world that He sent Jesus My Brother and now has sent me, and God shall not cease from sending until the world ends."

"But that is like Petran Confession," said another, "for in this assurance humanity can do what it likes and there will always be a safety net." "God is not a safety net but saves absolutely. Humanity was created to love and even when it is dark, people still struggle to love, but God Our Parent will not ask of the children more than they can bear. When earthly life becomes too difficult because of the accumulation of cruelty, the coarsening of the spiritual sensibility, the balance needs to be redressed and that is why I am here now, to bring you back to where you were after the Resurrection, ready to begin a pilgrimage which will last for hundreds of years towards a new, high and deep understanding of the relationship between the Creator and humanity."

Some of the younger people began to be restless as the discussion continued and so Perpetua politely and smoothly brought it to a temporary halt. She turned to the young people and said: "What did you expect to see when you came here?" "We only came for a bit of a laugh," said one of the gang leaders. "True," she said, "I laughed when I saw you and your rivals standing next to each other without a harsh word or a violent gesture." "No, I don't mean that; I mean that we saw all these people and we thought something was going on and we might be able to have a bit of a laugh..." "...Disrupting what was going on?" "Yes, you know." "What is so funny about making life unpleasant for other people?" "Well, everything is so boring that you have to have a bit of a laugh. But then something changed and we helped to make the cross and put our stuff down there as a kind of offering." "Yes, the first thing I should do is thank you because you are usually not thanked for anything. The second thing is to say that blaming other people for what you don't like is lazy; and saying that the only things that matter are violence, sex, drugs, fashion and football is not only harmful to you and to those you hurt or simply disregard, it is also lazy; it discredits you in every way. I am not here to tell you what to do, I am here to tell you that I care about you more than I can express and you can fully understand, but my love is not mixed with judgment and harshness; I do not believe that you can be cruel to be kind; I believe that the only way to be kind is to be kind, and the only way to love is not to judge."

"Lots of words there; what does it really mean?" "It means that you will do much better if you are loved than if you are judged, but in the beginning this might mean that you make a fool of those who love you and hurt them very badly. Look at it this way: if love is making space for others in which they can exercise freedom to choose, every time you make a wrong choice it will hurt the person who created the space. It is really difficult creating space for others, as most people feel that they do not have enough space for themselves and they wrongly believe that there is only a limited amount, so the more they create for others the less they think they have left for themselves. That is not true. But the point here is that if you misuse space to hurt those who have created it for you, you tempt them to turn back to judgment and away from love. You know this; you do it yourselves and you feel it yourselves, and yet you lie to yourselves, saying that the whole world is against you and that you can only handle the world by descending into self indulgence, victimhood and cruelty.

"In the days of Jesus My Brother, people showed they had promised to make a new start by being washed in water; it was a sign of cleansing, and it still takes place in Christian churches, mostly as the excuse for a party afterwards. What I want you all to do," she said, raising her voice, "if you want to make a new start in life, to turn back to God, whether you have been baptised or not, is to take a piece of the cross away with you. Be careful because some of the glass is sharp; each piece represents a broken life, but we always need to be careful when handling pieces of the cross or a broken life. Take a piece home and put it where you can see it, and remember that it started out as a window and became a fragment but then it made a cross and now it is with you to remind you to remember the Cross."

She carefully picked up some pieces of glass and wrapped them separately in tissues and went to the edge of the crowd where there were old people sitting on benches, or chairs which people had brought outside, and she gave each one a piece of glass. Then the rest of the crowd brought her their pieces of glass to wrap; but she gave the children tiny, finished glass pieces that she had brought with her.

Then she spoke to the whole crowd and said: "Receive a small fragment of the pain of the Cross to remind you that it really was painful; by what you think and do, try to lessen the pain caused by the failure to love Jesus My Brother."

"I suppose," said the Priest, "that this is some sort of spiritualism like the things people do with crystals." "No, Father, this is sacramental; it is using what we do to bridge the gap between the human and the divine. This is the Sacrament of Healing, of taking the broken and using it to invoke Grace, not the sacrament of anointing the dead but of healing the living. The glass is sharp because that elicits voluntary, careful behaviour; you do not need other people to tell you to be careful with broken glass. You know yourself. The glass is sharp, it requires care. But much more important than that, we have to see brokenness as something that can contribute to the renewing of lives, otherwise how would broken people ever mend? They cannot be mended by others, they can only mend themselves. Yet if we care for a small piece of brokenness it will do good in the world through us with God's help. On the Cross it was the brokenness of Jesus that saved all humanity which had broken him. So much of contemporary religion pretends that to be broken, to make wrong choices, is some terrible aberration but it is not; it is the natural state of most of us for most of the time. The Church should stop judging and condemning and turn instead to working and living with brokenness, to see brokenness in itself and to be humble enough to know that its place is with the broken."

"But these thugs will attack each other with this glass," said a worried old lady. "I do not think so. If they wanted to hurt each other with pieces of glass there is plenty of it about—look around now—and if there were not then I am sure they would easily find something to break. I want to show people that the ordinary, even the potentially harmful, things that we have around us can be turned into symbols of hope if they are treated in a different way. You could say the same thing about fire, about water, about almost anything. We see some things as good and some things as bad; we see some people as good and some people as bad; but everything can be put to the good, and every person can become good. Then the problem for us is to stop forcing our definition of what is good on other people so that we stunt their goodness. I want people to learn to be good from inside their own experience, but I will not tell them how to be good. I will not give them a set of rules. I want to speak to them with the objects that they understand. If I went to them with the sacramental para-phernalia of the local church they would be bewildered, but they understand broken glass; they make it all the time."

"Leave the cross where it is," she said, "but pick up those weapons you have offered at the cross and make sure they do not do any more harm in your hands or the hands of others." "You should have confiscated them," said an angry man. "It would have made no difference. They could easily get more. The point is for these young people voluntarily to renounce weapons. Confiscation will not work."

A young man pushed through the circle around her. "That was really im-pressive," he said, "but what can I do about it?" "I seem to remember you." "Yes, I'm Dexter, the gang leader 'round here, but I'm giving it up. I'll do anything, I'll even give up the scams and just stack the shelves at Hypo to make an honest living after hearing what you said." "What did you hear?" "That it's up to me and nobody else. I keep hearing people 'round here talking about role models and special initiatives, saying that colonialism and even slavery, are excuses for the mess we've made. No: the mess I've made. I'm going to give it all up and join your gang." "Well, we have not got a 'gang' for you to join at the moment and I would prefer to think of it as a family. Tell me when you have given up the scams at Hypo; that is the kind of place where I would like to find some followers. It is a place of hidden talents." "I don't know, but I will be in touch as soon as I get sorted. Here's my knife and my gun." "I do not want them." "Nor do I. If you really are going to change it has to be just a little tough, so go to the Police and hand your weapons in and face up to the consequences. Technically you should be sent to court, and possibly prison, but my guess is that you will get off with a severe caution; but you have to go through with it. Handing the weapons to me is just a soft option." "True. How do you know what I had hardly thought through myself?" "It was not very original. There are millions like you. The Police; then Hypo; then call me."

As she walked up and down the aisles of Hypo, putting small items into her massive trolley, Perpetua scanned the faces of the shelf stackers. She saw Dexter before he saw her, lifting cartons of beer onto a shelf at a furious rate. "I am sure you do not have to lift such large loads so rapidly." "It's good exercise. I'm no longer a gang member but I want to keep fit." "Why? Is it some kind of vanity?" "No. I've thought about it. Look at these people 'round me who are shelf stackers. Most of them shouldn't be lifting anything, they're not built for that kind of work, so I can work faster and do some of their lifting, lighten their load." "How were the Police?" "I was going to say a nasty word but actually I was lucky. They seemed more relieved than anything. They asked me whether there would be a fight to fill the vacuum. There will be." "And here?" "All cleaned up. Price was bearing down on it, anyway."

After she had chosen some followers and squared it with Annie Price, she went to a coffee shop and they talked for a while. Then she found some more followers who were hanging around doing nothing.

When they were gathered she said: "I am not going to make an inspirational statement about changing the world. I am not even going to talk about God. I would like us to make some rules for ourselves. I have asked Trina to take notes and come up with a list."

After almost an hour Trina read out the results:

1. Respect. We must respect each other even when we disagree.
2. Courtesy. When we disagree we must do so gently and courteously.
3. Belief & Rationality. Disagreement must be on the basis of what we feel as a matter of God in us; but on many matters it should be based on evidence or personal experience, depending on what is relevant.
4. Trust. We need to be able to discuss difficult matters in an atmosphere of absolute trust; this means that we must all observe an absolute rule of confidentiality.
5. Support. There should be no sniping behind the backs of group members.
6. Good faith. We must assume that everything that is said is said in good faith; we should always assume good motives for behaviour and speech we do not understand.
7. Establish terms. We need to know whether we are solving a prob-

lem, trying to make a compromise, or trying to get a deeper understanding of a mystery. All these kinds of discussions are different. We should never use the 'devil's advocate' technique unless we are testing a solution against a likely hostile reception.

8. Motive. Discussion is to help us negotiate minefields not use arguments as ammunition.

9. Honesty. If we work in trust we can be honest; honesty includes saying when we have been hurt by what is said; it is better to say something than bear a grudge.

10. Perspective. We need to remember how small our decisions are in God's scheme of things.

11. Promises. If we make a promise to do something we must keep it.

"That is much better than sentimental poetry about love," said Perpetua. "If we try to follow these rules we will have established a strong platform of mutual love."

It was evening and the sun rose.

II.

And out of the air, as if from nowhere, unimpeded by walls, unconfined by technol-ogy, untainted by romanticism and ego, the music of Bach filled us with pure hope. We felt our hearts lift towards heaven, freed from the guilt and care, from the chronic cor-rosion of contaminated lives. In a miraculous transformation we were no longer hearing Bach's world through the soundscape of Mahler which we inhabited, we were inhabiting Bach's soundscape and viewing the sadness of Mahler as a life episode we had left be-hind. We climbed with Dante, we studied with the Angelic Doctor, we reached out for the heavenly summit in the bright, clear day. We were like angels except that we were free. We knew of the night but we did not fear it.

Our anxiety footprint shrank to almost nothing. How much anxiety and guilt we produced and consumed. How much nervousness we expended in the hopeless quest for self-reliance. How much spirit we wasted, because we thought we had been abandoned by God Our Parent.

Looking back, it is not difficult to see why so many people talked about the death of God. Only when she came did we begin to realise how bad it had been without her. Through ignoring all that Jesus said about freedom in love, about our helplessness without God, we had made ourselves prisoners of ourselves, locked away from light, locked away from hope, heads in the machinery, hearts heavy.

Wherever she went there was colour and choirs. It was as if her passing gave added lustre to the flowers, as if the grime of centuries had been removed from a Poussin pas-toral, so that there were always flowers in the grass, as if the ravage of the wild flowers had ceased and the imprisonment of the bordered flowers had ceased so that there were flowers everywhere. The colours were radiant not garish, giving out not a reflection, an artificial smile, but a light from within, taking us up to Dante's Paradiso, a time before the world went dark. How beautifully she would have made snow sparkle, but by the time she came its beauty was more or less a memory.

And the music. Often she performed marvelous acts which some called miracles but the greatest miracle was the sound that went around with her. Now we know how the heavenly choir must have sounded when the shepherds were given the good news of Jesus. She moved in an aura of divine music, giving lustre to everything around her.

She went to a wedding with her followers and the food was disgusting. It was trays full of compromises undermined by an inadequate budget. They had been careless with the guest list and even more careless with the caterers, so that the old people thought it was nasty and American and the young people thought it was nasty and foreign. What had started in familiar chaos at the church was now becoming resentful and ugly. What warm beer there was ran out and the food, first criticised for its scarcity, lay half eaten on discarded pa-per plates. Somebody said: "Ask that Perpetua to do something as she's so well connected." "What do you think this is?" came the reply, "the Marriage Feast at Cana?" "I am certain you can do something," whispered Dexter, just slightly doubtful. "Yes; but not yet. I'm not ready yet."

Dexter went to the gate and said to the very grumpy best man: "Whatever Perpetua says goes, all right." A few minutes later she came outside and said to the best man. "There's a van coming from Hypo any minute now. Get the driver to unload it. Here's a tip for him. You can say there was a slip-up and orders were mixed up. As this was Hypo's fault there will be no charge. And there's a bottle of single malt in a box with your name tag on it, but remember: do not say a word more than you have to."

She went back into the house and two minutes later a huge Hypo van arrived with hot and cold Caribbean, English and American food, chilled beer and white wine, red wine and rum, juices and fizzy drinks, plates and glasses; and, when they had finished unloading, the driver handed the best man a smart bag containing a single malt in a fancy box. Perpetua helped her followers to clear away the rubbish and when the groom asked what she was doing he was interrupted by the best man who said the real catering had arrived with an apology from Hypo. There would be no bill. The groom looked relieved and when he was offered a glass of wine he said he had never tasted anything like it in his life.

Dexter said to her later: "That was special but why didn't you say anything?" Trina added: "You can't spread the word of God Our Parent if you do special things and say nothing. I'm not asking you to take credit because I know you won't, but you could give God credit." "I can and I will, but people do not want systematic theology lessons at wedding receptions. There is a time and a place for everything and, contrary to what many devout people think, there is a time for being entirely with God alone and a time for being with God through each other. If we get too overwhelmed with the idea of God—I mean the idea, not the real relationship which is what we should really be pursuing—then we relegate the gifts of the earth to a secondary place. We can be so alienated by the wickedness and greed that we see, the corruption and degradation, that we think that physical things are inferior to spiritual things instead of believing that the whole of existence is one in the Creator and that the gifts of creation are not to be ranked. On this day of all days everybody there, from the bride and groom to those who opposed the marriage, needed to be deeply conscious of the beauty of the physical, of the appearance of the couple and the children that took them to the altar; and, most of all, aware of the beauty of their physical intimacy.

"After the need to eat, sex is the most powerful human driving force but, because it is such a force, it is always subject to abuse through the exercise of power. People use physical power to commit rape, inside and outside marriage;

they use physical and economic power to establish brothels, and they use economic power to market pornography, and force people into relationships or to stay in relationships that they would not be in without money. Yet psychological pressure is even more dangerous because everybody can exercise immense sexual power through manipulation and mind games, threats of violence and threats of self-violence.

"At the other end of the spectrum, because of the development of contraception, humanity has been able almost entirely to separate 'sex' from the procreation of children. This has taken the 'risk' out of it. Contrary to what many moralists say, society has handled the impact of contraception rather well. Yes, there has been greater promiscuity but society has not fallen apart—well, not for that reason. Interestingly, too, there is no relationship between going to church, social stability and sexual fidelity. Contraception has coincided with the declining need in rich countries to procreate children to maintain society and this has turned 'sex' into a recreational activity. 'Sex' is 'fun' and there is nothing wrong with that, but it is more than 'fun'. It has a lot to contend with, being so vulnerable to power plays and trivialisation, but there is no need to be downcast because when people search for human love the place they will find it most tangibly is in a physical relationship. That is not to say that there are not other kinds of love but we must be careful never to rank sublimated physical love above physical love. When we look at our lives we will always remember the look of falling in love, the feel of falling in love. Sometimes a physical relationship can disappoint—like coffee or bacon, it might be better anticipated than enjoyed—but because we were all created to love it is, in the end, what we do best. We are better lovers than we are criminals and no amount of exploitation and trivialisation has robbed physical love of its magic for every generation.

"The world is full of love stories, many of them unhappy because we are imperfect; but imperfection is the only condition in which we can choose to love. I keep saying this because Christians keep forgetting it; love through freedom is our purpose and to love is to create space in which others can exercise their freedom, to love us or somebody else, or not to love.

"The world is so full of love stories, so here is my favourite.

"There was a woman who really loved a man. When they met she had so much to say but she let him to talk. He had so much he needed to do so she let him do it and remained tranquil. He was unsure of himself and she let him explore his own feelings for himself and for her. Her love spoke most to him when she was silent. He went away from her because the space she made was daunting; she would not let him dominate her and she would not dominate him and so, sometimes, the space was too much for him; but she had made such space in his life that he kept coming back, fleetingly, for a day or a week, never quite near, never quite far; and, in the end, he realised that the only way he could live in the space she had made was to recognise that it was the space she had made and he could not live without it. But that was not enough. He still agonised and tried to make structures for them both which were superficially attractive to him but which ultimately cramped him; and every time he tried to make a structure for her or for them both she resisted and he drifted away.

"Then one day, looking from his bedroom window, he saw her walking across the field towards his house in the early morning, occasionally stooping to pick a flower. She did not walk in a straight line but stood still, slowly looking around, before picking a flower and then moving on. And he knew in a moment of inspiration for which he had waited all of his adult life that the only way they could be happy was if he created space for her in the way that she had so faithfully created space for him, so that she could walk about the field and beyond it, never in a straight line, looking at the world and picking flowers in no particular order.

"I would like to say that they lived happily ever after but I think they did not—space is a very difficult reality in which to live—but I can say that when they were happy they were more happy than those who try to control each other."

"But if we are all the children of God, why can't we all live happily ever after?" asked Dexter. "Because," said Perpetua, "that is for after. For now we have to keep remembering imperfection and freedom. When people ask why God Our Parent allows suffering there is no point in evading the obvious answer which is that suffering is a direct and inevitable consequence of the exercise of freedom in conditions of imperfection. Perhaps a more difficult question is why poor people generally suffer at the hands of rich people in such contexts as global warming, to which the answer is that those with most power can do both most good and most harm. If we could do neither good nor harm we would be nothing. God Our Parent is responsible for suffering because it is part of Creation; there is no point pretending otherwise. And although it might sound somewhat clever and recursive to say this, without freedom, and therefore without suffering, there would be no way of asking why there is suffering; a world without suffering would be a world without a question. There is the further question about earthquakes and other natural disasters that kill people. Again, Christians tend to be rather squeamish in answering the question. In this instance it is not the freedom of choice that causes suffering but the physical variation in the amphitheatre of our choices. A totally benign environment would not present us with material for choice. Look at the choices we face every time there is a natural disaster: will we help the survivors and will we help to avoid the consequences of a similar catastrophe? Do people live at the foot of volcanoes because they really want to take that risk or because they have no choice because we do not give them a choice? The world has enough resources to ensure that everybody can possess the basics but it means that those of us who have more than we need must choose to give.

"But what about small children dying of terrible disease?" said Jo. "This is another issue that Christians find difficult. Every time you see a child suffer, remember that it suffers for your choice and that, therefore, you have a terrible responsibility to that child when you choose between loving and not loving; and the other part of the answer, which Christians ought to recognise but seem not to, is that Jesus My Brother is the special companion of the suffering; He said that He was, and He still is. He is with all of those who suffer from wrong choices and all of those who suffer from the variable world in which we exercise choice. God Our Parent would never create children and then be 'unfair' to them; as Jesus said, theirs is the Kingdom of Heaven.

"Imagine a world without suffering; where would the beauty be? How could we ever look at a sunrise of hope without remembering the night of despair? What people are most often worried about is not the existence of suffering but its distribution, as if this was some kind of sacred distribution system that people pray to God to alter. It is not God Our Parent that distributes suffering in the way that we now experience it; that distribution is managed largely by the exercise of individual and collective freedom; but those who do not suffer do not know beauty. It is the combination of suffering and joy, of despair and hope, of vulnerability and generosity, of limitation and space, which condition us to create and recognise beauty. Beauty is the defining gift of humanity to itself; it has made beauty and learned to recognise beauty. God Our Parent made a world where humanity could live and beauty was not part of that creation. If we look at the old Jewish theology of creation in Eden we can see that there was no beauty in the Garden of Eden; there was nothing. Beauty was born when Adam and Eve looked at each other outside the Garden.

"It is the characteristic of being the children of God Our Parent, therefore, that we exist to exercise freedom and that this both requires human imperfection and physical variation, and even unpredictability. Some people would argue that this makes our life some kind of game. Yes, it is the only game, the serious game. People will quarrel with this but then people often quarrel with what you call something instead of looking at what it is. It is the game in which we test ourselves against ourselves, our choices against the gifts we have been given."

"So what has gone wrong with Christianity?" asked Trina. "It has turned God Our Parent into a member of humanity. The intellectuals of the eighteenth century Enlightenment demanded proof of God and Christians, particularly Torans, turned the numbered verses of the Bible into a book of proofs, like Wittgenstein's *Tractatus*. God Our Parent is no longer the ultimate sacred mystery; instead the whole phenomenon of Godhead can be explained and its existence proven. Torans have no theology at all, they are scientific Christians whose quantity and quality of doubting about God is identical to that of their faith that the sun sets in the West. They do not understand the degree of difference between God and humanity, and they are deeply suspicious of mystery; they use Enlightenment methodology to contest the Enlightenment. Because they have no doubt they can have no faith. What they have is a scientific certainty of their own superiority by virtue of their self-conscious relationship with God."

"What about Petrans?" asked Andy. "I was brought up among them and it all seemed to be mystery." "For Petrans the idea of mystery is central but they have made a nonsense of that idea by insisting that there must be, externally at least, a uniform way of trying to penetrate the mystery. Petrans fully understand the theology of free will and its relationship to mystery but that understanding does not inform what has come to be imposed: perverse discipline, as if the discipline were the point rather than the mystery. Everybody knows that the Pope is the head of the official Petran Church but hardly anybody knows that Petrans are subject to him (and, sadly, it is still always 'Him') subject to their proper exercise of free will, which they call 'conscience'. Petrans are quite properly criticised for distorting humanity's reason for being, but at least they question our reason for being.

"You have asked about Torans and Petrans but there is a large, third group of Christians to whom no convenient name is given, so let us call them Extrans. They are like the Laodiceans, neither too hot nor too cold. They are too languidly self-willed to worry about conscience and too self-satisfied to consider the idea of Godhead as mystery. They believe that pleasing themselves without doing anything that appears to be harmful and believing whatever they like without any need to think about it, much less to pray, is the epitome of civilised religion.

"But how can we ever begin to penetrate a mystery without the exercise of freedom? Can we penetrate it by imitating a peer? Because she approaches the mission in a certain way does that mean that we must? As no two people are identical they must necessarily approach mystery in different ways." "But why is there a Church that Jesus is supposed to have left?" asked Kylie. "Because the Church exists to provide a safe space of love in which people can exercise their freedom to explore the mystery that is God. The Church does not exist to make exploration rules or to set exploration standards but it can provide exploration handbooks, tools to help people, individually and collectively, to penetrate the mystery." "But how can we ever penetrate the mystery of God while we live here?" asked Heather. "Because Jesus My Brother and I are bridges between humanity and the mystery. The essence of the mystery is not the existence of the Godhead but the unending love which it has for humanity. The colloquial way of putting this is: 'Why did God bother?' to which the answer is that the loving economy of the Godhead, although self-sufficient and containing all love, needed a richer way of expressing that love. Humanity is the enriching of the love of the Godhead; it does not add nor subtract from that love but it gives it a different form and shape, a different purpose." She said: "Let us go and see what I mean."

They said goodbye to the people who were still listening to Her and walked to where some children were playing. "If you look at the children, the older they are, the more calculations they make, the less space they give each other to choose, the more conformist they become. There is a kind of holiness which comes from facing difficult choices but there is also a fundamental holiness which comes from generosity, the generosity which says 'here is a gift, enjoy it.' That is very different from a gift which comes with a manual. Children often collaborate to make new games, new gifts, mutually agreed manuals which allow for both freedom and structure; but as they grow older the structure becomes more dense and the freedom is narrowed." "But isn't there chaos without structure?" asked a teacher who was standing nearby, watching the children. "Yes, there would be chaos, but that is because humanity substitutes structure when love fails; and because, as imperfect people, love must fail, we realise what love we can through structure; and the looser the structure and the wider the bounds, the more the love corresponds to the Divine Love." "I think I see. Do you mean that we limit children's growth through being too authoritarian?" "I warm to the way the question is put. We are too apt to confuse freedom and danger. Quite often when children make up their own minds and exercise their own freedom it makes them more open and loving young people but it also endangers our authority. When we think about structure we often really mean authority, not some system of channels. Those who want to join in the singing, why not stand where you can hear each other because you cannot sing well unless you can blend with your friends."

Most of the children stood quite close to her. "What should we do about the few who have not come over?" asked the teacher. "Give me a moment. I am just going to talk to your friends over there."

She went over to a little boy who was sitting, looking anxiously at the rest of the children. "Do you want to be over there?" she asked. "Yes." "Well, why are you not?" "I can't sing." "Everybody can sing better than they think they can. You cannot sing without practice." "They will laugh at me." "They will be too busy concentrating." "All right."

Then she went to a little girl who was almost in tears. "I can't sing because I'm deaf," she said before Perpetua could ask anything. "I thought so," she said. "That is a very stylish hearing aid, though. I know, if you stand next to me you can use your lip reading skills to see if they are all beginning and ending their words at the same time. But you must tell me quietly and gently so as not to embarrass yourself and them."

Finally she went to a boy about eight years of age. "Do you mind being the only person not wanting to sing?" "No. I prefer my book." "Sometimes if you exercise a freedom to choose that way you are improving your individual gifts but not improving the gift of companionship. Think about what you will gain from the book and what everybody, including you, will gain if you are all together. Life is not simply about exercising individual preferences." "I know, but they make fun of me because I read so many books." "Well, that is quite a different reason for not wanting to join, so how honest are you being with yourself? Is it best to join to cut down how much fun they make of you or is it best to be brave and stick to your book and let them make fun of you?" "I don't know." "What about saying: 'I am not joining you to stop you making fun of me but because I like being with you'?" "They wouldn't believe me." "Try it."

Nobody, particularly the teacher, knew where the skill and beauty came from but they sang like angels. It was as if Perpetua was conducting them with her eyes. The little deaf girl stood, watching, but had nothing to report. She said their mouths formed the same shapes at the same time. Perpetua thanked them and asked if they had enjoyed themselves. "Yes," one said, "because we could see you smiling. You looked like you were in love with us." "I am," she said.

When they had said goodbye and were sitting in a circle on some scruffy grass Dexter said: "You talked for so long about freedom and then you took us to see a choir where everybody joined in." "That is because the modern idea of freedom is confused with exercising individual, autonomous choice regardless of the people around us. We can exercise our freedom to do what will please others, or exercise our freedom, paradoxically, not to exercise it but to love instead by making space to enable the choice of somebody else. The idea that freedom is about 'I' is also false. Frequently freedom is about 'we', about pooling our choice with other people so that we generate solidarity." "But the world is becoming ever more inter-dependent," said Trina. "Yes it is but that does not make us any more loving. There is no virtue in paying your taxes unless you vote for a generous level of taxation and pay your tax cheerfully. The reverse side of inter-dependence is collective exploitation. We are all trapped in this massive, complex structure of inter-dependency and the tendency is for people to try to dominate the structure. Sadly, when people become richer one of the first things they buy is privacy and, if they can afford it, exclusivity. They want to buy their way out of inter-dependence, just as many people prefer to pay to put their relatives into nursing homes rather than looking after them. Nursing homes are full of very brave people who humble themselves so as not to embarrass those who put them there. By accepting confinement they are giving space to their children; that is a practical expression of love that is no less wonderful for not being recognised.

"There is a wonderful paradox between exercising freedom and making space for it to be exercised which can never be resolved because that is the condition of humanity."

She left them to pray. "Sometimes, Lord, I become depressed that I have to use all these words instead of just being able to transmit love. I know that I have to explain because humanity is a linguistic creature and language, too, is a kind of choosing. They have so much in front of them that could make them happy but they spend all their time closing down options for themselves and for others. I thank you God My Parent that you have sent me so that I may re-open their eyes to the prospect of loving through freedom, that I may re-open their hearts to the transfer of suffering from others to themselves, that I may re-open their wholeness to the prospect of love in freedom instead of the love they crave through power and structure, through the gratification of the self and the other. May I help them to see beauty. They are so good at seeing what is pleasing or pretty but they have lost the real sense of the beautiful, of the wholeness which comes from learning how suffering and freedom are part of the same human condition that makes humanity what it is."

She saw a young woman walking down the path towards her, humming as she carried a baby on her back. "Hello," said the young woman. "You look nice calm." "Thank you. You look very happy." "Today, yes. Yesterday, no. Tomorrow, probably no. Today, yes." "What is your name?" "Marta." "Well, Marta, would you like to sit for a few moments and tell me about yourself." "Yes, I like you. Your name?" "Perpetua." "OK, Perpetwa. I came from the East but not like a star. They told me about the exploiters in the West but said if I came here my own people would look after me; but my own people made me leave my lovely little country farm and come to this nasty housing estate; but now I like it better because I learn more here than at the farm. And they said I would be working in a nice hotel but the man who met me said that if I did not work for him he would kill me. So he allowed his horrible friend to rape me but look how beautiful she is, lying there." "What is her name?" "Perhaps she English Lucy. Out of darkness come light. So out of leaving farm and wicked man and rape come learning English and Lucy. I do not know yet. I do not know how God works but it seems like we are sometimes sad and sometimes happy and when we are one we don't know whether it will bring the other." "Are you angry?" "Was very angry but no point. It happened. If there was no leaving the farm there would be no here; if there was no nasty man there would be no baby. This man, Max, he says that I am very naïve but I have not found other way to think. Max was very rich and now is very poor and so he, like me, knows how it changes; but he has all kinds of reasons and says how it could be different.

I am naïve; but was not the Blessed Virgin naïve?" "Oh, My Auntie Mary, yes, she was very naïve." "Your Auntie Mary?" "Yes. You see I am the Sister of Jesus." "Everybody sister of Jesus." "Yes but in a special way. What if I said I was God." "What did Your Auntie Mary say when the Angel ask her to help God?" "She said yes." "OK. I say yes. You look like God and you smile like God and you say you are God; and I am naïve. So, what must I do?" "Jesus My Brother used to ask people to worship him if they believed but times change. I do not think I want you to do anything except go on loving God and humanity, particularly your Lucy, or whatever you call her. And pray for me." "Why should God need prayers?" "Because God likes gifts and prayers are the best gifts of all: prayers on your knees, prayers with your hands, prayers with your heart; prayers of charity and prayers of restraint. Oh, and I need prayers because my life will become very unpleasant later on." "Yes, like Jesus. I always find the more good the more suffering, like the Psalm. Wicked seem to laugh. Never mind. I pray. I am happy now and can do nothing about tomorrow being happy."

As she went away down the path, humming, Perpetua cried. She had seen the beauty which God had enabled.

III.

And as if a great cloud of doubt and confusion had been lifted to reveal the clear sky of salvation, decisions which had once been mired in confusion became simple. Not that they became easy; many of them presented themselves with a stark clarity that was frighteningly unfamiliar. Self-deception gave way to self-enlightenment; theoretical philosophy was replaced by an urgent sense of a search for truth in the self; the obfuscations and pusillanimities, the committees and compromises, the multiple factors and fears of ramifications, the whole superstructure of distributed responsibility where everyone was responsible so that no-one was responsible, fell away.

Time seemed to speed up. The numbing delay of indecision and irresponsibility was dissipated like the smothering smog from the coal age and figures began to emerge from the gloom. There were thousands of time servers who had no-one to serve; there were compromisers and fixers with nothing to settle or fix; con men were exposed; liars stood out clearly. The inner mind had migrated into the eyes of dealers and dodgers. It was amazing how many equivocators there were and how few simple, holy people.

She walked through the garden of fresh, wild flowers with music all around her, gleaming with truth, clear as crystal, sure as gold. In the councils and committees and seminars and workshops and consultations and questionnaires and market surveys and declarations, nobody could resist her. She said where there had been moralising there should be morality; where there were resolutions there should be solutions; where there were frameworks there should be works; where there were aspirations there should be inspirations. She knew that she would make enemies but in those early days her way was clear and undisputed.

She went to an official summit meeting on drugs. They talked about complex causality and the economics of heroin, of the farmers in Afghanistan and the dealers on the streets, of alienation and despair, of knives and guns, of poverty and hopelessness; and she said: "Look at us. We could make the farmers of Afghanistan prosperous without poppies; we could provide closer, personal, loving support for the desperate and alienated, accompanied by better prospects and more reasonable benefits; we could gear the education system to the least gifted and least motivated and set the gifted and motivated free from rigid structures; we could encourage the well-off suburbs to twin with their neighbouring slums as well as with the charming little towns of France and Germany; and, most of all, we could take personal responsibility as individuals and groups and as tax payers."

The usual response would have been lengthy explanations and excuses, the suggestion of working groups and another summit, a plan for some pilots. There would have been complaints that the country could not sustain any more taxation, it would frighten international business away and there were no votes in it.

But instead she was congratulated on her foresight. Everybody said that something could be done; it might take longer and be more difficult than Perpetua implied, but it was their duty to work together to see that everything was done.

"But will it?" asked Dexter. "No, of course not," she said. "I did not come to perfect the world nor to make difficult problems go away but to give hope, to give people a new start. There will be a falling away over time but what people need is a clear vision of where they are going and why. They need to be confronted with, to revel in, the choices that lie before them, to see the clear challenge. After a while the old ways will assert themselves and the people who see the new vision will have enemies, and I, too, will have enemies where there are currently none, and, in the way of human affairs, the enemies will overcome my body, but I will have brought the new hope. That is for the future. Today we are going to bring new hope to those who really need it, those who are the subjects of the summit, those who have been the sad sufferers from the procrastinators, waiting until there is nothing worth waiting for. Let us gather a few of those businessmen who talked about community partnerships between major companies and run-down areas and see how they react to the places where the partnerships will take place. I said 'businessmen' but of course we will take our old Hypo friend, Annie Price, as well as her boss, Sir Pluto."

They crossed the river from the glittering buildings of church and state to the streets where both were regarded with some suspicion but even more indifference. They picked up Father Bill Midway on the very edge of down-at-heel respectability and then plunged into the gruesome crucible of Grunge Park, to its very heart at the Hollow. If Perpetua had not been one of the party, there would have been trouble. People in smart, conventional clothes, if they brought anything at all, brought clip-boards or trouble.

"Hello," said Perpetua. "You are Max, are you not?" "Yes." "Tell us your story. My friends would like to hear it." "I know one of your friends. That one. He fired me from my bank; and look at me now." "Good God! It's you. I had no choice." "You had no choice," said Perpetua. "I keep hearing that." "I will try to help you," said the embarrassed man. "No thank you," said Max. "I don't want to go near the bank again. I'm a mess but I am beginning to work out a way to get out of the mess. I want a simple life and I think I am falling in love; but I still have terrible times when I hit the bottle." "So what is the essence of the story," asked Perpetua, "just so these people can get it clear?" "I was the head of my bank and there was a corporate takeover and I was sacked by text message without a kind word or even a tiny amount of money—tiny by the bank's standards, anyway—to allow me to sort things out. One minute I was rich, the next minute I was facing poverty. I was living right up to, and possibly beyond, my means, but I never imagined." "That, then, is a relatively simple message," said Perpetua. "With a little consideration and compassion we could stop people falling into desperation. Did none of the senior managers see it coming?" "I am afraid we had more important things to think about like the net assets of the new venture and the reaction on the international markets." "What about those people in the Human Resources division?" "We fired the head of HR in Max's bank and kept the other one and she was kept busy limiting our obligations to employees to a minimum." "Yes. I think we all see. Have we not all noticed how short-term this is, how it transfers trouble from well equipped perpetrators to victims, how it is careless with lives?" "Yes," said the banker, "looked at that way you have a point; but we have shareholders." "And do you not have a whole mass of shareholders in the country where you live whose shareholder value you exist to protect as a brother?" "I suppose so. It would have sounded a little far-fetched in those days but today you have helped me to see things in a new way." "Well, Max," said Perpetua, "all is not lost; be brave. I know you will have black moments but if you work hard and exercise the muscle of your choice it will strengthen."

An even more decrepit and scruffy man than Max struggled across the bruised and broken grass. "Oh, Brod," muttered Max. "Max," whispered Perpetua, "be patient with him as many are with you. Hello Brod, these friends of mine would like to hear your story." "Not much of a story. Give us a cigarette. I don't suppose you have a drink?" "Afterwards," said Perpetua, "not as a bribe but as a reward and a comfort." "My dad beat me and my mum up and my mum ran away and then I ran away. Thieving, booze, drugs, this. Short story." "But you have still got some lucidity and you have got Max." "Not much of either." "Hang on to what you have, choose to stay with Max and, now and again, choose to stay off the booze. Could you possibly introduce us to some other people?" "Oh the druggies, no, we don't deal with them; they're scum." "Brod," said Perpetua, "don't say that. Without Max you would probably be with them." "All right. Over there. What about the drink?" "It will be waiting for you at the *Down & Out* after seven when I will join you and Max. A starting point is to drink in public with friends rather than alone in private. If you are going to drink, at the very least you should enjoy it a little."

They went towards a burned-out building which had been a drop-in centre. "I will go in," she said. "You just discreetly look on. Hello." "Who are you?" shouted a boy about fourteen years old, aggressively. "Perpetua. I am sure we have met before. What is your name?" "None of your business." "Everything is my business and a good start to a relationship is using your name." "I don't want a relationship." "People say that people like you want role models and relationships." "They don't know what they're talking about. I just want to be left." "To die?" "Of course not." "But do you not think that heroin will kill you?" "Only if

I get unlucky and there's a dodgy score; but I could get killed by a skidding car. I will be all right as long as I am careful where I get the stuff." "Tell me about how you ended up here? Are there many people who are interested in you?" "Only dealers and the police are interested in me." "Wrong: I am, and my friends are." "I'll tell you if you give me some money for food." "I will give you nothing unless you tell me your name, and after that I will gladly give you money for food." "They buy drugs with it," whispered one of the businessmen. "Not if I pay the tab at the cafe," said Perpetua, "and you do not need an MBA to work that out." "I'm Calib. My nutty Bible mother called me Caleb but it got made into Calib, short for Caliban." "You know the Bible and Shakespeare, then?" "Of course I do. Why do people think that because I'm on drugs I'm stupid?" "Well, one reason is that they find it difficult to see the person behind the drugs; but we will come back to that later." "Why did you abandon these interesting books?" "Mum and dad split up. Dad just disappeared and mum gave up the Bible. She said it had done nothing for her. She started drinking and then took drugs and then she died. I started on booze and glue and anything and now I'm here." "How do you get the money to live?" "Odd jobs." "What is the last odd job that you completed?" "Bits and pieces." "You see, so much potential, and it broke down so rapidly, and we are here. Who is that?" "Ruthie. She's sleeping." "She looks to me as if she might be dying." "No, she's often like that. Takes more than she should and gets angry and then it blows out and she sleeps. I look after her." "Yes," said Perpetua, "the loving instinct, the caring instinct, it never quite dies in anyone. Most people looking at Calib would reject him completely but we have seen the good in him along with the careless."

Annie Price came through the door. "I can't stand outside there when this is happening. Let me look." "Leave her alone, she's all right. She's my girl." "She is a girl but we do not own people like that, particularly if they are weak and helpless. The weak belong to all of us." "What about the money?" "If she really is somebody you care for, think about Ruthie for a few moments and we will then talk about money." The girl stirred under Annie's hand. "Go away! Don't touch me! Leave me alone." "It's all right. I want to help." "I'm thirsty." "Here's a water bottle. What a poor, lovely face you have, Ruthie. How do you feel?" "A bit weak but it will pass. I'll be all right." "How did you get here?" "Same as everybody else. Abusive step father, indifferent mother who didn't care what he did to me. Ran away. Tried a bit of sex work but I was gang raped by some so-called customers and was threatened with worse. I ran away and I'm here." "But can't you do better?" "Calib looks after me. He's the first man I've known who hasn't tried to have sex with me." "Do you want help?" asked Perpetua. "Ask Calib." "No. Calib wants what you choose, so you must answer." "I will try to answer." Calib looked doubtful. "Look, Calib, I am not foolish. I know that your attention span has almost ended because you need your next fix, but you do not

430

need to worry." "Why not?" "You will see. I want you to come along with my friends and me." "What's in it for me?" "Shut up," said Ruthie. "Give it a try."

All day Perpetua talked to broken people, passive past desperation except for the next fix. Annie took Ruthie to a refuge for which Hypo had provided some funding and she arranged for all the people Perpetua found to be given food and drink. She took the businessmen to the *Paradise* cafe for lunch which they thought was far from paradise and far from lunch. "I thought they were different from us," said the banker, "but they look pretty much the same underneath. It's the clothes and, above all, the eyes, the empty eyes, wandering about looking for the next opportunity. When my boy looked like he was going off the rails with his studies I sent him to a private school. I suppose if Calib had gone to a private school he would have been all right."

While such conversations as these went on, Perpetua sat back and enjoyed their voyage of discovery and self-discovery. They were intelligent; they had just not addressed this problem rationally. Dexter came in the late afternoon to say that almost everything was ready. He wanted to go to the gang headquarters, but Perpetua would not let him. "You do not need to worry," she said, "Kish will turn up when he hears what is going on and then we will see what happens."

Perpetua, Dexter, Trina, most of the other *god4u* leaders and Father Bill somehow shepherded a huge crowd of addicts into Bill's church. Again, there was plenty of food from Hypo and the smell of high quality coffee seemed temporarily to have suspended the addicts' usual concerns.

Perpetua said: "Just so that everybody knows. I have broken my usual rule of simply giving people a push in the right direction by giving everybody here a new start by curing you of your cravings. Some of you will take the chance you have been given more fully than others, so the first thing to say is that Jesus My Brother and I love you regardless of how successful you are at taking the chance. What I would like us to do is to tell each other some stories and then see what conclusions we might draw. We are not telling stories, as people do so often, to compete, to show we are braver or brighter; nobody knows what each of us has had to confront in our lives and so the idea of competition is foolish. We want to learn from each other and I think that stories are better than theories."

Meanwhile, there were extraordinary scenes outside being monitored by Dexter with a certain degree of amusement. Kish and the gang had heard about Perpetua's meeting. They had already suffered a loss of prestige and trade from her frequent interventions and they were determined this time to stop her in her tracks. They had planned to do a little shooting in the air and some serious knife wielding, together with a special drugs discount. When they had all finished planning at the headquarters they had gone to their motor bikes. None of them worked; not a spark. They reached for their mobile phones; they were dead. Without transport and phones they were disoriented. They walked towards the church, looking as if they did not really know what to do. "Kish walking!" said Dexter. "Come in, my friend." He hung back. "No, friend, you are really welcome; just hand me that weapon and you can have a nice cup of Jamaican coffee and an English muffin." Kish dropped his pistol and Dexter flicked it up into his hands without relaxing his watchful gaze. "I presume the others have knives; to cut the cakes, I suppose. Well, we can do that for them as good hosts. If I were you I would only bring in a representative sample. The rest can go. We will security check them together, shall we."

Perpetua saw Kish coming in with Dexter. "Just the person," she said. "Kish, tell us your story." He came forward, pushed by Dexter. "Rotten home, no money, crazy parents, truancy, glue, drugs, stealing. What do you want to know? Most of us are like that." "I do not think so," she said, under her breath. "but it is too public to contradict."

There was then a succession of very similar, short stories, most of which ended with: "That's just how it was," or "That's just how we are," and at last Perpetua said: "Are we?

"Some of you will have noticed that we are telling these stories to some people who do not know us and I particularly want to thank you for that. Now I would like to hear something different from one of our visitors; Annie, what about you?" "Some of you know me though you pretend not to. And I must admit I try hard but I sometimes pretend that I don't know you. When I grew up here there were plenty of poor white people who were living very similar lives to black people but it's usually the blacks that get picked on by the *Toxic Times*. My Welsh dad beat up my mother and then beat me up. He tried to sexually abuse me but I fought him off. I told him I would blow his cover if he touched me. I should have blown his cover to protect mum and me but it was too much. All the same, the behaviour somehow seemed to rub off. I began to drink Export until it made me sick so I switched to hash, stronger and stronger. I missed school and nobody cared: my parents were past caring, they were so messed up in their alcohol and violence, and I was so troublesome and articulate that school didn't want to find me. I was too much trouble. Then one day my best friend took an overdose and I thought she was dead. My first instinct was to abandon her, just to run away, but in the end I took her to the hospital with the money for my next fix and as they took her away I thought: 'I never want to be like that'.

"The next week was terrible. I was on my own. I couldn't communicate with my parents. I didn't have my best friend. I had nobody else to talk to. And before you get the wrong idea, I didn't get a flash of light from God or anything spectacular. It wasn't a priest or somebody who did something. It was me. I simply lived from one minute to the next refusing to buy any more stuff. I went on stealing but this time it was money to buy cigarettes and alcohol and food. But I soon got sick with the alcohol and stuck to cigarettes and food. A week later I saw my friend before she saw me. She had obviously let herself out of hospital and she was out of her head. I thought: 'I don't want to be like that. It does not matter how bad I feel, I don't feel that bad.' I went over to her and offered to help but she was rude and threatened to beat me up. My best friend."

Meanwhile, Kish's main supplier was waiting for his regular payment. He tried to start his Jaguar but nothing happened. He tried to use his mobile phone but it was dead.

"I had been well enough for long enough to need help and losing the friend shook me into action. I went to the local government office and said if they didn't look after me properly I'd report them to the papers. I said they had no right to neglect people like me when they were receiving loads of money to care for people like me. I stayed at school, though I hated it, just long enough to scrape some exams and then went in as a shelf stacker at Hypo. They didn't mind who they had. I didn't do anything spectacular, I just made thousands of small choices, more often than not the right choices, just doing an extra hour or refusing another glass of wine."

A man who was attending a conference on global drug control tried to reach the man in the Jaguar but his phone was dead. In half an hour his President would get in touch to request a final statement on the cash transfer to his private bank account. If anything went wrong the diplomat would be put on a hit list.

"One of the statements which makes me most angry—and when I think about the misuse of drugs I become very angry because of the collusion between the rich and powerful who could do so much more to reduce the problem—is that addicts just need to pull themselves together. They have been pulled apart by society, they have been weakened so badly that they cease to make choices. They turn to drugs because this keeps them away from choices. If human beings stop making choices they cease to be human beings. All of you were victims of one sort or another but all the time that you were being abused and led astray you still had choices. How many of you never once knew you were making a wrong choice?" All hands stayed down. "All right, how many of you knew on at least one occasion that you were making a wrong choice?" More than half the hands went up. "How many of you knew you could reverse the choice?" Almost all hands went up. "But at that point I guess it was just too difficult to turn around." Near unanimity.

"Turning around is the important thing. I have turned you all around today to face yourselves as children of God Our Parent, but if you only remember one thing let it be that you are capable of turning round after you have made wrong choices. I do not want us to put Annie up on a pedestal but she has described how she made some choices that made a difference. Some of us become so discouraged that we do not want another choice. What kind of choice is it to be either hungry or beaten up by your own father? This is where our friends from international business come in. Rupert is going to tell us what he plans to do in the Business Regeneration Assistance Group."

"Well we thought that it would be really helpful if a coalition of world class players got together to build an IT centre for Grunge Park. I know there will be a few friction points because of our competitiveness but we think we can solve these because the PR dividend is so great and we can get the funding out of our Corporate Social Responsibility budget on which we get a generous Government tax break. You can't buy that kind of PR." "And I thought I had convinced you earlier today to act in the best interests of disadvantaged people. Now it seems that the main purpose of BRAG is to enhance your PR profile using taxation. I suppose you will also use end-of-line equipment as well? No; you do not need to answer that question.

"What you have heard so far is that people who end up in trouble make a whole string of wrong choices. Sometimes the first of these is trivial but people feel that they are then pushed into smaller and smaller spaces. Now, Rupert, the reason why your corporation is so successful—including your company sailing so close to the wind over taxation—is that you spend all your time making thousands of choices, small and big. If I ask you what the consequences will be of deciding in favour of one choice over others you will be able to give me all the pros and cons of all the choices on offer; and, unlike most people, you will not make the mistake of thinking that you only have two choices which are diametrically opposite each other. You will know that you can make a third or fourth choice, or take pieces of different options and put them into a package. These are precisely the skills that these people need and all you want to do is dump old kit on them for your own PR. What I propose that you do is to set up a life choices laboratory in Grunge Park with information technology as one of the main features but not as the end in itself.

"Before we close this meeting I want to say two things. The first, following my short discussion with Rupert, is that I will press for everybody to have the chance to learn about making choices, how to distinguish between real options and false options, how to distinguish between peer pressure and self-interest, how to assess junk opinion and sound advice.

"Much more important, I want all of you to remember that you are no longer alone. You never were alone—God Our Parent would never abandon you—but you thought you were alone and now you know that you are not. I broke my own rule by curing many of you here of addictive behaviour but that was to give you the chance to start choosing again; without the cures it would have been so difficult for you to break free. Now you are free, remember: you are not alone. I am with you and so is Jesus My Brother, and you are all back within the reach of God Our Parent.

"This has been a difficult day for us all. Those of you who do not know where you can sleep tonight, please report to those wearing *god4u* t-shirts at the back of the hall and we will try to sort you out. It will probably not feel as if you have been cured as you will be forced to make all kinds of decisions and some of them will be difficult. Now," she said, turning to the business party, "we need to have a de-brief over in that corner.

"What have we learned today?" "I thought it would all be more dramatic but these people aren't very different from my kind, just living in a scruffy area and getting lost. It could happen to anyone." "Yes and it does," she replied, "and there are children from all kinds of backgrounds who get trapped in drugs and never escape but you can see that the root of it is desperation and a kind of mental entrapment." "On the other hand it looks as if sorting this out is going to be very difficult; just passing more laws does not seem as if it will work." "You cannot legislate happiness and responsibility and both of these are crucial to solutions." "What about de-criminalising drugs?" "That is one pragmatic way of dealing with the problem; it would decrease some of the evils, but the basic evil is that people feel that they need to escape from making choices, that what they confront is so beyond their means that they cannot live with themselves. One possibility is that drugs simply widen the choice difference between the rich and the poor, the privileged and the down-trodden, because drug abuse affects those with a mission much less than those without a mission.

"Have you missed anything out?" she asked. "We don't think so." "What about the link between poverty and a lack of choice which leads to drug taking which speeds up the flight from choice. Do you think you have any responsibilities to the poor or will you just complain about higher taxes? I did not mention this in front of our audience because it would not be fair, but I would like you to think about this. You have heard enough from me for one day. It is time for you, who are experts in this field, to go away and make some choices."

She left her followers to sort out the cured but homeless people and went to a quiet place to spend the night in prayer. As usual, the prayer was not straightforward. She saw the cured people with their hope restored, their eyes bright; and then she saw the hope fade and the eyes become vacant. This was not supernatural foresight, it was recognising the inevitable. She was tempted to pray that this would not happen, that they would somehow be saved from themselves but she resisted the temptation. All that she could honestly pray was that God would give them strength to resist but, of course, it would not be that simple. As a parent, God would provide the means but could not direct the choice. So many people were paying such a high price for freedom of choice and yet it was a freedom that society took for granted, almost certainly because most people did not make a strong link between choice and suffering.

She cried.

The inevitability of the falling away was almost too much to take. It was not only humans that suffered because of choice but the God who had given it. She would always be with them.

As she prayed, a President was arrested, followed by a diplomat and a man in a Jaguar.

She had given the people new life but she knew that most of them would waste it.

She would always be with them.

IV.

And she made all things fair. The space between Heaven and earth was full of movement, and the gap between the spiritual and the physical, the divine and the human, disappeared. The effect that great music has, of unifying the human frailty of orchestral execution with the sublime vision of the composer and transmitting this in a holistic way to the listener, applied to all areas of human endeavour. No longer was there brutal materialism and sublime spirituality; physical labour was a natural part of God's purpose and the spiritual dimension was no longer some distant aspiration, only open to the obviously holy and the painstakingly philosophical. It was as if the whole world again realised that it was the sacrament of the Creator.

She walked in an aura of heightened colour and mysterious music, personifying in herself the new unity. Wherever she went the environment looked different; she did not transform it temporarily from greyness to gold, she helped us to see everything in a new golden light, the light that she transmitted as a channel from the Creator who had made the world in light before wrong choices made it dark. She made everything clear and uncluttered as if, for a short time, there would be no cloud in the sky, no dimming of light, no distortion of sound, no coarseness of tone, no jerkiness in movement.

She made all things fair and all things simple so that humble people who had read nothing understood what she was saying about their revived hope. Everybody who met her knew that she had brought Heaven to earth as surely as she promised that the people of earth were destined for Heaven. The commentators and columnists, opinion formers and pundits, the tabloid simplifiers and the 'Berliner' amplifiers, the clever broadcasters and the cunning PR companies, the spinners and the sinners, those who sailed close to the wind and those who sold flimsy craft, those who risked everything they had and those who risked everything that belonged to others, did not know what to make of her. A familiar way of life was passing away before their puzzled but enchanted eyes. There was corporate stress as believers, formerly dismissed as a minority of cranks, made their views known at the head of solid, polite but firm, delegations of workers in advertising, newspapers and television. Even though its roots were buried deep in foreign soil out of the reach of regulators and revenue officers, internet pornography shrivelled and died. There was corporate upheaval as fraud and venality was exposed, as the old ways gave way to the new. There were still pockets of resistance, particularly in the Christian churches and such media phenomena as the Toxic Times, *and government, beset by vested interest and complexity, stubbornly resisted the reform which brought openness and simplicity to what had been closed and intricate.*

She made all things fair. Wherever she went she brought hope. People no longer thought of hope as something for others but not themselves. What they called 'Heaven' no longer seemed out of reach. Where the priests had called for penance all she asked for was penitence; where the clergy had asked for obedience she asked for self-criticism.

Wherever she went she spread a moral revolution which made a nonsense of all the false walls and restrictions that had divided people and ideas from each other.

She said to Father Bill: "I think I should talk to a clergy conference so that they can understand what we are trying to do."

It took place in the magnificent Church Corporation headquarters, under the watchful and proprietorial Presidency of Archdeacon Varnish. When she arrived she was completely ignored by the large gathering of clergy clustered round the coffee and biscuits. She was a woman and she was not formally dressed and so she could not have anything important to say or do. To avoid embarrassing them, she looked at the plaques, coffee in hand, until the Archdeacon arrived to greet her. "I am sorry," he said, "but some of my colleagues are just a little awkward with, er, people." "Women?" "Oh no. Please don't take this personally; they would not have behaved much better with any other kind of stranger but they find young women particularly, er, challenging." "Sexually?" "God forbid, no. Almost all of them, except the Petrans, have wives, you know. No, it is female opinion that they find difficult. I daresay most of them make allowances for their wives—I know I do—but they are not being that biased. After all, they do not find lay opinion of any kind easy to digest but strong ideas expressed by a woman are particularly, er, challenging." "Repugnant?" "Oh no, I think not; they are much too generous for that but change takes a good deal of getting used to. Some of us find it very difficult to adjust to falling standards." "I hope you do not include the vocations of women within that terrible fall." "Pardon me. Of course not. It is just that we seem to be losing our sense of beauty with churches being torn apart." "Yet they are not museums, Archdeacon." "No, quite." "That is what I wish to talk about today." "I didn't know you knew about architecture and, anyway, we asked you to talk about spiritual renewal." "That is what I will talk about, transforming churches from museums into places for the future." "Quite." "Although I am not sure how you can have spiritual renewal in an architectural museum. How can you ask for renewal in one area and ultra-conservatism in another?" "Conservation not conservatism, my dear." A sharp look. "Pardon me. Conservation, quite."

When she climbed onto the platform and switched on the microphone, the main doors creaked wide open and stuck fast. Under the gentle supervision of Dexter, Trina and other followers, people began to come into the great hall and sit down as she said an opening prayer. The archdeacon first looked puzzled and then angry. He could not leave his place to talk to her. She saw his difficulty and sent a pencilled note: "Everything that we do not specifically shut must be open. There is no point in a secret God. Our mission is to reveal the secret." She asked the organist to play something light and popular. "I like Bach," she said, "but people tell me it gives them a headache." Again, Varnish looked upset but did not intervene.

"Today I want us to think about the idea of Sacrament which is central to most parts of the Christian church. Let us start at the beginning. The world is a Sacrament. It is the special Sacrament of God Our Parent. It is the form in which the love of the Godhead has been made physical. That is why it is so important for the Church to concentrate on the contemporary global crisis, not because of what it will do to us—although that is naturally important—nor even what it will do to our brothers and sisters all over the world—although without much more help from the whole world that will be catastrophic—but because we are defacing the physical manifestation of the Godhead with our greed and neglect. Imagine if I told you that it did not matter how you treated the elements of the Eucharist? You would be scandalised. Well, if the earth is a Sacrament we must treat it with the same respect with which we treat the elements of the Eucharist; As the created gift of God the earth should be treated with reverence. The idea that the earth is a lump of resource that we can plunder and fight over is totally wrong. The idea that because we are God's children we have a right to be selfish and to mistreat animate and inanimate resources is preposterous. In many ways scientists show more respect and wonder at our world than theologians. We can learn a great deal from their observations and how they transpose them into elegance and poetry. Theology is not superior to physics; it is a totally different kind of enterprise. Just as scientists are mistaken when they say that God does not exist because the existence cannot be proven scientifically, so we are mistaken when we elevate the theological probing into the mystery of God over understanding what God has created. This is another form of elevating the spiritual over the physical instead of seeing them together. Think of what we can learn about the Godhead from the combination of three colours—red, blue and green—which form the basis of every picture everybody has ever seen. Think of what we can learn about mystery from anti-matter. Think how much we can improve our awareness of the link between the divine and human if we think about the relationship between the virtual and the real. Also remember that familiarity with scientific research is necessary for an informed conscience when making personal decisions about, for example, the use of human tissue and the nature of gender.

"Next, the Christian Church is the Sacrament of Jesus My Brother. The Church has taken pieces of what My Brother said, together with some of the wisdom of the Fathers, and created pieces of sacramentality but in doing so it has not seen the shape of the mission of Jesus My Brother but only some partial realisations. The Church was to be the constant presence of Jesus on earth after He was enfolded back into the wholeness of God Our Parent. It was to be a constant celebration and love and a support for the weak; it was to be an alternative focus to the civil power, neither subject to it nor seeking to subject it. Those who exercise civil power who are of the Church should behave according to their precept of love without institutional wrangling between Church and state. The Church is the space for promoting perfection, the state is the space for managing imperfection; each has its proper function. To the extent that imperfection is intrinsic to humanity, the state is intrinsic to human need; yet the Church is still the place where perfection in love is the single focus. The Church, as Sacramental, is the earthly presence of God existing in all those children who have consciously recognised their life in the gift of creation. Because it is a sacrament it is to be revered but it must also be worthy of reverence. This means that those in the Church who are called to special ministries through their gifts must not treat the Church as if it were the state, as a sphere where imperfection is managed. They must operate in a trusting environment, vulnerable to imperfection. Their job, as the leadership in love, is to create space in which others can exercise their gifts; it is not for them to create ministry monopolies.

"Just as God Our Parent is the celebrant at the Sacrament of creation so My Sister the Spirit is the celebrant at the celebration of the Sacrament of the Church. Nothing is possible without Her.

"Jesus My Brother is the celebrant at all the Sacraments of the Church. Currently the Church is confused about this and believes that My Sister the Spirit presides at the Sacraments. In one way it does not matter—the explanations are in metaphorical language—but our understanding would be much clearer if we saw that while the Spirit celebrates the Sacrament of the Church, My Brother celebrates at the Sacraments of the Church. Why? Because the humanity of Jesus helps to make the purpose of Sacraments clearer. We cannot know what it 'looks' like if the Spirit pours the water of Baptism but to know that the baptiser stands in the place of Jesus makes it all much simpler. To know that the human celebrant represents Jesus at the Eucharist, in the Reconciliation, at Marriage and in the Sacrament of the dying, touches our sense of how the divine and human are fused. The celebration of those rites where My Sister the Spirit is said to preside tend to be given a strange *de facto* superiority over the Sacraments of My Brother. It is absurd and disrespectful to rank sacraments, to think that Confirmation is somehow superior to Baptism and particularly to think that commissioning servants at Ordination is somehow more important than Marriage. Insofar as there is a distinct Priesthood it is the priesthood of My Brother whose life is known and whose teaching is spoken. To call upon the unseen, unknowable Spirit and claim to know what She advises is a piece of power-wielding hocus-pocus, reducing the clarity of My Brother's message to self-empowering magic. How can the Church of My Sister the Spirit, founded by Jesus My Brother according to His teaching, exclude half of its members from representing Him at the altar? How can a small group of narrowly gifted and self-referential men turn down the vocational callings of Church members by claiming that they have special powers granted by the Holy Spirit when they are exercising personal preferences or resorting to contemporary academic, cultural and presentational yardsticks? Nobody needs to invoke a mysterious ritual involving My Sister when it is easy enough to see when a person is following in the footsteps of Jesus.

"The Sacraments of the Church have grown tired. Take Baptism: how exciting is it now to admit a new Member into the Church? Does your heart race at the prospect? Does anybody take it seriously? It does not matter if the young parents and their friends want a good party, but do not call that Baptism. Baptism is being admitted into the space where there is room to love and grow and the opportunity to create space for others. It is the purpose for which humanity was created. To be in the Church is the highest form of human opportunity. Water and light are lovely symbols but they are too tame; the trickle of water and the demure candle. They are not symbols of space. As the Church is the collective enterprise of the people of God, initiation need not be in the enclosed space of a church with best clothes and tamed symbols. To carry a swimming pool into a church, as some do, is a preposterous distortion; take the people to the water. Sadly, too, the Eucharist has been tamed. Here is the body and blood of Jesus My Brother given to us in all its fullness and generosity, in all its spontaneity and vulnerability, and we have chosen the solidity of bread and the elegance of wine. Where is the sacred risk in receiving My Brother? Where is the wildness of the sadness and joy of it? Bread might be a perfectly good symbol of stability and reliability, for the solidity of flesh, but wine should be its opposite; it should stand for the fluidity of blood, for risk and courage, for spontaneity and rejoicing, for crying and pain; the sacrifice of My Brother is the point at which the human and divine is most flawlessly fused and it is, too, the place where all the great emotions are combined, as if the elements of the rainbow have been speeded up to re-combine into pure, white light.

"I have come to bring you new Sacraments. Some of you will already have heard of my Sacrament of Community in Christ which involves all the people of God bringing symbols of their brokenness and combining them to make a beautiful object out of fragments. You will remember that we made a Cross with fragments of broken glass and decorated it with the surrendered knives of gangsters and a gun; and each person then took away a piece of broken glass as a remembrance of the act. They might take the same piece to another Sacrament of Community where it will be taken home by somebody else. We are all givers and takers of the brokenness of each other; it is not something we suffer alone or hand over to a single person. The Church is a corporate body which spans the world; it has the strength for all our brokenness, but what do we do? We shy away from our imperfection which is our human lot and we condemn those who are not perfect when everyone must stand condemned, including those who condemn. What a futile way to live as a gift of God Our Parent. Do you think God does not know and 'understand' the necessity of human imperfection or do you think, as I half suspect you do, that God made a terrible mistake which made some people better than others with you, in particular, being some of those who are better? When you read stories that My Brother told, do you always think of yourselves as the rich man or the poor man? The Sacrament of Community is a vital ingredient in the life of the Church because it complements the only existing Sacrament which is collective and not focused on specific people on a specific occasion. The Sacrament of Community is a sharp humanity-based balance to the sacrifice of Jesus My Brother in the Eucharist. Where we have been accustomed to receiving Jesus in Word and Sacrament in the Eucharist we must now begin with a complementary Sacrament of surrendering our brokenness to Him and to each other. It is too difficult to beg forgiveness and promise repentance in an abstract prayer which is why the custom has become almost redundant and so we must act out our brokenness and penitence Sacramentally, together. Until we understand the idea of brokenness we can never fully understand the idea of creativity, of taking different elements and changing them or fusing them. The idea that we will always fail because we cannot make perfection is creatively crippling and fundamentally incorrect; only God can make something that is perfect and humanity is therefore outside that kind of expectation, but humanity can bring so many different elements together to create. In a strange way which I cannot explain in language, humanity and God bring different elements together which make up Sacramentality; that is what is so wonderful about it, it is the partnership between the divine and the human.

"Instead of embracing this partnership with the divine which must be entered into by all the people of God, the Church is being destroyed by clericalism. I am sorry to say that to you, but deep in your hearts I think you know it. You know that you are trying to do the work of many different people while denying those people the right to do the work. To separate Confirmation from Ordination is a stark expression of hierarchical self-importance. If Baptism is the Sacrament of Christian Citizenship then adult affirmation is the Sacrament of Ministry. Who would dare say that there is anyone in the Church with no Ministry? Who is to say that the Ministry of Priests and Bishops is more important than the Ministry of someone who visits the sick? Who is to say that the witness of a Christian in a factory is not more difficult and needful of the Spirit than the Ministry of a Priest who lives in a comfortable churchy box? All Christians should be offered the opportunity to make one or more public affirmations of their Christian commitment and those whom the people designate to act on their behalf must in turn show good cause why any person should be denied. Christianity has been far too involved in the absurd enterprise of limiting risk; it is part of its unhappy sojourn in to the State, where it does not belong. Let the Church be the Church and take the risks that love requires.

"I have almost said enough but there is one final, major point which I want to make. We must work together to be a more Sacramental Church. We must not be content to accept the elements of bread, wine and oil bequeathed to us by an Eastern Mediterranean agricultural economy, no matter how nostalgic. We must not settle for the jug of water and the candle. We need to construct contemporary Sacramentality with elements of God's creation which speak to people now about brokenness, the fusion of the divine and human—which is the essence of Sacramentality—and the risks of love. I have already brought one new Sacrament and there will be others, involving the running of water and the leaping of the flame; but we must also use the beauty of flowers, not as incidental ornaments but as central. To do this we must understand love yet again as a risk, not a passport to earthly bliss. We must understand that creating space for others—the essence of loving—is a high risk strategy that requires a Sacramentality of risk."

There was complete silence for what seemed like a long time. Then the Archdeacon shifted slightly in his chair and the tension relaxed. "If I might start the questioning," he said smoothly. "We in the Church recognise the necessity—I do not think that is too strong a word—for 'cutting edge' theological thinking, for speculation, but we do not expect those who undertake this very challenging work to claim that they are sacred instruments of reform, empowered to overthrow the traditions of the Church, long established by the discernment of the will of the Holy Spirit. I do not wish to be offensive in any way, of course, but we must be very careful to sift the wheat from the chaff." "I suppose, Archdeacon that, in spite of your politeness, you classify me as 'chaff'. So be it. I would only say this: the Sacramentality of the Christian Church has never been fixed and it is not fixed now. There are some who think that Sacramentality depends upon replicating the actions of Jesus My Brother and others who think not. My claim that we need a reformed Sacramentality is separate from my parallel claim that I am God Our Parent's Special Vessel. That is quite another matter. You might refuse my second proposition without abandoning my first."

"We could resolve this easily enough if you were to give us some sort of sign," said a Toran at the back of the church. "I could quite readily perform some sort of sign but it does not follow that this would persuade you or anybody else that I am of the Godhead. I know you have already accused me of blasphemy and I am not sure how big the sign would have to be to overcome the objection." "You could imitate God by, for example, turning time backwards…" "…In some sort of conjuring trick? I do not think so…" "…or, even more usefully, you could bring peace to the world or restore its depleted resources." "Even if I could do these things, it would be wrong. I have not been sent to usurp human responsibility. Now and again I make little gestures, like healing sick people or curing addiction, because some people just make me so sad; but humanity has to live with the choices it has made. It has chosen war, it has chosen greed. If I were to put everything right it would never learn that behaviour has consequences. In a strange, reflexive sort of way, if I were to put right that which is wrong, God would be blamed for what has gone wrong. That is the atheist's claim, that if God exists, God must be responsible for all the ills of the world; that is like saying that if music exists it is responsible for crop blight. The two phenomena happen to share a common interface which is humanity, just as God and suffering share a common interface in humanity, but it does not mean that one causes the other." "But," said a very clever academic, "God cannot somehow evade responsibility for creating everything because that defines Godhead; and so, in some way, God must have created suffering." "To create is not to dictate. If you create a cake you do not necessarily know who will turn up at church to eat it after the service and you have no power to force people to eat it or refuse it. The idea that God created human conditions is to see God from an entirely human perspective. It does not matter how often we go around this set of arguments, we come back to the same place. Creation is a mystery: humanity wants to blame God for its imperfection but only imperfection can generate choices, including the wrong choices, for which humanity is responsible; and so, in a strange way, God is definitely responsible for imperfection but not for the way it operates through choice. I think that the problem here is that we spend too much time thinking of Christianity as a philosophy instead of a relationship based on Sacramentality as the bridge between the divine and the human and so, with your permission, we should undertake a Sacramental act although, of course, I recognise that many of you would not use that term in an official sort of way. Nonetheless, I know how committed you are to your beliefs; it is not integrity that is usually at stake but a failure of vision.

"I would like us to perform a variation on a process we already know. Many of you encourage people to write their prayers or their concerns on pieces of paper and offer them on the altar or put them on boards around the church. I want us to begin by writing our concern, our request, our brokenness, and we will amalgamate all of these; and then we will call down My Sister the Spirit to be with us before we come forward again and each take a concern that we promise to pray about and think about. You see, the Sacramentality of Community often involves people being collectively responsible, in an abstract way, for the troubles of others but I want everybody here to know that somebody else has physically grasped each individual concern. Community is about specifics, not principles. It is about personal responsibility as well as communal recognition. Is this acceptable?"

The Archdeacon smiled almost benignly. It could have been worse. The clergy formed an orderly line and walked towards Perpetua, putting their pieces of paper into a bowl. When the last one had finished, Perpetua led prayers for the community and all its individual people and concerns. Then the line formed again as each person took a piece of paper at random from the bowl.

From the Archdeacon's point of view it had been a successful occasion which he thought he had handled very well. Perpetua had had her say, no doubt of that, but it did not seem likely that she would rock the boat. A little dabbling with bits of paper and prayers was hardly revolutionary; there were plenty of experiments in churches, particularly in pursuit of youth, that came and went without causing any real harm. Yet there were many on that day who thought much more deeply about what it was to be a Sacramental church than they had since they were undergoing training. This was probably the moment when Father Bill Midway finally committed himself to Perpetua, prepared to face whatever consequences might follow. No doubt one of these would be the withering disregard of the Archdeacon before a final referral to the Bishop. It wasn't so much the person of Perpetua, although she was very engaging and, inasmuch as he could think about it at all, he found it possible to accept that she might be part of the Godhead; it was her willingness to engage with the idea of brokenness that really hit him, for he felt broken. He had always felt broken. Sitting among the rows of clergy who were individually broken in different ways made him feel uncomfortable because when they came together there was a professional bond of self-satisfaction which the admission of women to the Priesthood had not yet dented. He did not shove through the crowd at the back to talk to her; he knew there would be a right moment.

Dexter said: "That was all rather difficult. Can you simplify it for us?"

"Yes, I can. Everybody knows the same story. There are a group of people on an island who have been given the opportunity to make a new start. There is plenty of everything, including food, drink, desirable partners, occupations and recreations, but they are not all equally well endowed physically or mentally; but instead of making rules which do not take account of their own situation, they very foolishly make rules which favour the powerful and the gifted. This is all right at the beginning because there is enough of everything and so the not so powerful and not so gifted do not feel threatened; but, as time goes by, the powerful become more powerful and the gifted become more gifted. And when the weak and vulnerable protest, asking for a fairer share of resources, they are told that they are welcome by all means to share what is left once the rich and powerful have reserved what they need for themselves because only by reserving resources can they guarantee the proper governance of the island; without these special privileges, everything will collapse."

"I see that," said Dexter. "That is about freedom to make good and bad choices; but what about natural disasters, which you didn't deal with?" "On the same island there are many hazards, notably volcanoes and diseases; and matters are so arranged that the poor live at the foot of the volcanoes and have the poorest health care." "But what about really big disasters that can't be avoided?" "There have been species-obliterating disasters and one day there might even be such a disaster that wipes out humanity but that does not take away humanity's responsibility to behave responsibly within the limits of its competence.

"One of the cleverest tricks of the powerful is to turn discussions about individual responsibility into abstract, philosophical propositions which claim to show why the proposer cannot be held responsible for anything in particular. There is always somebody else to do everything, or some reason why nobody can do anything; either way the individual making the proposal is clear that he cannot do anything. It is just how things are. Yet, if we think about it, the idea that anything is just the way that it is when there are so many of us capable of making individual and collective decisions is clearly an evasion."

"So what does that have to do with Sacramentality?" asked Trina. "If humanity was simply a collection of creatures with language skills and large brains it would face the same choices that we face but, having no notion of the divine, it would have no horizon nor perspective. Although Sacramentality is mysterious it is also deeply explanatory and strengthening. It not only affirms that all humanity is created by God and that, therefore, all humanity will ultimately be enfolded back into God, but it provides a way of involving God in, but not making God responsible for, the way in which we are human. Without God our risks would be simply punishing but with God our risks, our Sacramental risks, are enlivening. We are not punished for taking a risk for love that fails."

She left them to pray, and as she prepared she cut herself on a piece of glass. "Yes," she said, "sacramentality is risky."

V.

And in all she did she gave a new meaning to the life of Jesus her Brother. When she walked among the poor it was as if He was walking; when she celebrated the Eucharist it was as if He was breaking bread. She revitalised the reality of His incarnation in herself. In her membership of the Godhead she reminded the world of His incarnation. She transformed the message from one of historical obscurity to one of contemporary immediacy. Where Jesus had walked by a lake, she walked in the aisles of the supermarkets; where Jesus had told parables of sowers and shepherds, she told parables of brokers and technicians. And although she was respectful of tradition, with one mighty sweep she set aside the esoteric arguments of Byzantium and the Magisterium and brought belief to life in a new way of looking at doctrine. Her reception was generally polite on the surface but there were forces at work which sought to undermine her message and, in doing so, to undermine the message of her brother. There was a dreadful confusion between the essence of what she taught about the nature of Godhead and the way that the teaching of Jesus had come to be understood after two thousand years of speculation and philosophy; and this led good people to think of curtailing her mission for the purest of motives; but curtailing the mission without contemplating some violent action became ever less possible as the extreme opponents of her message began to coalesce.

On the Second Sunday of Advent she took a short break from city life to visit a country church where she had been invited to spend the weekend, leading a discussion day and preaching. She took Dexter and Trina with her to help with the discussion groups but also to show them what the countryside was like. Trina had some intimation of it from her study of English literature, and both of them had seen the countryside on television, but neither had any direct experience of it. As luck would have it, there was a freak fall of snow as they arrived which made the fields and cottages look like the pictures on Christmas cards. "I wonder," said Perpetua, "what people would think about Christmas if they thought that there was no snow in Bethlehem. Jesus My Brother was born before Passover when the weather was wet and windy. There is nothing wrong with transporting images into our own culture as long as we know that is what we are doing, just like the pictures of Jesus which make Him look like a Renaissance sage. Still, I wish we could spend less time on the set and a bit more time on the characters." "What do we know about the characters?" asked Trina. "Well, your average Christmas card buyer, particularly if he does not go to church, would be scandalised by this but the only characters we can really vouch for are My Auntie Mary and Uncle Joe. It is one of those strange paradoxes of modern Christianity that only the non-believers get upset when you tell them that there were no shepherds and kings and, of course, many people get upset, particularly British people, when you say there was no ox and ass, no sheep and no camels. The crib would look very bare, particularly if it was simply a small, damp cave with just the three of them. There was a King Herod and he was known to be very cruel, as well as learned, but the story of the massacre is just that: a story, a kind of parable to illustrate a point; and they did not go to Egypt in spite of the attractive lesson this could teach us about the way we treat asylum seekers. That is bad enough but when we dig deeper I do not think my Uncle Joe would have been pleased to be told that Auntie Mary got pregnant without his assistance; My Sister the Spirit works through human beings rather than going round them; the accounts should say: 'And the Holy Spirit, working through Joseph and with the specific consent of Mary, caused her to become pregnant.' There is a strange myth that the pregnancy was attributed to the Holy Spirit because it could not have been attributed to Joseph, otherwise the baby would not have been legitimate; but in those days not all peasant Jews went through formal marriages and Mary was almost certainly living in Joseph's house when she decided that she was bearing the Son of God." "How do you know all this?" "Most of it is reasonably simple but we have allowed ourselves to develop layers of myth and misinterpretation. The most outstanding is this persistent down-grading of the physical, particularly of physical love." "Does that mean there wasn't an angel?" "Well she might have had a vision in her sleep but the sequence in the Gospels is all wrong; it was after she became pregnant that she knew she was bearing the Son of God. The question was not whether she would bear a child but whether she would rec- ognise the reality of what she was bearing. In a strange way, St. John is nearer the truth of the Nativity without describing it." "So if you take away the nativ- ity stories in the Gospels what is left?" "St. John says that the Word became Flesh; Mary recognised that in herself and she and Joseph brought up Jesus in that belief to such a degree that He believed from quite a young age that He was a special child of God; how special He never knew; we know now because the Evangelists, particularly John, wrote in the retrospective light of the heady days after the Resurrection." "You don't have any special knowledge?" "No. Like Jesus My Brother, when I was sent by God Our Parent, I lost any vestige of divinity which might allow me to have special knowledge of the past or the fu- ture. This is very confusing for Christians because Jesus says all kinds of things about His death and about the sending of My Sister the Spirit when He cannot possibly have known. If we only remember one thing it must be that Jesus was human, as human as me. He was also divine but that does not in any way cancel out his complete humanity." "We are getting close to the Creed." "Yes, that is what we are going to tackle in our discussion groups tomorrow."

She went for a walk over the snowy fields in the moonlight. Far from being "deep and crisp and even", the snow was only deep enough to form a light cover and would soon disappear. "I find Christmas very difficult," she said, "because people are so muddled about it and the collective muddle generates a great deal of anxiety. Above all, we suffer from nostalgia, but it is not even for a time that has been but for a time that never was. True, there were winters of heavy snow which have now largely gone with climate change; but is it just that which makes us disappointed? In the condemnation of commercialism and consumerism there is surely a seed of deep regret; but what for? Perhaps it is regret for the loss of Jesus My Brother in so many lives. Behind all the pretty images which so easily grow melancholy or sentimental, there is a real sense of loss. Perhaps, too, it is the decline of real contrast. It is not only the climate that is losing contrast. Today Christmas is another lavish meal, not one of the few lavish meals of the year. Now we are so rich we have lost the sense of fasting and feasting, of delayed gratification." "Then should we fast?" asked Trina. "We should. That is what Lent and Advent were set aside for; but there are much more important things. Simply thinking about what the birth of Jesus means is important, giving ourselves time. It is better to get out of the rat race and the peer pressure of consumerism for a few minutes than to glibly condemn a thing of which we are part and in which we take pleasure in spite of the stresses. Jesus fasted but He also prayed; He set high standards of behaviour but advised people to be gentle and to take their time, to think rather than to do too much talking."

"So how do we get back this real sense of the baby Jesus?" asked Dexter. "We keep coming around to the same point again and again," she said. "Here is My Brother as a tiny baby, born into a hostile world and a poor family. But we have surrounded Him with thickets of doctrine and institutions. I do not wish to say that all of this is wrong, but it too often gets us away from the central truth that humanity has to establish a personal relationship with God. Yes, it can and must be mediated by the Church, but the Church does not own the idea of God, let alone the Godhead itself. People relate to the baby and then it all gets too complicated, so they are frightened by the effort and the ideas, and so they lose the point of the birth because they never travel all the way to Easter. It is like somebody who sees a sign and knows he has to go on a journey but is given so much information about the route, the rules and regulations for passing through borders, the equipment for climbing and descending, the dietary and dress customs of those on the route, that simply getting through from day to day becomes the point, not the end. And then the journey becomes the thing and it does not really matter whether it follows a direction or goes round in circles; and then many people on these journeys stop travelling and become experts in writing the travel literature that became the problem for the traveller."

Perpetua said to Mother Mary, the Parish Priest: "I hope you do not mind but I want to take the Apostles Creed to pieces and see if we can get something better." "No, Perpetua, that is fine; after all, we have had to dismantle the doctrine of Male Headship, why not go the whole way?"

"Today we are going to think about the Creed; I have chosen the simplest version. The idea," she said, "is to empty your head as much as you can; forget all the half-understood bits of Greek and Latin, all the formularies and catechisms; and then let us see how we get on."

The thirty or so people were split into four groups: the Father, the Son, the Holy Spirit and Etcetera. Perpetua moved from group to group, encouraging, smiling, questioning.

They reported back in order. "We don't like the idea of a Father very much. We accept that there is a phenomenon called a Creator and, therefore, in a sense we don't quite understand, we were created. So that initial idea seems to work. We thought about God being a partner or even a lover but in the end that seemed to describe an equal relationship and if you're created by something else it's hardly equal. Then there was the problem of whether this phenomenon had anything to do with what was created, and we decided there wouldn't be much point in creating something just for the sake of it, if you weren't really interested in it. So," the spokeswoman said, smiling just a little sheepishly, "we opted for your idea of God as a Creator Parent. Then we went on to consider how that parent might relate to us and we had the idea that Godness was a state of unbroken communication forever, to everyone; God transmitting Godness. Which led us to the idea that we exist as created people to try to tune into that communication. We want to come   back to how this might be different for Christians and non-Christians when we have heard what the Son Group says, but we think that God could not have created anything that would not return in some way to the Creator. How would a creator create something that was unwanted? We also wanted to say something about freedom because there's no point being a creature if we simply do what God wants; there's no creativity in it, and, as you say, there's no love unless there's choice." "And what about the second part?" "Oh, 'Creator of heaven and earth' is rather narrow. Creator of everything seems more coherent but we don't like the idea of heaven. It sounds too much like a place. I know it's the Etcetera Group's responsibility but we think that we return to the Father and at that point we get outside time and space."

"The second group had far more material to work with and so its task in getting rid of baggage was more difficult." "The first idea was easy; although the word 'incarnation' is silly Latin for God became human, we accepted the basic idea. It's the most mind blowing idea that there has ever been but we are so deeply ingrained in our Christianity that that is the bit that sticks. We wondered about 'only son'. We wondered why God couldn't have other children. I mean," the spokesman looked embarrassed, "you seem to be claiming that you are a child of God in a different way from the sense in which we are all children of God. It's all very well to say that Jesus is the only son, but if we are created and are God's children aren't we sons and daughters too? So on your account and ours, we didn't like the language. We accept that Jesus was the Son of God in a unique way because He was also God; but we thought about you and we also thought about other planets we know nothing of where God might have wanted to send a child." "What about Jesus My Brother?" "Well, we don't like to admit this but none of us actually believes in the Virgin Birth." "That's a relief. My Auntie Mary will be pleased." "I mean, if the Holy Spirit acts through humanity why couldn't he. . ." "She." "Sorry, why couldn't she act through Joseph instead of going 'round Joseph?" "A very good question. What was your answer?" "Something to do with clergy not liking sex." "Well, liking it and not liking it at the same time. It's the problem of ranking the spiritual above the physical. If God had thought that the spiritual was higher in some way than the physical, why a human Jesus?" "Well, anyway, we didn't like the lines about the conception or the virgin birth." "Good." "The next three bits were easy, really. I mean Jesus did suffer under Pontius Pilate, was crucified, died and was buried." "Why?" "We talked about that for a while but were divided. Some of us think that Jesus died to take away our sins—for all of us, forever—but some of us thought that Jesus died because imperfect humanity just couldn't face how good He was." "Do you mean this group of people thought that He didn't die to save people from their sin?" "If I may," said one of the group, "I was the leader, if you like, of a minority faction and what we believe is that the key to this is the Resurrection which tells us that we may all be returned to God, overcoming death. We don't really see why Jesus had to die to do anything about our sins; in a sense there's nothing He could or can do about that. We are imperfect and therefore we make wrong choices or, as you might describe that, we commit sins, mostly of omission, of turning away from God. Anyway, for us the cross is the visible sign of our imperfection, that we, who were created by God, could, through our wrong choices, murder God." "That sounds a little harsh," said Perpetua. "Well, there is no gentler way of putting it." "What do you think about the next part?" "We didn't understand it very well," said the spokesman. "We don't understand hell but we did think this might symbolise the idea that the people who lived before Jesus were equal to those who lived after; in other words, although Jesus lived in time, God's relationship with all humanity is the same whenever it takes place. We were far more excited about rising again although we have problems with the idea that Mary Magdalene was told not to touch Jesus but Thomas could touch him. It's all a bit odd." "But what does it mean?" "It means that God's promise that we should all be complete after death is real to us through the life and Resurrection of Jesus. Again, we had a problem with ascending into Heaven, but accept that Jesus re-joined God in a way that we will." "That is difficult but it might be best to leave that for the second round.

"Now the Holy Spirit." "We had even less to go on than the Father Group. There's just this one line. We accept that God communicates with everyone, as the Father Group said, and we suppose this to be the phenomenon of the Spirit, but we can't grasp why this phenomenon, to switch to the other creed, should proceed from the Father and Son nor be called a 'person'. We got a bit radical, probably because we had so little material to work with, but we thought that the whole idea of the Trinity and of 'Persons' wasn't very helpful. We accept that God is a Creator and that Jesus was in some way our Saviour and part of the Godhead and that God communicates through what we call 'the Spirit' but these are such different phenomena that trying to call them collectively anything is very difficult." "Very good. We always have to remember that theology is provisional.

"What about the theology, then, Etcetera group?" "Well, we believe in the Holy Catholic Church but it's a bit forlorn. We can't even agree among ourselves what we need to agree among ourselves. We like the Communion of Saints in a vaguely ancestral sort of way but wonder whether it matters much. We had real problems with the Resurrection of the Body but not really much of a problem with life everlasting."

"All right. I am going try try and sum up round one. We believe in a creator God who made everything, is a compulsively communicating parent whose children are free to love or not to love; this Parent sent Jesus as a son to become human but this physical manifestation might not be unique. I claim, for instance, that I am one such manifestation. Jesus came to bring hope to the world and His Resurrection confirmed that hope. We are not very sure about the Crucifixion. Some of us think that Jesus died in order in some way to mitigate human sinfulness; others stay with the idea of hope. We accept the idea of My Sister the Spirit but are worried about the talk of Persons in a Trinity. We were very weak on the idea of a church, so we will give that more time in the next round. Finally, we like the idea of life everlasting but are puzzled about our own Resurrection. Good.

"Now we will split up into different groups so that we do not get into a rut. What I would like the Groups to consider is the following: What is God's purpose and, therefore, what is human purpose? What is special about Jesus? What is the Church? And is anything missing from the Creed that we would like to include?"

These second round sessions were much more difficult. There was not so much animated talk. People looked puzzled and sometimes bewildered. Perpetua wanted to be in all four places at once and, even with the help of Dexter and Trina, it was difficult to keep up the momentum. But gradually thoughts began to emerge and people looked more comfortable.

"All right. We will start again with the idea of God." "It's very difficult to think of God having a purpose, so we started with the idea that God is love because there is no other explanation of why anything is made; you would not make something out of nothing to hate it, or for no reason at all. So, God is love and God's purpose, insofar as there is a purpose, is therefore to love. Our purpose, as creatures of God, exactly mirrors God's purpose; we exist to love. God would not have created anything to do anything different from what God does, although we do it differently. So our love as creatures can't be the same as God's love as a creator. We call that imperfection but we might also call it freedom; they are the same thing. It's startling, that." "I know. You have done well.

"What about Jesus My Brother?" "We were back in the problem of the Crucifixion. We didn't have any problem with the birth; the idea that God sent a Son who was both divine and human is difficult but, as we said, we can't shift that out of our psyche. Still, we had real problems with the Crucifixion. We couldn't really get past our part in it, and we found it significant that the Creeds don't say why Jesus was crucified, although Paul spent a long time on it." "What about this idea?" said Perpetua. "Jesus was sent by God to make the idea of Godhead more concrete; and that concreteness included startling humanity by showing it how wrong wrong choices can be, such that humanity, in a collective way, killed Jesus?" "Yes, so far so good, but what about this idea of wiping the slate clean which divides this group as well as the previous group?" "Well, frankly, I feel that Jesus My Brother in some way absorbed the world's sin, tried to take a lot of guilt away and replace it with hope. I am trying to do the same thing. I feel like God's Sacred Vessel but to me that is like collecting all the remorse and guilt I can find to free people to make more loving choices. I don't like the thing about slates. You have done very well to face up to this, what about other issues?" "We wondered if one way of understanding the Crucifixion and the Resurrection would be to say that we now know there is no wrong choice that we can make, including killing God, that will limit God's love for us." "Intriguing." "The rest was very similar to the group that considered Jesus. We think that the real way to understand the Spirit is to think of it as our raised consciousness of God as the communicator."

"So, what of the Church?" "We found ourselves wanting a different kind of Church. I mean, we like what we've got now; don't get me wrong. We like our services and we love our Vicar—and I'm not just saying that because she's here—but we wanted something more radical; and that's when your colleagues combined us with the 'What else?' Group because it was discussing the idea of the bridge between the human and divine, the idea of Sacramentality which you have been promoting so much; and it's only fair that somebody who started talking about that should go on."

"Thank you. Yes, we thought that the Sacraments, as constituted, are a bit tame and a bit lame. They do not express the vitality of the fusion of body and spirit. We want the whole Church to be a Sacramental thing, to live sort of suspended between the two. It's all a bit earth-bound and doctrinal. If we are to be enfolded back into the Godhead, as you describe it, then our life on earth should be something about doing some of that enfolding now, practising for heaven, you might call it. One of our members put it a different way, she said—but she doesn't want to say it herself—she said that we are the only race we know that have had the unique privilege of trying to love God freely and that that is why we are here and it is more than enough. It isn't an ante-room to heaven, she said, it's a unique thing to be able to do; the whole of life, then, is Sacramental because it's physical beings encountering the divine." "That is very good. What about those who are not in the Church?" "We accepted the work of the first Group which said that God perpetually communicates with all humanity but that some people, through the encounter with the Spirit, are better attuned; that brings added responsibility. What makes Christians different is not that we will be re-united with God—everybody will—but that we have a unique responsibility to give people that hope; to tell them that is what is going to happen because that will actually make them understand better their purpose for being on earth, like that lady said."

"Which rounds everything off. We have had an excellent morning and you deserve your lunch. This proves what I have often said, that people who are loyal Christians can discuss theology without the need for formal training as long as they give themselves time to think clearly."

After lunch they came back together and Perpetua said: "This will be the most difficult part of the work. I want us to boil down everything we agree on into a single, short new Creed; and where we disagree, as we do on the Crucifixion, we might have to leave things out."

All through the afternoon, past the deadline on the agenda, they worked carefully and respectfully. Perpetua hardly pushed at all. They were fully aware of what she taught and they had thought about what she had said. Trina wrote down agreements, statement by statement, tidying up the grammar, always checking that she had fairly represented what was said, before moving on.

This is what she wrote:

We believe:

- That God who is love created everything out of love and created humanity as imperfect so that we might freely love.
- That in love God Our Parent sent a Son, Jesus Christ, as God to share our humanity; by such sharing He brought new hope but His perfection was too much for imperfect humanity to bear and so we killed Him.

- That He absorbed all humanity's wrong choices and gave it new resources to love through our consciousness of our Sister the Spirit which attunes us more closely to God's communication in love.
- That by His resurrection Jesus confirmed that, because no wrong choice, including killing Jesus, will limit God's limitless love, all humanity will be enfolded back into the Godhead from which we came.

We affirm:

- Our earthly purpose of living a Sacramental life of physical encounter with the divine through the Church and accept the privileged responsibility inherent in that encounter to bring the news to all humanity that it will be re-united in God.

"So far, so good," said Perpetua. People looked disappointed. "Do not worry. There are only two important items we need to think about. I am sure we left them out because they are so obvious; but a Creed has to be obvious if it is to succeed. That is why our current creeds are failing; they are no longer obvious enough. We need to humanise the rather dry statements we have made. I suppose it is inevitable that committees will come up with documents that sound rather official, but we should think about the personal nature of our relationship with God; it is not a philosophical state of mind but a direct personal relationship; the second idea is that the whole of what we are talking about is deeply mysterious.

Where they had been tempted to hurry when Perpetua summed up, people settled down again and worked with Trina to put the final draft in order:

We believe in the mysteries:

- That God who is love created everything out of love and created humanity as imperfect so that we might freely love God in a personal relationship and love each other.
- That in love God Our Parent sent a Son, Jesus Christ, as God to share our humanity; by such sharing He brought new hope but His perfection was too much for humanity to bear and so we killed Him.
- That He absorbed all humanity's wrong choices and gave it new resources to love through our consciousness of our Sister the Spirit which attunes us more closely to God's communication in love.
- That by His resurrection Jesus confirmed that, because no wrong choice, including killing Jesus, will limit God's limitless love, all humanity will be enfolded back into the Godhead from which we came.

We affirm the mysteries:

- Our earthly purpose of living a Sacramental life of physical encounter with the divine through the Church and accept the privileged responsibility inherent in that encounter to bring the news to all humanity that it will be re-united in God.

"You have been wonderful," she said. "Let us stand and say this Creed together."

"That is enough doctrine for one day," she said as she waved goodbye to all the smiling people. "Look, the moon is out; Mother Mary, let us go for a walk."

The four of them walked through the fields in silence for a while until Trina said: "It is sad but the snow is melting and soon the fields will be green again. I like them when they are white." "Yes," said Mary, "snow is pretty and there is room for it as long as people don't mistake it for what lies beneath. I thought that the work we did today was rather like seeing Christianity without snow, stripping off all the pretty coverings we have got used to." "People need pretty things from time to time," said Dexter, "otherwise it's all too serious. I found today very difficult." "I know you did," said Perpetua, "but your reality was that you went on encouraging other people when they reached a deadlock, not with doctrinal fixes but with goodwill. Yes, we all need things that are pretty as long as they do not come to stifle us or make us sentimental. I was once in a guest house that was absolutely covered in ornaments: jugs, teddy bears, boxes, thimbles, dolls, glass animals, plates, dried flowers, photographs, feathers, screens, ash trays, china cats; tables of chess pieces; baskets of wool; a flock of sheep; a menagerie of soft toys; a collection of butterflies; a calendar of elephants; a library of prints. The whole time I was there she was dusting and I was so frightened of knocking something over that I could not move. Often I think that the church is like that; the clergy spend all their time dusting a mad collection of theological objects and the congregation are frightened of knocking something over.

"Oh look. The snow is melting, the moon is behind a cloud. It might rain as it did on the night that Jesus My Brother was born. We are getting back to reality."

VI.

And the earth grew more quiet as people learned of the renewed Word through radio and television; and as Perpetua walked among the people they, too, were quietened; and racial tension declined as people learned to give each other the benefit of the doubt, to assume good unless there was contrary evidence, to renounce demagogues and fear bred of ignorance and to listen. And she walked in every place, encouraging the poor and downtrodden, bringing the Good News to all who would listen; walking through the markets, sitting in slums, visiting women behind the high walls of their isolation, joking with prisoners and always comforting the lonely. She walked in radiant light with the mysterious, noble music all around, bringing fresh life to what had faded, to paint and stone, to clothes and shoes, to fruit and vegetables, to faces and to eyes; wherever she went there was brightness and lightness and smiling faces. She went to markets where poor white people looked for the cheapest food, she went to markets where people from the Caribbean, South Asia, Africa and Eastern Europe looked for food that would remind them of their homeland or their ancestors; and she told them that their true home was with God, and it did not matter which route they took to reach that home as long as they tried, as long as they travelled in faith, as long as they persevered. She talked with Muslims, Sikhs, Hindus, Christian charismatics and Pentecostalists, and with people from an almost unimaginable number of sects and people with an endless variety of pick-and-mix spiritualities. She always smiled, she always listened and encouraged, she often said a few words and sometimes even preached but she never judged.

And she brought a sense of optimism to the lives of everyone she met, damping down pessimism and cynicism, opening a world of promise and fulfillment. She moved in a world of good but anchorless people and gave them a new sense of self and purpose.

She stood at a stall of vegetables and fruit from all over the world and a man said: "Why do you bother to come here? We are Muslims, not Christians." "Because... I am sorry, what is your name?" "Yusuf." "A nice name, I had an Uncle called Yusuf. I am here because I want to encourage everybody to be with God." "But what can you tell us that we cannot learn from the Koran?" "I do not think that there is anything I can tell you that you cannot learn from the Koran but to read and 'be told' is not enough, is it? If reading and instruction were enough the world would be a peaceful and happy place but it is not. Do you really gain enough from the Koran to enable you to be happy and to be close with God?" "Not really, but that is because I am poor." "So the Koran does not help you to be a poor person?" "No." "Nor does the Bible or any other book. Books can help us to realise why it is spiritually acceptable—and perhaps even necessary—to be poor; there is a philosophy of poverty but that only solves the intellectual problem. As a good Muslim you know both what you must do by giving to the poor and you know what you must do as a poor person; but is that really enough? Do you think that Muslims are happier than other people?" "No, but I think we should be." "I think Christians would give you the same answer." "Because we have the truth we should be happier." "And what truth is that?" "That Islam is the way to God." "The only way?" "I think so." "Christians say much the same thing." "Are they wrong?" "It is not a matter of being wrong the way that we are wrong if we say $2 + 2 = 5$. You are wrong for making a mistake about the nature of what you are thinking and feeling." "I don't like to be told by a woman that I'm wrong." "Wait just a moment, Yusuf, that is quite a different issue. If there is only one way to God, what are we to think of all the people who have never been told about that way?" "I don't know, really." "What about all the people who follow different ways?" "They are wrong." "And then I ask Christians the same question and they give the answers you have given. Then where are we? Surely there is some truth in the idea that there are different ways to the same God and that all travellers on these ways have much more in common than any of those poor people who have not seen the necessity to travel?" "I suppose so." "Have you ever learned about Christianity?" "No, except that it has three Gods and we know that there is only one God." "All right, look at it this way. If you said to me that you had three children but you were all united in one happy family, how would you feel if I said that that simply could not be true? What if I argued that perfect unity between your children is not possible?" "I would have to accept that because any human unity would be imperfect." "But Christians say the unity of the Trinity in one God is being undertaken, if you like, in a 'perfect' context. Why would you want to assume that Christians are saying there is one God in bad faith?" "Because we can't understand this three-in-one." "Nor can Christians understand it; but religion, Muslim or Christian, Jewish or Hindu, is not about understanding, it is about establishing a dynamic relationship with God where we try to move towards God."

Yusuf grudgingly accepted. "Look, Yusuf. You do not need to take my word for it; just think about it, and think what a better place the world—no, your world—would be if you reduced the number of hostile people in it by giving Christians the benefit of the doubt."

"Well, we've formed a Bengali Islamic Association." "Just men, just Bengali Muslims? What about other Muslims from Nigeria, say, or Indonesia?" "Well. . ." "Never mind. I know all the reasons why people need to bond; but we need to think about living in two different kinds of organisations, not just people here, but all of us, including white people who think that this is their country and that we are somehow invaders or, even though I was born here, outsiders. We need to enjoy the security of our own kinds of organisations but we also need to form organisations where we meet people who are not like us, where we are even a little uncomfortable. Have you noticed how white people form twinning arrangements with other white people in pretty little towns in Germany and France? I think it would be better if parts of London twinned with each other, white parts with black parts, rich parts with poor parts, suburban parts with central parts. It would also be good if people from very rich towns twinned with people in very poor towns.

"On the other issue, it is impossible for me to talk with you honestly about the way you treat women, without causing some hurt, and so I can only refer you to my questions about women. Can I stand up on your stall and talk to all the people around now that the market is getting ready to close?" "Yes you can; but it's the woman thing," said Yusuf. "It is difficult just to let you stand on top of this stall and start making a public speech which is what you are going to do." "I am sorry, Yusuf, yes I am. I am worried and hurt about the way you treat women but no doubt you are worried and hurt about the way my people behave; but if we are not able to talk about it we just sink into mutual recrimination instead of building a society together. This needs hard work. It would be very rude of me, and wrong, to think I know why Muslim people have such different attitudes from Christian people to the place of women. I am not going to tell you or anybody that your religious and cultural ideas are wrong but I think I might ask you—not the whole world, just you—a few questions that you can think about. First, can you honestly say that the way you treat women is a direct result of Koranic teaching or is it cultural, something that has grown up by tradition through the centuries? Secondly, does the isolation of women—I am sorry if that sounds harsh—have anything to do with women as property, women as possessions? And, connected with that, do you suspect all your fellow men of lusting after the wife that you have married? And do you suspect all men of lust and rape? And are you one of the men you suspect?" "I can't take any more of this." "I am not, as far as I can tell, giving you anything; I am simply asking questions. I am interested in what, from the outside, looks like a complex love-hate relationship that men in your culture have for women." "Psychological nonsense." "Fair enough; but ask yourself the questions."

Her followers bought most of the fruit and she asked again if she could climb on the stall. "As you have bought most of the fruit I suppose I have to let you." "No. We bought your fruit because it looked nice, because you asked a fair price and also because it looked as if you had not done so well as some of your neighbours.

She climbed onto the bare boards of the stall. "I want to talk to you for just a few minutes," she said, "about our lives. For a beginning, I recognise that our lives are difficult but God is not an escape route. We do not escape from poverty by turning to God; we escape from it by joining together in the power of God to call, courteously but firmly, for change."

A man from Pakistan and a man from Romania began to look at each other curiously. What had caught their attention was the fact that each of them was listening carefully to an English-speaking Perpetua. They could not exchange a word with each other but they knew that each of them could hear what she was saying.

"Here is a problem that we need to overcome. Take a community like this: many of us halve our strength by denying the support of women; next we halve our strength by denying the authenticity and comradeship of people who believe the same things as us but have a different language and culture of belief; then we halve our strength by believing that everybody we do not know or cannot understand is hostile; then we halve our strength by limiting our understanding because we will not learn to communicate with each other, so 'multi-culturalism' for all means a single culture for each."

"Blacks!" a man shouted at her as she left. "Why don't you all go home." "Home is in Grunge Park," she said, "where I was born; but I do not suppose you mean that. The point, as you know, is that immigrant families come here because there is work that most indigenous people do not really want to do. Did you want to import people to drive your buses, run the health service and then send them back? Did you want the workers to live in camps without family love? To an extent, that is what is happening now and I do not suppose you like it any better. Of course, sorry, what is your name?" "Charlie." "Of course, Charlie, you are a decent man to individual black people but you cannot help repeating these sad prejudices. Do not worry about black people, immigrants, exiles, asylum seekers, just worry about each person you meet."

She said to her followers: "Poor Charlie. The world is like that, full of people who generalise bitterness but are actually decent to individuals. There are people who are content with the services they receive at a personal level but think the service in general is bad. We have reached a cultural position where people are automatically pessimistic and cynical, almost beyond content. Either it is centralisation or a post code lottery; either it is the nanny state or the uncaring Government; either it is red tape or carelessness; either it is moralising Christians or Christians who have abdicated responsibility; either it is wasteful choice or not enough choice; either it is too much competition or too little. We have got into the habit of being discontent about everything in general but usually pretty content about things in particular. This is because most people now are still very decent but they have lost a balanced world view anchored in a relationship with God. Even their spirituality is generated by themselves as consumers. Now, let us go to see the rich people in their fastness."

She was addressing a lunch-time gathering of business people in a city church. "I want to begin by saying that what you do for a living, making money by making money, is not wrong. I say that because you are frequently accused by people of being immoral just for what you do when they are happy enough to enjoy the fruit of your labours in their pension plans and other forms of investment; but I want to give you a big warning, to say something that you know in your hearts but which you keep pushing away. You are the people who can change almost everything and you change almost nothing. You could be the engine of social justice, the engine of climate justice, the engine of world justice, but you look at the 'bottom line' and shove the problem onto politicians, reformers, whomever you can see except yourselves; and then you even have the nerve to make fun of the reformers onto whom you have shoved the problems, either because they are ineffective or because they are effective enough to make a tiny pin prick in what you are doing. We are asked to give to this world in proportion to what we have. Why is it that as incomes go up, the percentage of giving for justice goes down? Why is it that you will not give but neither will you advocate higher taxes to match your higher wealth? Why is it that many of you think it is acceptable to pay no tax at all? I know that you can appeal to the law but is that not what the Pharisees did at the time of Jesus My Brother?

"You care too much for the world and too little. Here are two people, Bob and Jim. Bob answers every letter as soon as it comes in, every email and voice mail. Bob lives in his own frenetic soap opera, eighteen hours per day, making sure that the business gets done, making money he has no time to spend; throwing it at the feet of his wife whose feet he has no time to kiss; throwing it at his children as the only story they ever hear. Jim, on the other hand, was born into riches and he never bothers. He never answers the phone, never answers emails, never answers his wife or his children but just lives in the cloud of his own luxury. Then, one day, Bob breaks down. He has made all the money you could imagine but he is not happy. He asks colleagues for help but he has screwed the last penny out of each of them; he asks his wife for help but she does not know what to say; he even asks his children to listen but they do not hear his voice. At the same time, there comes a day when Jim has no money. He has not answered letters from his lawyers, from his bankers, from his financial advisers, and it is all gone away.

"Bob and Jim meet at a bridge from which they intend to throw themselves, when a man comes by with a dog. 'This is a strange place for two men such as you,' the man says. 'We don't know each other,' says Bob, 'so we are two separate men.' 'That,' says the man with the dog, 'might just be your problem. Now why would you want to be standing on this bridge as if you might throw yourselves off?' 'Lonely and rich,' says Bob. 'Lonely and poor,' says Jim. 'Put together," says the man with the dog, 'that could be either two men dead or two men no longer lonely and somewhere between poor and rich.'

"I do not say this kind of story will change your minds but you are supposed to be pragmatic people, devoid of sentiment and yet you do not value society; you think you are above it. You think you define it, and in some ways you do, through financial instruments and a massive superstructure of inter-dependency; but we expect more of you, as you should expect more of your-selves. I do not need to re-tell the stories of Jesus My Brother; you know them all but, sadly, you have forgotten what they mean. Perhaps they need to be told in new ways but I doubt it; I think that is one respect in which 'trendy' Christians are profoundly wrong; I do not need to dress up the story of the Good Samaritan, the Prodigal Son, or Dives and Lazarus for you to know what is meant.

"Let me end by being constructive. You cannot forge social justice through aggressive competition, and so neither can you forge it through aggressive, competitive self-denial. You can only achieve justice through collaboration, through sharing values of social justice and seeing them reflected in the work you do. If you all halved your profits, shareholders would move elsewhere be-cause, I do not need to tell you, the people who buy your services and think your prices excessive are also shareholders through their pension funds. Your job is to work together to change the social climate, to make social justice re-spectable, to make yourselves good citizens through mutual support, to change the minds of those over whom you have influence.

"Finally, you cannot do this alone. God is reaching out to you, to each one of you, forever; each of you was made to hear God's communication with you but you have turned off your receivers. Listen to God, together, alone, in silence. Practice the silence of the open heart."

"I am not sure," said the first questioner, "but I think we got off quite lightly. Most people just want to slag off global capitalism." "I do not see the point of slagging off anything. When you think about it carefully, you know that what you are doing is disproportionate, that is the word I want you to take away. Bob and Jim were disproportionate in different ways. To lead a good life is to live in balance with your neighbours and yourselves but most of all with God. There are a few people who live in extreme relationships with them-selves, their communities and God; some of them are saints and others are vil-lains but the majority of us are neither; as creatures, we need to live in balance with our Creator."

"But we give millions to charities." "I recognise that, but surely that is putting the problem somewhere else, pushing it off to other people. I know that taxation is a form of pushing away but at least it is socially coherent. It is the way we have to work in a complex world. We should ask ourselves what we really think of the people who work for charities. Would you be happy if the chief executive of the biggest charity in the country was earning as much as anybody in this room? I doubt it. You want your charity and social justice on the cheap to assuage your guilt, but the main purpose of social justice is not to assuage the guilt of the unjust, it is to provide dignity to the victim. I do not doubt that many of you are very generous, particularly when there is a major natural disaster, but, as you would say of your own professional concerns, you cannot solve a deep-seated problem with a quick fix."

"But there are problems, like ecology, that we cannot fix as business people." "We all have to fix the ecological problem, but you are so influential. You know that the poor will be damaged more than the rich by natural disaster; those of you, particularly in the insurance industry, know the benefit of insurance and the disaster of not having it. Certainly the ecological crisis has arisen because of collective greed and short termism, the inability of society to delay and modify its self-gratification; and you need to ask how serious is the criticism of you that the only factor that curbs your greed is fear. Would you be more greedy if the risks were fewer? To the extent that civilisation is built on self-denial—or what you would call investment—our civilisation is disintegrating. In your own sphere, you know what happens when people simply spend and stop saving; it works for a while and then there is a disaster; well, that is what we have done with the world's physical resources and, closer to home, that is what we are doing with social capital; greed and short-termism erode social capital because people have nothing and nobody to trust."

"What do you really want us to do?" "I want you to use your brains to work out ways of re-engineering social justice without a collapse of the structures which you operate; justice without revolution, not because revolution is necessarily bad but because, practically, it always hurts the poor, in whose name it is carried out, disproportionately; full justice without collapse. I recognise that you live in a dynamic both of solidarity and competition; harness this wonderful tension for the benefit of others. Perhaps it may sound strange, given what Jesus My Brother used to say, but give yourselves, not your money, to the poor. Give to institutions that can work with poor people for their balanced development.

"We must never allow subtle get-out arguments to obscure the central truths:

- people who are poor need money
- people who are ill-educated need education
- and, most of all, people who are unloved need love.

"I want you to show your personal and collective commitment in personal action, by working in difficult environments; we need to make real contact with real people, but at a more institutional level, we need to build institutions that can channel personal commitment and large quantities of money; the institutions can channel your money, they can secure education, but only you can give the love.

"Let me finish with some questions to you, your wives, your families and your class:

- What do you know about poverty, misery, suffering, want, hopeless-ness, despair, addiction, nihilism, emptiness?
- Are you personally doing enough to help your brothers and sisters overcome their problems in terms of brain power, time, money and love?
- Are you collectively putting the same effort into social justice that you put into personal well-being?
- Are you avoiding this problem by asserting that it belongs to some-body else, to "them"?
- Even from a selfish perspective, how long can this go on before it wrecks your lives but, more probably, the lives of the children you say you love?

The chairman, closing the meeting, said: "I think if we are honest it is time for us to put our hands up and admit that we have not been doing enough. We give to charities, yes, probably less than we can afford, but we steer clear of the poor. With the help of our Priest here, who tries to moderate our aggres-sive capitalism during lunch-time worship, we will set up a cash and contact association. I will put my hand in my pocket, and I daresay all of you will too, but next time, when you're asked out to do a spot of business on the golf course or at Lords, give it a miss and save the day for a contact visit to whatever poor area of London Father chooses."

As they went away, one of her followers asked: "Why were you so gentle with those rich people who cause all the problems?" "I was as gentle as I could be because, like the rest of us, they are not so much wicked as thoughtless, and those who are opposed to what they do are too apt to come up with mindless, heartless solutions. Western civilisation was almost wrecked by mad Marxism which put ends before means and ruined the very people it was supposed to help. If you force people to be good, compulsory altruism, that is not be-ing good at all. I would have thought that that was obvious. These people are no worse nor better than anybody else, it is just that their weaknesses are magnified in our eyes because of their wealth. Look how they reacted when they were made to think. Like all of us, they will begin with enthusiasm and then lose it but I am nominating Andy, as our financial man, to be their special helper. Now let us go and see the politicians."

She had been asked to address the Forum for Social Justice which was full of policy makers, advisers, think tanks, authors, journalists and politicians. She said: "Why have you handed over all the challenges to the sensible shoes and the safe hands? It seems extremely churlish to begin by asking why we think that movements for social justice have yielded such poor results. Look at all the money that has been ploughed into social programmes in our country; look at the funding that has been poured into poor countries. Do we really believe that failure is a matter of quantity; that if we did twice as much there would be half as much of a problem? Do we really think that if we doubled the number of fire engines it would halve the number of fires? Do we really think—*really* think—that if we doubled the number of policemen it would halve the number of crimes? Do we really think that doubling the number of places for drug addicts will even increase slightly the number of addicts that finally break free from their addiction?

"I have just been to see the rich people in the city and asked them to think about their role, so it is not simply a question of looking elsewhere. You may dislike what happens in the financial sector but I doubt that there is anybody here who does not benefit from what these people do, so let us draw a line under that.

"What I want to talk to you about is the clash between system and passion, between care and love, between professionalism and emotion. There was a time—it was not a golden age, but there was a time—when people lived in family units. Like or dislike the people they lived with, they had to get on with it and that made their love strong; it has to be if you find that you cannot like somebody. Occasionally people needed help from outsiders such as doctors, if they could afford it, and, increasingly, children went to school and were partially brought up by teachers; but there was still that family core. Now there are millions of people who do not really have a family core and yet the conventional wisdom is still that professionals must not become emotionally involved and that there should be a boundary between caring and loving. That is partly because our society thinks about sex when anybody says the word love which is why, disastrously, men have been driven out of our primary schools, but the underlying assumption about professionalism and caring on the one hand and emotionalism and loving on the other, needs to be thought through. Professionals are no longer social add-ons who can afford to stay aloof, they are, for many people, all that there is. That is not to say that it should be this way. Many people have extended their consumerism into their dealings with people, even close family members; they have given up on people and handed the 'problem' to professionals; but just because they are selfish in doing that, it does not mean that professionals can go on pretending that things are the way they were. Otherwise the weakest people in our society get pushed away by their own people and are greeted with cool care from professionals. What kind of a life is that? This is a very difficult area because you will rightly say that it is dangerous for professionals to become involved with people. Yes, love is always dangerous but we cannot afford to say: 'In these circumstances I will love but in those circumstances I will withhold my love for sound professional reasons'. Love is about professionalism, not one of its tools which you can choose to use or not use, remembering that this love, this vulnerability to the other, is quite distinct from care."

"Would a high-level committee help?" asked a senior civil servant. "Yes it would. I know people are glibly critical of committees—and sometimes they are used to delay decisions—but this is a difficult area. Getting society to re-introduce love as a civic virtue which has been absent from it since the supposed Enlightenment is a major enterprise."

"But are we the right people when our reputations are so tarnished?" asked a Junior Minister. "I think you are. It is very easy to attack politicians because you take the difficult decisions which we will not take for ourselves and then we feel free to attack you for it. We have made a pact with you; you must not tell us the truth and, in exchange, we will pretend that you are really liars when you are only doing what we ask while, at the same time, letting the truth come out sideways. We know when a politician is lying for himself rather than lying for us. Bishops are good people but they think that their goodness allows them to make disastrously bad decisions; they also think goodness always lies in compromise, although how you reach a compromise between a round earth and a flat earth is a mystery to me. As for journalists, they lie for their bosses, hiding under the completely bogus umbrella of the Fourth Estate. They survive by making people unhappy and by switching wildly between points of view, often in the same issue of a paper; so you will see a picture of a nearly naked teenage girl opposite an editorial raging against sexual abuse. If I had the choice of being marooned on a desert island with bishops, journalists or politicians, I would take the politicians every time."

"What might the Church do to help?" asked a Member of Parliament. "I do not know," she said, "but I am about to ask."

On the way out she passed between two lines of protesters, the one to her right holding banners reading:

FIGHT TERRORISM

the one to her left holding banners reading:

NO WAR

"Please could you stop shouting for a few minutes?" she asked. "How many of you have read about the grounds for just wars?" "There is no such thing as a just war," returned one of the protesters on her left. "I think you are only entitled to that conclusion when you have thought about it, dare I say prayed about it? We are all too apt to pick and chose our wars; the 'Left' was in favour of the Serbian war even though it was not sanctioned by the UN but it is against the war in Iraq, saying that that is because it was not sanctioned by the UN." "But if we don't fight," said one to her right, "our way of life will be destroyed." "Only you can destroy your way of life," she said. "I think it would be much better for all of you if you held a seminar where you discussed a little philosophy and said a few prayers." "Religion is the opium of the people," shouted one to her left. "Sadly, religion is trying hard but failing to combat the real problem; heroin is the opium of the people. There is plenty for the Church to do," She added, "but at least it has its humble side. That is what I hope to see."

VII.

And she was called upon to address the mighty Synod, with all the power of the Church arrayed, the purple of the Bishops and the wigs of the lawyers and the suits of the legislators with their amendments to amendments and their points of order. She had been called upon by friends but there were many who were hostile and even more who were indifferent. And as she spoke, a faction began to wonder how she might be curbed.

"Even if I were inclined to it—which I am not—it is too late to be angry. You have brought the Church which Jesus My Brother founded to its lowest point, to its point of extinction in the form that it has been known since Constantine. And we will need to make a new church for a new age, proclaiming the Third Testament for the Third Millennium.

"I have seven charges against you. The first is that you have become obsessed with structure. As the world reels from injustice and degradation, as greed eats up the life of the planet, as the name of Jesus My Brother is strange to the lips of most of the people of this land and other lands which you call Christian, you are locked in an argument about structure. You use words like 'Communion' and 'Covenant' to describe an esoteric process to try to bring the order of statecraft to the Body of Christ. If you were arguing about the Creed, I would understand the passion of your words, although no Creed would be worth a single word of reproach, and certainly not of recrimination. If you were divided over the nation of the Godhead, I would understand. If one said to another: 'Is Perpetua God? And does this mean we must abandon the idea of the Trinity?' I would understand. If you were divided over such great matters and had searched your consciences and thought that there was some merit in deciding who is to be part of the Church and who must be left outside, I would not agree with your process, but I would understand. Instead, you have taken a matter of conscience—I will come to the substance of the issue later—and have tried to impose structures so that consciences are beaten or worn down. There are those who say that Scripture requires them to be brutal, Torans who claim the authority of God to be brutal—a strange and horrible perversion— whereas Scripture requires them to exercise their conscience for themselves. If those of a like conscience wish to band together, to gather in the name of Jesus, then so be it. If there are those who say that Scripture guides them differently from the Torans and wish to gather together, so be it. If there are those—and they are many—who have nothing to say, then let them go where they will go. There are many of you who say that our brothers in Islam are incorrect when they wish to establish a theocratic state but you have done the opposite, which is much worse: you have made for yourselves a political Church.

"It would be unfair of me to say 'you' as if you were the only ones. The

Petrans began this process with Constantine but now, as the love of Jesus My Brother seems to grow cold in the world, you are becoming more extreme in your politics. When the monarchs of this land interfered with the Church it was bad enough, but when bishops and clergy and lay people who claim to care for the welfare of the Church try to construct systems to retain some believers and expel others on marginal grounds, the time for the end is close. I have noted that some have refused to share the Eucharist of My Brother with others, withholding their Christian solidarity because they believe that those with whom they disagree are sinners? Who knows who is a sinner? And who knows the 'mind' of God Our Parent? And who are you to draw up a guest list for the Lord's Supper, deciding who is worthy?

"You say that you know from the Bible, but the Scriptures do not free you from the exercise of your conscience and they do not entitle you to impose the conclusions of your conscience on others. St. Paul demands mutual respect between conservatives and liberals; but, most of all, Scripture does not tell you to abandon love in order to prosecute some different aim which you think higher. You might think that it is more important to impose your orthodoxy than to love your brothers and sisters, but you are wrong. The church was not founded by My Brother so that it should develop and impose a set of doctrines: such should not be imposed by one man, or a College of Cardinals, or a bench of bishops, or a Grand Synod, or a king, or anyone; not even an obvious Saint should impose. You are here for two purposes: to love God and to love one another. You know this. Every day of your lives you remind yourselves of this; but how can establishing tests for orthodoxy be part of either of these purposes?

"The obsession with structure and doctrine is bad enough but you are indulging yourselves at a time when there are many tasks which are more urgent and, worse still, you know it.

"My second charge is that in following this direction, you are going against your own principles. Whether or not the principles that you have established are the best you could devise is not the point; the point is that you have decided that your Church should be Episcopal, that your Bishops should enjoy a high degree of self-determination, that no Church in the Communion can exercise authority over another Church in the Communion. So, what are you doing? You are seeking to establish a hydra Papacy. You are raising a body of special bishops or 'Primates' above the Communion to pass judgment. Remember, these bishops are only special because of the way in which secular states arrange themselves; no bishop is above another. Your claim when the Church renounced the Papacy is that you would never go back to a system of ecclesiastical dictatorship and that is precisely what you are doing now.

"My third charge against you is that you have clericalised the Church. You might argue that in an imperfect world the sheep require shepherds; and I accept that that is a reasonable case. You might then argue that where there are so many shepherds there needs to be a structure of governance; I think this less good a case but I accept it has some credibility. But the rest of your proceedings are inexplicable. If Jesus My Brother had wanted a priestly succession He could have arranged it. He could have taken all the Apostles from the Tribe of Levi. What has become of Peter's 'Royal Priesthood'? You do not emerge from the people; you are not put forward by the flock, you are not elected. You are a class apart, a self-perpetuating oligarchy that imposes itself on the people. You presume to know who has a calling and who does not and you assign this decision not to yourselves but to My Sister the Spirit. You thought for centuries that half of the people, women, could not have a calling. I say to you, that you must re-dedicate yourselves to trusting the people of God; what you must do is to show strong evidence why someone does not have a calling. Instead of setting your Priesthood apart, you should combine Confirmation and Ordination so that all may be publicly confirmed in their various Ministries which they have voluntarily undertaken and for which they have received training; but who are you to say that such-and-such cannot be trained to Preside at My Brother's table? Do you think that you have bottled My Sister the Spirit so that you can dispense Her when you have a mind? Do you believe that My Sister the Spirit is a weapon which you can brandish, using it to beat fellow Christians over the head?

"My fourth charge against you is that you are cold. There are many people here who lead good, honest and holy lives but you lack passion. You cower in your fortress churches and wait for people to come in. You say that it is your physical presence in every community that makes you what you are. What does it make you? How many of you can honestly say that your churches are havens for the poor and down-trodden? How many of you can honestly say that you trudge the dirty streets, carrying the message of Jesus? Is this massive superstructure of the Grand Synod, Diocesan Synods, Deanery Synods, Primates' Council, Bishops Councils and parochial Church Councils the way to bring good news to the poor?

"I started house groups. There were only four rules: that everyone in the group was equal; that they should consist of long-time believers and either new believers or non-believers; that they should be made up of people from different social classes (which frequently live apart but which live within walking distance of each other); and that they should choose their own group leaders and those who should preside at the Eucharist. Many of you opposed me but you never gave me any good reasons why, except on the last point where you said that only ordained Priests, on behalf of Bishops, could preside at the Eucharist. In other words, you did not address my first three rules and simply gave me an empty procedural argument against my fourth rule.

"My fifth charge is that you want to turn this Church into a private club. Instead of opening the doors to all, based on the will of Jesus My Brother, you are forever thinking about entry tests. You presume to know what love is but, much worse, you presume to know what is in the hearts of people, which only God knows. You presume that you are right; you presume that the Word is explicable and not a mystery; you presume that you have the power to exclude."

"And that leads me to my sixth charge against you that, whether you know it or not, you have built the Church of Christ on power not love. You are accustomed to wielding power and some of you have become so used to it that, without thinking, you use it to hurt people. What else but power drives you to make rules, to exclude and to bully, to write documents that few people can understand, to get yourselves tangled in obscurities?"

"All these lead to my final charge, that you have put judgment over love. You know what I am going to say but I am still going to say it. All the above six charges concentrate in this one, 'Presenting' issue of whether people who are gay (a foolish word, incidentally) are fit persons to be leaders in the Church. Setting aside the point that there are more important issues, setting aside the problems of understanding Scripture, setting aside your presumption that God Our Parent made a mistake with gay people during the creative process, the central point is that even if you were right on these three introductory points—which you are not—you would still be elevating judgment over love. Are you saying that you can define precisely to what degree a person must or must not be a sinner in order to be ordained? Are you saying you can rank sin? Are you saying that somebody who says he is called to Preside at the table of Jesus My Brother must be forbidden, no matter how much he loves My Brother, because you think that the way in which he was created bars him? That is precisely the same mistake you made with poor people, black people and now women; and you persist with this mistake in the case of gays. How many more times do you think that rational, educated people like you should make the same mistake before you learn from your wretched history?

"It is somewhat harsh of me to generalise. There are some people here who oppose the structuralist power play, there are some of you who prayed and argued for women to become priests; there are some of you who are committed to the Priesthood, ordained or otherwise, of all God's people; but even you—*even you*—have made one terrible error because you are wedded to the ways of statecraft. If you believe that love is more important than judgment; if you believe that it is for God to call and for all of us to respond; if you believe that Christianity is a religion of mystery; then there are no compromises to be made with those who believe that the exercise of power is more important than love; who believe that they have a veto on who is called; who believe that they know precisely what God means and wants. You must elevate your conscience above structure, you must elevate honesty of speech above formulae to keep others on board, you must elevate the needs of those who are being oppressed above the desires of those who wish to exercise power.

"I look at Christ's sad Church: the Torans are snarling, the Petrans are sulking, the Medians are withdrawing and the fixers are fixing. Is this all that is left of Pentecost?

"I want to end by proclaiming the new mission, the Third Testament for the Third Millennium. I was sent as God's Sacred Vessel to contain within me, within my life and within my death, all the wrong choices which Christians have made. I proclaim that the Sacrifice of Jesus My Brother was full but not final, that the same sacrifice can be undertaken at different times and in different places. I am certain that I will soon have to undergo that same sacrifice in a different time and place but it will be the same; it will be my Calvary, somewhere in this land. But I want you to know that this is the beginning of a new age, of a new opening of the channel between humanity and God's endless, perfect, universal self-communication with all those who have been created to worship fully and love freely. In this new age there will be a role for physical churches and for leaders in the Church but the old ways must go. You are the inheritors of a conforming Church, I am the proclaimer of an affirming Church. You will have to dispense with your Synods and your purple clothes; you will have to dispense with the pomp and the procedure. You will keep the richness of worship but remember that it is worship and not a theatre for your own pleasure. You will have to learn how to walk in suffering with the people, to walk with them and by their Grace to lead them.

"God is love. Jesus My Brother came to bring a Gospel of love. In two thousand years you have forgotten. I am the new manifestation of the Godhead, come to remind you as Jesus reminded you, come to make a new Covenant, as Jesus made a new Covenant. You will put me to death but I will rise again."

A questioner asked: "If we follow your advice there will be chaos. There is already instability because of disagreements and you will split the Church." "Jesus My Brother came preaching revolution and the Priests of Jerusalem asked the same question. They were waiting for the Messiah but they had no mechanism for knowing when the Messiah had arrived. Jesus brought the good news of the Kingdom and asked the people to believe. I am bringing the same news and asking you to believe. You know that every time the good news is proclaimed, as it was with Abraham and Moses and Jesus, that everyone is filled with My Sister the Spirit, and love is preached, and then love is seen to fail and people build institutions and make laws which they think will shore up the institution; and then the laws become the institution. So with Moses, so with Jesus, so with me; we have come in different generations to begin anew, to bring the message afresh. No doubt in thousands of years to come God Our Parent will have to send Another; that is why this doctrine of the Trinity you have proclaimed is incomplete; it is a doctrine of closure whereas God is the essence of openness of possibility. You cannot close down the 'options' of God."

"When you say you are like Jesus, even saying that you will die like Him, you are just a cheap copy, a self-proclaimed crank." "I know you feel more comfortable with the Bible than with the wind of My Sister the Spirit blowing; but you have built yourself a religion that has no risk. Love is a risk; the Bible, once nailed down into a rationalist textbook, is no longer a risk. You want certainty, I proclaim afresh the mystery of the love of God."

"Very interesting," said the Chairman, "and I am sure we would like to have asked many more questions but time presses. May I thank Perpetua for her provocative presentation. I am sure it will make us all think. The next business is the consideration of the Covenant of Uniformity for the Anglican Communion."

Archbishop Hawthorne, Chris Smoother, the Church's media chief, Archdeacon Varnish, representing the clergy, and Lady Broadparks, representing the Laity, met late in the evening to discuss the day's proceedings, with a theological student called Damian to take notes. They went through all the procedural items and arranged the line for *Church & State* and then spent some time on the controversial issues of the Covenant and the still vexed issue of gay bishops. Then they finally came to Perpetua.

"I suppose," said Archbishop Hawthorne, "there is something in what she says. After all, the idea that God can perform the same act at different times in different places is coherent." "You have a bad enough problem as it is," said Smoother, "as speakers repeatedly pointed out. You have almost lost the American Church and it is far more important to sort out that problem than to enter into idle theological speculation which might split us further." "On the whole," said Varnish, "I would favour a long view of the situation. There are a wide variety of approaches which we might bring together in the Faith and Uniformity Commission to provide some kind of framework in which the idea of the Trinity could be refreshed." "Well, it wouldn't worry the media," said Smoother, with a self-satisfied look. "On the whole," said Lady Broadparks, "the Laity are not very interested in theology, they just want to worship in their own quiet way as their parents worshipped. They have not liked all the change of the last thirty years and they need a period of calm. They are not very worried about the Covenant and the idea of Communion; they are suspicious of hierarchy but they have enough deference left to trust the Archbishop if he will only assert himself. They would not like to think that he is meddling with the Trinity. They are, incidentally, bored by the gay issue and even the more conservative, of which I admit I am one, are getting used to women priests. They are, in any case, more willing and much cheaper, and in an increasingly impoverished

Church, that is something."

"My conscience is very much stirred by this woman," said Hawthorne, "because she clearly has something. She is not just some fraud. There is a depth and radicalism in what she says which must be addressed. We are to proclaim the Faith afresh in each generation; and I liked what she said about being an affirming and not a conforming Church." "You would," said Smoother, almost ungraciously, "because conformity is becoming increasingly difficult to arrange and there is a good deal of untidy affirming about." "And," said Hawthorne, "there has been so little love lately, it depresses me. I knew when I became Archbishop that it would be a difficult job and I would personally have preferred to stay with my books; but God called me to face up to my responsibility. I never dreamed how unpleasant senior Church figures would be to each other. I almost wept when some bishops refused to share Communion with their brothers and sisters." "It was a PR disaster, admittedly," said Smoother, "but the moral is that we must limit the damage and that means that you must go to America." "I suppose so; but it is against my better judgment nonetheless."

Slowly and sadly, Hawthorne left the room. "Now," said Smoother, "we need to get ourselves sorted out pretty quickly. This woman has to be marginalised. There won't be a church left worth the name if we don't get her sorted out. Do you all agree?" The other two nodded; they had completely forgotten that Damian was in the room. "Here is my idea. The *Cutting Edge Channel* is planning a reality TV programme on drug abuse and violence. It has chosen Grunge Park. I know this because my daughter Poppy is in line to make her reputation with it. What we need to do is to arrange for Perpetua to be featured in that programme, taking drugs. She has already been discredited because her followers are a bunch of ne'er-do-wells including at least one financial crook and a gay; and her right-hand man, Dexter, is an ex gang leader. Well, his successor can easily be persuaded to arrange a scenario for Poppy and there are a couple of Perpetua's people who can be turned because I gather they are disappointed that they are not already part of a royal entourage with the kind of lifestyle enjoyed by footballers' fancy women." "That sounds a bit risky," said Varnish. "On the contrary, Archdeacon, your son Rory and his mates are the kind of young men who could bring this off without any trouble; and keep their mouths shut." "I don't like the sound of that." "I don't like the sound of these fine young men being exposed for their current, er, activities. I don't suppose you would like the headline: 'Archdeacon's Son Is Porn King'. No. I didn't think you would. Your boy has not been altogether discreet; but I think Poppy and he can reach a satisfactory agreement on the way forward." "What about the police?" asked Lady Broadparks. "You are on the London Police Board and can ensure that *Cutting Edge* has a 'no-go' area so that the programme is properly authentic. We don't want Mr. Plod wading in with his big boots at the wrong moment, just before Perpetua makes a spectacle of herself. We want to see that everything goes smoothly. They would take your word for it, I think." "Well, I suppose so, as long as I have your word that it will be neat and tidy."

"You have my word on it. I don't like untidiness, which is why there are other measures we need to take: first, I will make sure that matters in America turn very ugly indeed during the next few days. The *Cutting Edge* programme is scheduled for Good Friday and I know old Hawthorne likes to be in Canterbury on that day but needs must. He will have to celebrate in some Godforsaken wooden church in the Mid-West. Secondly, I will make sure that the agreement on policing is between the bigwigs at *Cutting Edge* and the Chief of Police which will clear you, Lady Broadparks. All you have to do as a Member of the Board is to make the suggestion and say that the Board, if called upon, will be supportive. I doubt you will be called upon as the Chief of Police can't resist a bit of a gimmick: 'Chief Exposes Crime Wave' might be a nice sort of headline. Next, I'll up the pressure on the newspapers, particularly the TT, to see that Perpetua takes her eye off the ball, if it's ever on it. We could tie up a deal between *Cutting Edge* and the TT if that would make things sweeter. Last but not least, Varnish, you need to drop the hint to your boy that there's something in it for him or, rather, a couple of things: first, he can look forward to a really good night; secondly, this will buy him some time over the porn empire. I happen to know that the police have been showing some interest there and my friends at the TT would certainly like the story; but this little escapade will make up for a lot of his recent bad behaviour." "But," said the Archdeacon, shaking, "going on television is hardly a way of lowering your profile." "Don't worry, it will be dark. It's not really him we're interested in, it's Perpetua." "Isn't this all somewhat disproportionate?" he asked. "I don't think so. It is my job to protect the Church from harm and if that means that we have to use rather unpleasant means, so be it. I'll answer for it at the Last Judgment. All you need to do is have a quiet word and then lose yourself back in your church heritage campaign. Oh, Damian, are you still here? Hand over those notes. We don't want you causing any security breaches."

As he left, Damian wondered what he should do but decided that it was too big and complicated a game for him. His best course was to warn Perpetua, so he went into Smoother's empty office, under the pretext of editing his notes of a previous meeting, and looked up Perpetua's mobile number.

They met in a coffee bar near the river. "I know what you are going to tell me," she said, disconcertingly. "I don't know the details but I have a rough idea that Mr. Smoother is after my blood." "No, not at all, he just wants to expose you as a drug taker." "These things have a habit of getting out of hand," she said, "and I have no doubt that this will. If you get involved with drugs that means being in the company of some very unpleasant people." "So all you need to do is go away." "I cannot do that. I know that God is calling me to do what I have to do. What I need you to know is that you have done everything you can. The rest must take its course. I am in the hands of God." "That sounds fatalistic to me." "Look… oh, I am sorry, in my concern for what you have to say I forgot to ask your name." "Damian. I am a theology student acting as an intern at Church Corporate HQ." "Even better. Look Damian, you are a theology student so you know what it says in the New Testament about Jesus having to fulfill the Scriptures. Well, we all know that that was a little fanciful hindsight; but, nonetheless, the life of Jesus My Brother was grounded in Scripture and what He had to say grew out of its soil. I am in much the same situation. I know that I am being called upon, as God's Sacred Vessel, to absorb all the wrong choices of humanity and that means dying a rather unpleasant death so that I can, in my words of earlier, perform the act which Jesus My Brother performed on the Cross but at a different time and place. All I ask you to do is to wait upon the Resurrection. Oh, and by the way; thank you for being so brave. Be careful. Do no more and you will be all right until my time comes. Just avoid any opportunity to work for Mr. Smoother."

Lady Broadparks was not given to self doubt. She did not even doubt that she was a true representative of the Christian laity. It was not that she thought that Peers had an obligation to care for lesser folk; she simply thought that exercising influence, as she would have put it, was her role in life just as somebody else might be a banker or a farmer, and so it was with a sense of purpose but no trepidation that she walked the two blocks to Police Headquarters and ascended in the lift to the top floor. She knew the Chief would be there because he never left for his mid-town club bedroom until after midnight. "I know it's late and it's only a small matter," she said, helping herself to a small brandy and soda, "but I thought it best to come right to the top. We—the Church—need a bit of help in waking up the public to the dangers of drugs, particularly when they are used by celebrities." "Yes, pop musicians keep being caught." "Yes they do; but would not the impact be much greater if a person who claimed to be a religious prophet was implicated? Then people would know how widespread the danger really is." "Intriguing." "We have just such a person in view. You know Perpetua of course?" "Yes, she's cost me a fortune in overtime." "Well, we believe that she is implicated in drugs and we want to make a reality TV programme which catches her in the act." "And you want me to arrange to keep out of the way, I suppose?" "How did you guess?" "Well I did not suppose you had come here to ask me to get involved. We would not be permitted to witness a crime and ignore it; but we could make other arrangements for the greater good." "Precisely." "Get your friend Smoother to see my media people. I will have a word but I will not, as I am sure you will understand, write a formal note." "Thank you. You look tired." "I am. There are so many things to do that I hardly have the time to deal with crime. It seems to me that most really important people, and that includes journalists, don't care what I do as long as I follow the rules; or, put the other way round, they are only interested in claiming my scalp for breaking some point of process. What I actually do is irrelevant." "I know what you mean; but you can't trust anyone these days." He smiled ironically as she left.

Archdeacon Varnish was deeply troubled. He had known for some time about Rory's unsavory life but he had not wanted to confront him in case this completely destroyed their fragile relationship which could not stand a face-to-face encounter. He phoned Rory's mobile: "Rory, it's your dad." "What? At this time of night." "I think you're in danger." "So, what's new?" "No, I think people are on your trail over your, er, business." "Probably." "But you can get some time, time to change your ways, if you do a little business in another direction." "What?" "Could you talk to Poppy Smoother?" "With pleasure! She would make a great product! Sorry, dad. Yes, if you want." "Just do it quietly, she'll explain what to do." "Thanks for the tip. I could do with a bit of space and she's pleasing on the eye." "Good night."

Varnish was under no illusions; but it was the better of two evils. In life, religion, God, it frequently was.

VIII.

And she showed her Godhead to the whole world, to believers and unbelievers alike. She went into the palaces of the powerful and preached a Gospel of peace, choice and responsibility. She put down a marker that nobody who saw her would ever forget.

She said to her followers: "I will die very soon. I can see it coming. It is unstoppable. It is the inevitable result when imperfection and perfection collide; imperfection cannot survive with perfection and it is in its nature to choose to assault perfection whereas perfection, contained in itself, does not react to imperfection. I know you will be sad but I want you to know—I have told you this before but it has not really become part of your understanding of me— that after I have died I will still be with you. It will not be like the Resurrection of Jesus My Brother but you will know that I am with you. You will see me on television and some of you will see me in person. Meanwhile, I want us to do something together that will help you to remember why I came and who I am and also why you were chosen and who you are. Today we are going out into the world to show the glory and wonder of God to all people.

"Let us start with small things," she said, coming towards a dilapidated block of flats. Its rusting iron doors could only be released by a combination lock or a trigger from inside but she just took a handle and the doors opened. Immediately people began to struggle down the stairs and a moment later a lady in a wheelchair shot out of the lift, propelled by a friend. As if it was an insect colony where everyone knows what they have to do without being told, the whole block of flats emptied itself into the scruffy courtyard. "What brought you here?" she asked, smiling. "Telly. There was a special message on the telly—all channels—that you were down here and wanted to talk to us. Well, we know who you are because even though they've been trying to hide your heavenly powers we know about them. It doesn't matter what they do and how much we seem to be locked away in those horrible flats, we know what's going on." "I am sure you do." "Anyway, it came on telly, so what do you want?" "What do you want?" "Well, we don't like to complain, like, but these flats are pretty horrible and we can't get them repaired and we can't afford to do it ourselves and it's very depressing." "Would this be a matter of using what you call my powers to improve your material conditions?" "Well, we could ask you to use your divine powers to give us wisdom and understanding and to turn us all into saints but Jesus simply had compassion on the poor and needy. In those days it was illness that frightened them most, today it's loneliness and fear and the depression. I don't suppose people in the time of Jesus faced the prospect of living in a couple of tiny rooms almost alone for thirty-odd years." "I take your point; but there is more to it than that. Tell me, how did you all know how to sort things out so that the whole building emptied within minutes, wheelchair users and all?" "It just seemed to work." "Well, you cannot rely on that kind of luck again if, for example, there is a fire. But you are not really alone; you have each other but you have allowed doors and floors to divide you." "But we have no central space." "Have you ever asked for one?" "No." "If all of you ask, we will get somewhere. Now, I think you can all go back in now as long as you promise to live and work together instead of putting up with your loneliness and grumbling about it. Every time you look at the way your flats look new, remember what I have said. The outside of the flats still looked depressing but as her followers came out they reported that things looked much better inside.

"I know it's the glory of God," said Dexter, "but what was all that about, really?" "It was about doing something small and private to give people hope." "And what was that about television?" "I have a special way with technology, as you know. You will see more later."

They went to a school where the older children were working on computers. She said: "What do you see?" and a girl said: "I see a picture of you and underneath it says 'love is creating space for others'." "Yes. Have you seen anything like that before?" "I don't think so." "How many hours per day do you spend watching television or accessing your computer?" "Loads." "Well, it is a matter of looking carefully and not being distracted. I provide a simple message like this and some of you take a quick look but you do not have the patience to think of the words and what they mean and you go to the next thing. Some of you look at the words and think for a moment what they might mean but as soon as another image pops up you forget what you have seen. And some of you are really interested in the message and try to follow what it means but you become distracted by all kinds of pleasures and by money and jealousy and you forget the message. But a few of you, to use the modern phrase 'stay on message' and you are the ones that will make the difference. Part of the idea that love is making space is that you have to make space for yourselves; and when you induce this mass of information to swamp you, this is your deliberate act of losing yourself, of cutting yourself off from the space that love provides; you are escaping into a world of narrow self-indulgence. There is no such thing as 'information overload' any more than there is such a thing as externally induced obesity. You make all kinds of choices about clothes, shoes, hair, diet, drugs, alcohol, relationships, money, power, commentary and inclusion and what you live in is what you bring down upon yourselves." "But society is like that." "Society is like you." "But our parents are to blame." "Admittedly, parents have to take a great deal of responsibility for the way in which children behave; their complaints that children behave badly are pretty hollow when they are responsible for the upbringing of children. Yet you would not be here if you did not enjoy a degree of intelligence and you are responsible for your own choices. Anybody who is sitting here, fully self-conscious, can choose to remember my words or to forget them. However, I will make your lives easier. You can start again." At this point a message came over the public address system that all computers were to be turned off. Everybody looked irritated but complied. A minute later another message said they could be turned on. The students looked puzzled as they went back to their screens. "I know," said Perpetua, smiling. "Where have all those trivia sites gone? Where's all the gambling and pornography? I have no doubt you will be able to get them all back but every time you choose a trivial or harmful information source from now on you will have to choose it remembering me."

"Did you do that to the whole network?" asked a boy. "No, I only helped you to make different choices. You cannot spread love through a remote access system. If I cleaned up the computers of people I had not talked with they would simply be angry without understanding my purpose. A miracle is not a change in the environment it is a change in the person." "You mean when other people turned their computers back on they were the same?" "Yes. You are very special because you have been given a new chance to make the right choices."

She went to the office of the School Head. "I have just seen a plaque outside your office with the school values on it and I thought it was very good, dealing with respect and tolerance and helping each other and being constructive; but it seemed to me that there were two words that were missing. Love and God." "Ah well, that is because we are a state school and not a religious school." "Does that exempt you from the human propensity to love?" "Well, it is a word that has to be handled very carefully." "I am sure, but that does not mean abandoning it because a few people—not the children—might just think that the only kind of love is a physical relationship." "No; but we find respect a very good word for what we are looking for." "Surely that means allowing people to operate in their own space, their own milieu; love, on the other hand, is about creating space so that other people will have more room." "I see what you mean but I don't think the parents would be prepared to accept love as one of our school values." "What about the absence of God?" "Well, God is very controversial, you know. There are all kinds of religions in this school." "I daresay but I would be surprised if the 'all kinds of religions' did not find themselves closer together on this point than the people who say they have no religion; even the people who doubt the existence of God and those who attack God have more in common than those who simply ignore the reality. How do you know that your parents and children do not want the school to include love and God in its values?" "Because the Government would not allow it." "Now that may be true but it is a quite different issue. At the moment believers are being intimidated out of public belief by a few very aggressive atheists but mostly by officials who do not understand religion. Let me ask the question this way; how would it be if your educational values excluded discussing how children feel when they have heard a great symphony?" "We would never want to do that." "And yet everyone reacts differently to a symphony but there is some core reality about its greatness. God is like that only immeasurably bigger." "We have religious education." "But that is not a value, it simply communicates certain aspects of philosophy and history." "I still think that some parents would object." "As many as those who would object if you were open and asked them if they would like the school to be transparently secular?" "I don't know." "I did not think you did." As Perpetua was walking out of the front door, the Head Teacher noticed that the plaque of the school values had been changed.

She went into the offices of the *Toxic Times*, gliding through the security until she reached the Editor's office. "Mr. Sneer," she said "You know me." "I do, indeed, how did you get in here?" "God knows," she said, without apparent irony. "Well, what do you want?" "I simply want to show you something, just for you to remember when I am no longer with you, as I soon will not be." "Going away then?" "In a manner of speaking." "I've heard rumours that there's a plot to marginalise you." "Are you sure you have heard this rumour and not started it?" she asked, smiling. "I have my contact." "That works two ways, Mr. Sneer, you can either hear from contacts—which is what a journalist is supposed to do—or you can prime contacts to do something—which is what politicians are supposed to do—but I never can tell whether you are here to report the news or make it. Anyway, as I said, I came to show you something." "Just a minute; I need somebody to record what it is you are showing me." "It won't do any good." Nonetheless, Sneer picked up a phone and asked for a staff reporter and a photographer. While they waited he asked: "Are you not interested in this plot?" "I am always interested in what might happen, as we all are, but I do not think that there is anything I can do to stop the world doing what it will do. I just have to go on bearing witness to Jesus My Brother and bringing people new hope which is, as I know, directly counter to what you want to bring; you exist by bringing people fear, by making them discontent."

The journalist and photographer came in. She said: "I know you think I am of no account but it is not for that reason, which may be quite correct, that I am going to do what I do, but because it is not my account that matters. I am acting on behalf of God Our Parent to show you the power which I carry on behalf of the Godhead." Every communications device in the building shut itself off. "Do not worry; you will lose no data. I just want to show you that you work on sufferance; you exercise your free will as a gift of God; it is part of what you are to make wrong choices." People began running towards the door. "Do not worry," she said, "there is a temporary power problem that will affect all your systems, including your mobile phones. It will just give you a few minutes to think about what you are doing. Go back to your desks."

Suddenly she was on everybody's computer screen, somehow the photographer's pictures were being transmitted into the central system and out again. "I want you to think about one question. Are you happy earning a living deliberately making people unhappy? It is your individual and collective choice. I do not expect this newspaper to change immediately but I want you to remember this question when you look at your children who are becoming prisoners, who are only taught by women at primary school, who have learned to mistrust friends and neighbours, who sexualise everything physical. Our children are the most unhappy in the rich countries. Are you responsible for that in some way? You use these sad situations to beat the Government: would you not be better off beating yourselves? But, as I said, the central question is:are you happy making a living by making other people unhappy?"

Then she was gone. They were still looking at their screens as the lift doors closed behind her. "I'll get my own back," shouted Sneer. "She won't get away with this." After a few moments he called Smoother, then his daughter Poppy, then Rory Varnish. He was putting the pieces of a story together.

She went through Parliament's security with the same ease and, without any clear explanation, most of its Members of both Houses drifted into Freedom Hall. "You may wonder what you are doing here," she said, "but after I have gone I want you to think back to this day. You all know who I am, more or less; well, let me be explicit. I am Perpetua, the Sacred Vessel of God Our Parent, sent to earth to absorb all the wrong choices, the choices not to love, that humanity has made. I am here to share, at a different time and place, the suffering of Jesus My Brother. This may all sound mysterious but you all know that my statements are public, that I have followers. I want you to know that I will very soon die as the result of human imperfection but will return after my death. You are entitled to be sceptical; you see somebody like this every day. I want you, therefore, to think very hard about one person in your constituency, if you are an MP and one of your circle, if you are a Peer; or you might want to think of an organisation like a hospice. It is like making a wish but instead of that it is saying a prayer so that I can display God's power for you all to see and for you all to remember. Just think about what you want that is good, that is unselfish, that will give you no political or social advantage. Now stay silent." Grand Tom struck noon.

At that second, all over the land, there were strange happenings: a hospice in danger of closing received an anonymous donation which could not be traced; a youth team from a deprived area received a parcel of kit; a factory stopped emitting pollution; a little girl who had been lost for three days was found safe; an agreement over hospital staffing was reached; a Minister apologised and was not attacked as weak or for performing a U-turn; an ungiving woman smiled and signed an order for play equipment. All over the country, hundreds of tiny acts, each worthy of a local paragraph, none amounting to a piece of a national jig-saw, changed the lives of people in the way that their representatives had wished. Many remarked how curious it was that the acts took place dead on the stroke of noon, as the town hall clock struck, as the pips introduced the radio news, as jingles announced new DJs.

As she stood before them, listening to the chimes of Grand Tom, the huge chamber was quiet. When the chimes had finished, she said: "In your own way, say a little prayer for me, for what is going to happen to me; and say a prayer for yourselves and for the people you represent." As she was walking out, phones began to bring messages of good news from all over the land.

"Only one more job to do now," she said, "before we can go away and prepare for tomorrow." She went into London Minster and took control of the sound system. The place was seething with tourists from all over the world, taking pictures, talking about painting in Palermo, sick aunts in Sierra Leone, psychiatrists in Seattle, neighbours in Nagasaki, dancers in Dubrovnik, boy-friends in Berlin, architects in Adelaide, Buddhas in Burma, mosques in Mosul, temples in Tirupati, talking about anything and everything but the place they were visiting. "God bless you," she said. "Do not worry; all is well. Your cameras will begin to work again when I have finished saying a prayer. You need to be quiet. The place you are in is a church, dedicated to the worship of God Our Parent. Some people find such places terribly frightening but to others they bring great comfort as safe places to explore the self and to bring the self to God. I want us, for just a moment, to bring ourselves to God. Do not worry if you do not think you can do this, if you call yourself an atheist or an agnostic or if you are not a Christian but a believer in God through another religion."

The cameras had stopped, the turnstiles had stopped, the cash registers had stopped. Everything was quiet as she talked to all the people and each seemed to know what she was saying. "To most of you this will just be a strange moment in your visit to London Minster but I want you to remember it when you see me again after I have died.

"Now let us say a prayer to God Our Parent."

"That was enigmatic," said Varnish as he came over to her. "I am the senior clergyman on duty today and was about to lead the hourly prayers when you, er,…" "…Intervened?" "Well, spared me the trouble. What is this strange idea of seeing you again after you have died? Taken at face value it could mean that you are going to die and come back here; or we will see you when we arrive in heaven? I must say the latter explanation is much more credible. What makes you think you are going to die very soon, anyway?" "I do not think I said 'very soon' Archdeacon; but perhaps you know something I do not know." He hurried away.

The rest of the day was spent preparing for the Palm Sunday parade. Late in the evening, as her followers made their final checks, she prayed alone but found it difficult. First, she found it very hard not to concentrate on her own forthcoming death. She did not know how she would die but she thought it almost certain she would die on Good Friday, on the day Jesus Her Brother had died. She did not know how, but she knew it would be humiliating and painful. She did not hope for glory, she feared for misery. "I am not very good at this," she said. "I have had a comfortable life, always in Your care, Lord. I have hardly felt a pin prick and yet I will soon be cruelly treated. I know there is no alternative and that you will give me the resources I need to bear the pain but I am still frightened. Should I show my fear? Yes, I must show my fear of suffering but not allow this to be confused with fear of being abandoned by you."

Secondly, she was sad for the world she was leaving. She wanted to do so much more good, to smile at so many more people, to bring happiness, to bring relief; and although she had a strong idea—although she did not know how—that she would return after her death to encourage her followers, she did not want to die.

Fragments of her life and fragments of what might be her death, the real record of cinema and what she had gleaned from cinema, knit themselves into a sequence which made it hard for her to pray. "Perhaps watching the pictures is praying," she thought, "seeing myself as I am and trying to cut out the fantasy."

The next day, Palm Sunday, was the day on which she showed herself in all her divine glory to the whole of the world. She rode into London in an open-topped bus and commanded vast crowds in the Royal Park. When she spoke, everyone listened. She spoke of hope for the world, of peace and forgiveness. She said that there would only be an influx of new life into humanity if she could absorb all its wrong choices by suffering and dying; it was inevitable; nothing could be done about it. But she would never abandon them. They all shouted:

"Blessed be Our Sister and God."

She tried to calm them but they shouted ever more loudly. One group wanted to carry her away to install her in London Minster as the new Bishop. "No," she said, earnestly, "you know how much I am in favour of small house groups rather than big churches; I do not want to be trapped in a big church but, in any case, I think that bishops should emerge from the people by election or some other means." Another group wanted her to lead a political movement, a third wanted to make her the patron of a major charity. "I am so sorry," she said, "but you are missing the point. All these things are important but I came here to spend all my time in active, open, outward witness of Jesus My Brother and, besides, I do not think I am going to be here much longer." She said to Trina, who was making sure she was in the right place at the right time: "Why do they never listen to what I say? Why do they always think I am saying something I am not saying?" "They are so used to hearing what they want to hear, no matter what people say; it is like proof-reading your own material; you see what you want to see instead of what has been written."

She knew that it was going to be a very long day and so, to escape from the crowds for a few minutes, they took a cabin on the Wheel of Visions where they could be quietly together, looking over the vast expanse of London. "It is so beautiful," she said. "But it is so full of wickedness and sadness," said Andy. "All that money down there; and most of it in the hands of a few people." "Yes. Money, if you like, is a symbol of what goes wrong. However we start, whatever arrangements we make, the choices people make mean that it tends to gather in a few hands, leaving some reasonably well off but leaving many poor or very poor. It is not helpful to focus on the money itself—although I can see why people do—but on the choices that lead to where we are." "But sometimes people do not have any choice," said Kylie "They are just so down-trodden." "People always have choice." "What about the people who are persecuted and marginalised, those who live in prosperous countries but who know nothing but squalor?" "One of the problems of the society in which we live is that it confuses the scientific laboratory with the way we take moral decisions when we know from our personal experience that two people faced with the same situation will react differently. That is because no two people are the same and so nothing is inevitable; the situation they face may be the same yet as people they may be only subtly different but the difference will count. For some reason, a father may beat one twin on one occasion but not the other; not because he did not think that both should be beaten equally but perhaps the telephone rang. Whatever the cause, no two people are identical in their life histories and so they can be expected to react differently to a situation. So when commentators say that a country's foreign policy causes terrorism, or deprivation causes drug addiction, or excess wealth causes decadence, it is not the same thing as describing causality in physics or chemistry, but that is how it is presented. Those kinds of statements about causality begin to erode the idea of choice and, much worse, they let people off the hook who should be choosing; these causal statements tell people that certain behaviour is inevitable; and so, if people in a minority that believes it is being persecuted, are told that such treatment causes retaliation, they will feel justified in retaliating."

They were at the top of the Wheel's circle, looking North across the city. "Look at this city, full of choices, full of right and wrong, love and the failure to love. Do not accept that anything is inevitable." Then her face grew sad. "So lovely. Before the wheel turns down, let us look at my birth place to the South. She looked out on Grunge Park and said: "The place of my birth and I think very likely the place of my death not long from now. It never was a pretty place but I always found it to be lovely." "But there's so much wrong there," said Dexter. "Yes, but in spite of all the wrong, all the degradation, so many people, against the odds, have made choices in favour of generosity and love. When I look down there I can think of so many occasions when people were brave. Look at you, Dexter: you have bad cowardice attacks when things become difficult and there will be times when you will run away from a situation, but your hard upbringing has not made you morally cold, incapable of loving." "I won't run away from difficulties anymore," said Dexter. "I am sorry; but you will. However, let us not dwell on this, it is no time for an argument where I assert one thing and you another; events will show which of us was right. In the next few days I will be under severe pressure. Already two of our number have deserted us and I do not think they are up to any good." "Jo and Heather," said Dexter, "have been behaving rather strangely lately. I'll take care of them." "That would be easy and wrong in the way you mean it. I only wish you would take care of them by loving them whatever they do. I fear they have slipped back into their old ways." "Yes," said Kylie, "they were saying how they expected to stand on platforms next to you and be on television and have articles in magazines about them so that they would be famous. They said you promised that and then came up with nothing. They say you have stolen the show." "In one way, I suppose they are right; but I never did promise anything that was easy; and I have not really stolen the show because it is God's show and I must play the part in it which was ordained for me.

"This week you know that Wayne will be attacked for being gay and Andy will be accused of fraud and our whole mission will be attacked for undermining the Church. Do not be misled by tomorrow's headlines about the parade and the massive healing of the sick and the street party; forces are in play to destroy us. They will not succeed but we will all be under a great deal of stress. Do not worry if things go wrong; do not worry if you do not think you have behaved as well as you should. God Our Parent understands; and My Sister the Spirit will be with you."

As the cabin went slowly towards the ground she asked Jim to play a soft tune on his flute. They said a simple prayer. The flute died away. "Now for the great party," she said.

As they walked across the plaza before crossing the river, back into the crowds, Trina said: "I am not quite clear what you were saying. You said that nothing is inevitable but you also say that your early death is inevitable." "Yes, but my death is beyond my choice. Most people, no matter how subject they are to massive external sources, still are left with some kind of choice, even if the choice is to accept or reject, to respect or despise. Trina, my death, willed by God Our Parent, is inevitable because of who I am and what humanity is.

"The death of God made man in Jesus My Brother and God made Woman in me, is a mystery."

IX.

And she gave herself for the whole world, absorbing all the wrong choices, the choices not to love God and neighbour, which had ever been made, sharing the self-same sacrifice made by Jesus Her Brother at His Crucifixion, the self same-sacrifice but at a different time and place.

After a turbulent week which included a virulent attack by the media on Wayne, and an intensive series of public commitments—and sometimes confrontations—she prepared what she almost certainly knew would be her farewell meal with her followers. When the time came, all of them arrived, included Jo and Beth who had been away for some time, holding discussions with the gang leaders of Grunge Park. It was a borrowed house and so it had taken her some time to get used to everything but by the time they arrived there was something of herself in the lounge and dining room.

"Farewell parties are always difficult," she said. "There is the pleasure of the party and the sadness of the farewell both happening at the same time; and the closer we are to people the more the sadness takes over; but I would ask you at least to try to savour the moment, to think about now, because I want you to remember this evening long after I have gone away. Yes, I will come back to you, I will never leave you, but it will not be in the same way that I am here now." "Perhaps we should go," said Jo, looking at Heather. "No," she said, "you and Heather are welcome to stay as long as you like; I love you whatever you are planning to do. My only worry for you both is that you do not recognise what you have done, you do not see how easily something that you started can go in a wrong direction with unintended consequences." "What do you mean?" asked Heather. "I think you know what I mean. The kind of people you are dealing with are not to be trusted; and if you become involved in drugs again your judgment will not be trustworthy. But," she said to Dexter and Trina, turning away from the other two so that they would not hear what she said, "whether it is them or somebody else who resents what I am so much that they decide that I must die, the end result is inevitable; so do not think too harshly of them when I have gone. If they behave in the way that I expect, what they do will hurt them as much as it hurts me. If things go very wrong with me in the next few days—as I think they will—your mistake will not just be in abandoning me but also in abandoning each other." "What you are saying," said Dexter, "is that there's something inevitable about what's going on." "Yes, it is inevitable that something should happen to me because of who and what I am but the way it happens is not inevitable. I would not like Jo or Heather, or any of the rest of you, to think that you are human ciphers in a sacred drama with your free will confiscated. My death—if that is what is to be—will come about precisely because of the exercise of free will in an unloving way. The story of Jesus My Brother focuses so much on Judas, but remember how all the other followers behaved. The inevitability of suffering and death is not about divine will, it is about human self-will. However, let us put that into the background for now as we think about the blessed relationship between the human and the divine."

She had taken particular care over the table plan, putting Dexter to her right and Trina to her left. She put Wayne next to Dexter, not as a test but so that he would have the opportunity to provide comfort in a situation he still found difficult. Bob was next to Trina because he was still unhappy about losing his central role. Jo and Heather were near the door so that if they had to slip away it would not cause a fuss. Perpetua thought that they would not stay for the whole evening but she told them that she was particularly anxious that they stay for the Sacrament of the Mysterious Union. "You have learned," she said, "of the Sacraments of Eucharist and Reconciliation, but what they are both centred on is the mysterious union between the divine and the human. It is most obvious in the Sacrament of Communion when Jesus My Brother becomes present in the bread and wine; but people do not think of the union in the same way when they think about Reconciliation; they do not see that humanity can only be reconciled with God if there is a mysterious union confirmed through mending what is broken. Reconciliation mends, Communion nourishes; and they should not be separate but part of the same organic, seamless relationship which humanity, corporately and individually, is created to sustain with God.

"And so," she said, "my part in the reconciliation is to clean all your shoes; and your part is to think about why I am cleaning them and how you can imitate me in cleaning the shoes of others; how you cannot claim to love God but decide who is your neighbour."They were all uncomfortable as they sat in their socked feet as she knelt on a mat and cleaned their shoes but she said: "How can you serve with care and sensitivity if you do not know what it feels like to be served? It is supposed to feel beautiful but it does not. Those who serve are exercising all kinds of power and authority and those who are being served feel as if they are receiving a service which grows out of power and authority. It is only when you know what this feels like that you will learn to serve with love, to put your authority to one side."

"What can we do?" asked Bob. "You can offer those things which you want to be the elements of the Sacrament of the Mysterious Union." "Bread and wine?" "Possibly; but do not become fixed in one way of doing things. I have looked at the sacraments of the Church and I hope that I have given them new life and new meaning:

1. The sacrament of reception, of being received into the community

of God (which most people call church) and of beginning to receive God's self communication is fundamental; it is what was called Baptism but is much more about communication with God than simple membership in an earthly church. Like all Sacraments, it is a sign of God's presence with us, not a sign of our presence to God, which is why infants should take part in Sacraments as they do not primarily depend on the human affirmation.

2. The Sacrament of the Mysterious Union combines what was Communion (or Eucharist) and Reconciliation; it celebrates the mystery of the union of the human and divine but, again, it is God acting through the people that makes it effective, not the affirmation of the people no matter how important that is.

3. The Sacrament of Affirmation combines what was Confirmation, Holy Orders and marriage into a public and iterative statement of the commitment which humanity makes to perform its task of creatureliness in choosing to love God and neighbour in the corporate sphere and again, although personal commitment is fundamental to it, never forget that it is only effective through grace.

4. The Sacrament of Response takes disparate elements from creation, from our lives, and makes of them a whole which we offer in love to each other and the Creator, God Our Parent; it is the Sacrament of brokenness and healing, of God's healing, of self-healing through affirmation of our creative power, the affirmation that we are free to choose to love; you will remember how I celebrated it with broken glass at the beginning of my ministry.

"Here you have them: reception, union, affirmation and response, these are the Sacraments which give humanity strength to choose to love. If you are looking for elements for Union, Bob, you do not need to think of bread and wine which were the most highly prized elements in the time of Jesus; think about what you value, what would make the union real for you."

Bob collected different pieces of food from the people round the table and he said that, as this was a celebration, the wine should be champagne. "I wish," she said, half to herself, "he had chosen bits of the engine of the bus because that is what he really cares about; you do not have to physically eat the elements when they have been transformed; it might be better if you did not. Then you could hold onto things instead of having to go back to Church for another 'Eucharistic fix'."

She took a glass dish and placed all the pieces of food on it. She blessed them and said: "This food, this earthly richness, brought to God, is given back from God to those who gave it with the divine presence in it, in all the unity and diversity of God Our parent, Jesus My Brother, My Sister the Spirit and my own self, the Sacred Vessel of God; receive us all in one." She gave the plate to Dexter: "The only rule is that you take something different from that which you gave."

She then poured two bottles of champagne into a large, clear jug with a blood-red band at the rim. "The old symbolism of flesh and blood is difficult to discard," she said. "This is the wine of life, the wine of light, the strength of solidarity, the risk of dispersion, the strength of passion, the risk of excess. This is the wine of the free choice to love, which earth has made and which is offered to you from God as a symbol of all the good you might do and all the risk there will be in doing it. This is the wine of pleasure and pain; it is the wine that sums up in itself all the love of God Our Parent, the Brotherhood of Jesus, the Sisterhood of the Spirit and the renewed commitment I bring as God's Sacred Vessel; this wine is God in you."

As if they had reacted badly to the wine, Jo and Heather slipped out as soon as the jug had been handed on. Perpetua said: "Whatever will happen now, I have left you with the tools for survival in the difficult world: reception, union, affirmation and response, the four elements of your relationship with God.

"Whatever happens I will be with you. It will not be in the same way that Jesus My Brother returned because the world is not the same place. Jesus did not have the technology of ubiquity; we do. I will use that."

When they had finished and said a brief prayer, Jim played a tune and then all of them left except Dexter, Trina and Andy who stayed for a final, brief session; but they were tired and soon she was left alone.

She prayed and cried. She knew that she was about to face a physical trial and she was afraid. She had grown up with physical violence and, far from becoming used to it, she had found it more difficult to accept as she grew older. She knew enough of the knife and the boot, of the threat and the gun, of broken glass and broken promises, of double punishment and double crossing. She had seen women beaten and men pulverised, she had seen children terrorised and brow-beaten; she had seen the angry eye but, much worse, the cold, indifferent eye, the de-humanised eye, and she was afraid that it would soon be looking at her; and she felt terribly lonely now that they had all gone. For all their weaknesses, they were her people; they were what she had chosen and what she had kept. She loved them but she knew them too, realistically, unsentimentally. They had all lived hard lives and she knew that this did not mean that they would more easily tolerate punishment; just the opposite: "The foolhardy, the brave, if you like, can contemplate suffering and even imagine undergoing it but those who have been brought up in it only have two routes," she thought, "they can escape or replicate what they have suffered; better the first but it is not heroic." She knew why they would run away. Only people who had never had to run away did not understand, stood in principle for some more heroic view. Still, she felt lonely.

On Good Friday morning she found it difficult to concentrate on the Procession of Witness.

What made her concentrate most were not the prayers or the hymns but the expressions of the people as the procession went along. She thought: "These people are not hostile. They are sad and sorry and harassed; they need the Church but the Church has not met their need. If only it could suspend its internal dialogue and go out into the world and listen to its anguish. Surely theology is about listening; listening to God's creatures and listening to God. Surely the sadness of one person should be more important to the Church than passing judgment on the ways in which we try to express our human love."

She saw so much quiet desperation; not so acute as pain but a chronic condition of half-living. She detached herself from the procession and ran across the Plaza so that she could see it from a distance; about fifty people singing strange songs, following a wooden cross being carried by a man in strange clothes. She had seen the Church from this perspective before but on Good Friday it looked even more distant from its mission than it did on Sundays. "I think Good Friday should be the day on which we lay ourselves and our worldly goods at the foot of the cross and say: 'This is unconditional; take what you want'," but this brought her back to her premonition that when she lay down and did precisely that she would suffer terribly for it: "But, then," she thought, "what is my suffering to the chronic condition of halfness in which these people live their lives? They are not lively seekers who choose and do not choose; they seem to be oppressed by a kind of powerlessness. What sort of choice is it to choose between cars, cakes, cottages...". The list she was beginning to fall in love with was cut off by the shout of a man with a placard which read: "God is dead!" "Well," she said to him as she passed, "if God is dead then she wasn't God in the first place." She smiled. He smiled. "At least you believe something and that is better than believing nothing. I do not suppose it will give you any comfort to know that atheists and believers are much closer to each other than either group is to the indifferent." In spite of himself, he smiled again.

When the procession reached its destination and the Passion narrative was being read she thought: "I know how much I should concentrate on Jesus My Brother but I keep thinking about me and the time I am in, and the world around."

In spite of her usual discomfort with large churches, she felt comfortable in Bill Midway's church and it was easier for her to focus when she arrived there just before noon. "God Our Parent," she said, "if it pleases You, mark this day of my trial with some earthly symbols so that people may remember my final day and learn to relate their lives to my death. Not as a punishment but simply as a reminder. Make any damage temporary so that people are as amazed by the recovery as by the misfortune; just shake people out of their lethargy and indifference to Your Word. I do not quite mean this but I am prepared to do whatever You want as long as it helps people to have a relationship with You. My life has not been enough, there needs to be something more."

She took all the tiny fragments she had collected from the occasions when she had celebrated the Sacrament of Response: the piece of broken glass from the first occasion; a small stone; a bead; a twig; a piece of metal that had been melted on one of the occasions when the ceremony was centred on a fire; two Scrabble tiles. "In the name of all those who have joined me in Affirming You," she said, "show Your power that the world might know that You, through me, are still with those You have created."

As soon as she had finished there was a mighty downpour with thunder and lightning and a tornado tore through central London, wrenching the doors off churches, mutilating buildings, paralysing computer systems, disrupting the power supply. National emergency measures were triggered. At St. Simple's candles were brought out and Father Bill went on as if nothing had happened.

When the Liturgy of the Cross finished at 3 p.m the storm abated and many people testified later that order was restored as if nothing had happened. Only a very few places, it seemed, were permanently damaged, notably media organisations. She had asked permission to stay in church and encouraged her followers to leave so that she could be alone. When they had gone she lay on the floor in front of the altar and entered a trance-like state, being united with the Trinity in preparation for her ordeal. She took the Cross and held it to her in a dance of commitment, giving herself strength for the journey so that when the inevitable came she would be ready. There were no tears now; she was serene, almost other-worldly, as if she had already been partly 'taken up' from the earth that had given her so much joy but would soon hurt her cruelly.

Lining up the cameras, Poppy took a shot of Heather sending a text message. Damian, the observer from Chris Smoother's office, watched as the preparations were made. Unused to 'candid' television, he felt strange as Perpetua came into shot, not knowing she was being pictured as she walked towards the trap. Jo and Heather tried to slip past her as she arrived but she touched them both reassuringly as they passed her. The ritual dance of greeting and framing began as a voice over, being fed from the CEC studio, introduced the programme: "This is a live broadcast in which *The Cutting Edge Channel* will show the depths to which society has sunk. It shows gang leaders from a 'sink' estate entertaining middle class tearaways for a night of drug taking and violence and it explodes the myth of Perpetua, the self-proclaimed religious leader. Some of the shots may be difficult for some people but we are not showing these to shock but to inform in the public interest."

Poppy was restless because nothing was moving as quickly as she would like; it was a risk with live, unrehearsed documentary. She chose to use sequences featuring the worst parts of the estate taken by the roving camera, accompanied by an impromptu commentary, and ignore the 'trial' which was being filmed by the fixed camera.

"You are here on two charges," said Oliver O'Helly. "First, that you are a fraud; secondly that your so-called religion is a fraud. As to the first, you have claimed to be holier than thou but you are no different from anybody else. You have the same weaknesses and vices; you have the same needs. As to the second, the flaw in your religious outlook is that you elevate imperfection to a virtue."

She stayed silent. He hit her. She still stayed silent.

"I don't see how you can claim to be religious while trying to overthrow the Church. It's some perverted form of 'liberation theology'. Well, we like our religion solid and old-fashioned, something we can rely upon." "You can only rely upon God, not religion."

Rory hit her. She stayed silent. "The trouble with you is that you think that everything has to change; it's this modern urge for change." "God does not change." "If you say that you are part of the Godhead, as you do, then you are trying to change God." "God remains the same; the way we understand God changes."

At this point Poppy's boredom turned to animation as the discussion came to an abrupt end. She was soon frenetically occupied as she walked the tightrope between what she called "cutting edge actuality" and indecency. It was clear from the pictures that Perpetua was being gang raped. Poppy showed no signs of emotion other than excitement as the material became ever more degrading. Damian took his mobile phone out to call Smoother to get it stopped but she snatched it off him, removed the SIM card and stamped on the case until its tough plastic gave way to her stiletto. If he had not retreated into a corner she would have hit him. Later on he wished she had. He could still see the two streams of shots from which she was making her mix. "Dirty bitch", she said, working herself up into self-justifying rage, "all that pious cant and she's right in the middle of a drugs and sex orgy." Damian should have said: "It's gang rape," but he said nothing. Later he wished he had said something. "That's her cover busted," she said; but she soon lost interest in the broken figure on the ground as the gang and their guests became more crazed with the drugs they had taken. It made entertaining television for a short while as the middle class boys tried to act tough in imitation of their hosts. It showed clearly that drugs were not simply a phenomenon of social deprivation; but Perpetua had always said that there were other kinds of deprivation and desolation and it was these from which the rich youths were suffering.

It was the producer who signalled that the sequence of wild behaviour could not be continued. "It isn't the shots, Poppy. Just shut up for a minute and listen; and focus. I know we made an agreement with the police but that Perpetua woman looks as if she might be dying and we don't want to get mixed up in a murder investigation. It's not like a news camera covering a war where journalists are on the sidelines; this is our show; we're responsible for it; so we'll cut to a commercial break and then think about it." She retrieved a shot of Perpetua from early in the programme, lying in the mud just after she had been knocked to the ground, jeans removed, legs apart, and hastily concocted a caption from her lap-top and superimposed it on the face in the mud:

Perpetua

Daughter of God Our Parent

Sister of Jesus

Vessel for the world

It took them less than three minutes to clear up and leave. Poppy was reassured that she had some good material for future projects but she let out a stream of expletives as she stormed away from the makeshift studio. Later there were only memories to rely on as it was found that nobody could be found who had a copy of the broadcast. The material had been completely lost. Some people said it was one of Perpetua's technology miracles.

With the departure of the television crew came rumours of the arrival of the police and the gang were anxious to evacuate. Before they did so, Dexter came to the very edge of the Hollow, inches away from the light. Nobody from the scene was aware of him as he cowered in the shadows until Perpetua moved her head slightly so that their eyes met in a direct gaze across the mud and the debris.

She smiled.

It was probably much worse than if she had looked accusing. He ran as if it was the worst thing he had ever seen, which it was. He wished she had accused him with her eyes instead of smiling. As he ran, the thought crossed his mind that he could find a gun and shoot Roy but fear overcame revenge and he went on running.

Two tramps made their way unsteadily across the mud towards her. The first seemed sympathetic but the second was tetchy. The first bent down and offered her his beer can but she could not drink. The second tried to pull the first away but he would not leave. Then Father Bill and Jim appeared out of the shadows and went towards her, and Damian, with a little courage restored, went close enough to hear them.

"I'm frightened," said Jim. "Hold steady, Jim," said Father Bill. "This is the time for you to be brave. You have been under-estimated all your life; now you are going to show me—but most of all, Perpetua—that you are her brave follower whatever happens." She shifted slightly as a wave of pain crashed across her face; the move was timed so that by the time they could see her clearly, she was smiling. "Bill, Jim. I knew that not everybody would leave me here to die alone." "Dexter was here, too," said Jim. "I know he was. He was terrified. So would you be if you had grown up here and been the leader of a gang before abandoning it for me." "What can we do?" asked Bill. "This may sound a little peremptory, Bill, but what you need to do at the moment is listen because I have not got very much time and I am getting weaker." "An ambulance…" "… No, Bill, it is too late for that. Listen. The reason why I have placed so much reliance on you during the past few months is that I knew when my time came to suffer as Jesus My Brother suffered that my poor followers would lose heart. I want you to see that they are encouraged and, above all, that they recover their self-respect and do not start blaming themselves before going on to start blaming each other. They have a job to do which will be difficult and it will cost most of them their lives in due time. I want them to understand imperfection. You have heard me talk about it before." "Yes." She moved again, showing more pain, but when it subsided her face was crushed. Bill almost lay underneath her head, providing her with some support while enabling him to hear better. Damian edged closer. "I wish that humanity—no, I must focus on Dexter, Trina and the others—could learn to understand imperfection. Teach them, Bill; they will need to understand its purpose or they will destroy themselves." "I will do my best." "I know. You have got Jim now and he has got you and so you will be able to help each other. Jim has never told the others," she said, looking at him almost slyly, "but he has a gift of seeing in a special way. The new mission will need his gifts. Jim, when you see me again, as you soon will, but in a different light and from a different perspective, you can tell the others about your gift. They will need it and their need will make them more receptive. I am very weak now. Let me pray: God Our Parent, I come to You, having showed the union between perfection and imperfection, having absorbed the world's wrong choices in union with Jesus My Brother. The pain was surely worth it.

"What seemed to have ended, what Jesus My Brother started, has begun again."

She died.

And with her death the whole earth was revived as if her very blood had given it new life. Without the Christian schooling it would have been hard to see so much triumph in that terribly broken body, the burns, the broken glass, the gashes, the bits of torn clothing. Even without knowing what would happen later, there was a strange vibrancy in the sadness.

Bill and Jim believed in her so fervently that they seemed to think, as they carried her broken body, that this was an interlude in her triumph. They took her body carefully and without speed to the car and drove away.

Smoother was appalled, not by the programme content but because he was almost certain that he had seen Rory Varnish taking part in the show. There was enough on his plate without the extra complication of a compromised Archdeacon. When Damian finally managed to contact him, Smoother sacked him on the spot. "I don't mind," said Damian "because what I have seen is so appalling that I think it will wreck my sleep for the rest of my life." "Don't be stupid; if somebody is threatening the Church it's best that they are dealt with; what matters is the Church's overall well-being." "God?" "Don't split hairs; the only way you can know about God is through the Church so if there's no Church, there's no God, for practical purposes."

She was wrapped in a red choir robe and laid gently in the vestry until Father Bill could work out what to do. When they were about to leave he was so distracted that He did not notice that Jim had slipped back into the church. It had been a terrible and long day. Bill arranged a makeshift bed for Jim but, following his long practice, was not minded to try to tell him what to do. He dozed fitfully in his own hard, narrow bed as Jim dozed in the familiar warmth of the vestry. He was awakened by the sound of her ethereal music which she had carried with her right to the end. He was immediately aware of bright light in the corner where she lay. The light was so bright that he could not see clearly. He had seen such light before; it was what Perpetua had called his gift of seeing. He stayed still, knowing that it was her light. Perhaps this was what she had promised, that she would return in a different way. He did not know how long the music and light continued but it seemed like a very long time. At last, with the first appearance of dawn, it faded and he could approach the spot where she lay.

She was not there.

Only the folded robes provided evidence that she had been there. He knew what this meant; it was easier for him than the others. He would tell Bill and then leave the next steps to him.

X.

"There's something wrong here," said Smoother, tetchily, as he pressed the channel buttons on his television remote controller. "It doesn't matter which button I press I get the same stuff. There must be something wrong with the remote." "I don't think so," said Damian who had come in to clear his desk, "because every time you press the remote the channel changes. Instead of just looking at the pictures, look at the channel ID." "Oh, yes," said Smoother, slightly ashamed that his irritation had allowed him to make such an elementary mistake. "So whatever channel I turn to, I get precisely the same thing." "It could be a miracle," said Damian, half ironically. "Look," said Smoother, "this could be serious. If you help me I might re-consider my attitude." "Well, you said you had fired me but as I was working for nothing as an intern it doesn't amount to much, does it?" "Leave that until later. What does this current situation amount to?" "Well:

- First, we have a woman called Perpetua who claims to be the Fourth Person of the Godhead; she gets into an unfortunate mix-up which gets out of hand and she dies;
- Secondly, instead of going along with the obvious story, some of the press, borrowing out-dated theological language (they are all hopelessly shallow), say that she has "Risen from the Dead";
- Thirdly, she is on every television channel.

"Might it not be a good idea to listen to what She has to say instead of listening to me?" "I can get a transcript soon enough." "Yes; but just listen for a moment."

"When you think of the divine love of God for everyone, think only of returning God's faith in you, expressed in creation, with faith in God; God's hope in you, expressed in the Resurrection, with your hope in God; and return God's love for you, expressed in my space, through your love of God; and in all three, recognise the constancy of My Sister the Spirit."

"The first two seem all right, and the fourth, but there's something fishy about the third of those propositions." "She is simply saying what she has always said, that she is part of the Godhead." "We will need to be careful how we analyse this." "We?" "Well, you're a theological student, aren't you, so it's time for you to do a bit of praxis."

The screen showed the station logo and after a rather puzzled apology, its normal programming resumed.

"We have this woman," said Smoother, much calmer now, "who was dead, apparently appearing on the world's television screens still claiming to be the Fourth Person of the Godhead." "Correct." "So the first question is whether

She is alive or whether this is some kind of hoax." "It would be difficult for her and her followers to arrange a global television coup." "So is she alive now? That's a separate question." "Well, in a way that we seem not to know anything about, she seems to be; like Jesus was alive in a strange kind of way after His death." "Don't say that" said Smoother, getting agitated again. "Don't make the comparison." "We may have to." "I need to put out some sort of press statement." "What are you going to say?" "I haven't a clue. I suppose I better ask the boss." "You mean you're going to pray?" "No, I'll talk to Hawthorne." He dialled. "Good morning Archbishop. I suppose you have seen the news ... not surprised? ... Very impressed! ... Theologically coherent ... Could I just say that this will put the Church into an even greater turmoil than it is in already; much worse than gays or women bishops ... Yes, I grant you that the Church discussing theology would be a change from its current preoccupations but I would argue with your phrase 'a welcome change'. How has this manifestation gone down with our American friends? ... Split. I am not surprised. ... I suppose the liberals would find this very attractive, wouldn't they? All this stuff about choice and freedom to love. So what are you going to do to prevent the Torans and Petrans walking out? ... Nothing? So why did you go all that way? ... Look, Archbishop, I think it's a bit much to accuse me of forcing your hand. We were facing a crisis and it looks as if this Perpetua story has made that crisis worse. ... What do you mean, it's cleared everything up so that the former crises just fall away? Are you saying that the Church of England is unilaterally going to abandon the Holy Trinity? ... Well if not immediately, when? ... You want us to fix a meeting with the Pope ... and the leader of the American Baptists ... a global Petran, Toran and Liberal forum? ... Are you mad? Sorry, Archbishop, I over-stepped there. May we think about it? ... So you want an immediate statement saying that the whole Christian doctrine needs to be re-considered in the light of what we now think is happening? ... Well, be advised, I think the word 'know' is a bit strong here. I also need to warn you that you will probably lose your See if you go on like this. ... You only took the job because you thought God willed you to do so? ... This is impossible. No, please don't resign now. Give us some time. ... All right, later in the day we can see how events unfold, if they unfold." He rang off.

"We've managed to keep things together through years of turmoil and it's all being unravelled by a teenage girl." "I don't suppose that is very different from what the Pharisees said when they surveyed the impact of Jesus." "Don't say that. We have to stick to reality." "So what do you think is real?" "There is something we do not understand but we must not leap to conclusions. I think I better call my colleague at the *Stylus* to see what line they're taking. "Oh yes, He is risen indeed! Happy Easter. I had almost forgotten in all the rush. Yes. Alleluia. But has somebody else risen? What does the Cardinal Archbishop think about today's events? ... no, of course I don't mean that; I am well aware of his attitude to Easter; I am referring to Perpetua ... Nothing for at least a month? ... Yes, I know the Magisterium takes its time except in matters of a sexual nature but you would have thought that it would have something to say about someone who claims to have risen from the dead. ... Well, I suppose that is true. She hasn't actually claimed anything but that is what it amounts to. She was dead and now she isn't or, even if she is, she seems to be able to exercise power over global television. I suppose you could canonise her ... No, just a joke. Sometimes you Petrans take yourselves too seriously ... and, yes, I know, we don't take ourselves seriously enough ... So no full statement until the Bishops have held their regular Autumn meeting? Nothing in Low Week? ... The game could be up by then. ... You doubt it. Yes, of course you do. We will see." He did not quite cut the call off; but almost.

"Petrans are so bloody superior. I suppose they have been given confidence by this new infusion of immigrants. They will think they are the Church of England soon enough. I don't suppose it will do me any good but I have to ring the *Fortress*. Happy Easter. Christ is Risen! ... You do celebrate Easter, don't you? ... Well I know you are not so keen on it compared with Good Friday but the greeting was well meant. So what is your take on the Perpetua story? ... No story? ... I would have thought 'evil' and 'Possessed by the Devil' (always supposing there is one) is putting it rather strongly ... Well, I am surprised that you said that, it's verging on racism. I don't think you can bring her colour into it, can you? I mean, what colour was Jesus? ... I know The Bible doesn't say what colour he was but you can surely infer it. I mean, what colour are Middle Eastern Jews ... no, before the influx of European and Russian immigrants! ... I mean she's probably the same colour as Jesus; but that isn't the point, is it? ... So let me get this right. You are saying that Perpetua is exercising some kind of malign influence ... what? You don't mean that? ... You are actually going to put out an emergency statement warning Archbishop Hawthorne against being 'taken in' by her ... No. No. I am sure that is groundless. ... Almost immediately ... Don't you think you should wait until events unfold? ... What do you mean, 'What events?" ... Well, I don't know but if he can manipulate global television she's hardly likely to stop there, dead or alive." He did cut off the call.

"Damn! They've rumbled Hawthorne; it's obvious they would!"

The television channel seemed to flicker. The early afternoon sports preview was replaced by pictures from a market. "Look!" said Damian. "Up in the top right hand corner, the *god4u* logo." Smoother pressed remote controller buttons frenetically but wherever he went it was the same, market pictures with the *god4u* logo. "I suppose we will have to take this all in," said Smoother after a fruitless flurry of button pressing. "This is becoming serious. That's Dexter, isn't it, looking a bit phased by it all? While it's quiet I suppose I should ring up poor Varnish to see if he's in shock. I suppose one minor consolation is that *that* story will fade away. Archdeacon ... Oh yes! He has Risen indeed! ... On your way for a walk with your friend O'Helly who is going through some kind of emotional crisis. A very Christian way to spend Easter Sunday; but what about Rory? ... No. Really Where did you hear that? ... CEC told you that it has lost all its raw footage from last Friday night! ... A miracle! ... Well I know the Church isn't in the habit of using words to mean what they mean but it might just be a miracle! ... Enjoy your walk."

His face became suddenly preoccupied. He dialled. "Poppy, love, I am sorry it has taken me so long to get in touch today but, as you probably know, things have been happening. ... Yes, I've just heard about the footage ... I'm sorry ... What do you mean, you don't care? ... Seriously? ... Don't be silly. Sit down and think calmly, you didn't kill God ... I know she said she was God, in a way ... Well I suppose from some points of view it got out of hand but don't blame yourself ... Guilt as a starting point? Look I can't claim to have the detailed knowledge of Perpetua that other people have but the last thing she would have wanted is guilt as a starting point for anything. ... Yes, I can see him now. He looks as if he is about to say something. Take care of yourself and try to stay calm. There's nothing wrong with religious conviction as long as you don't take it too far. She didn't have to ring off like that. Just one more call. Sneer ... yes, it's Smoother. Just to say that if you don't leave my daughter alone you'll be in trouble if you aren't already."

They watched in silence for a while as Dexter and the other *god4u* people walked around the market place talking to people and handing out leaflets. "Pretty pointless television," said Smoother. "You're missing the point. It isn't the content that really counts it's the way you are receiving it. Like all human beings you have adjusted so easily to the new circumstances that you have forgotten how remarkable the pictures are that you are seeing. You are watching a group of people who believe that their leader, Perpetua, is in some way not dead even though you saw her killed with your own eyes—well, almost. You can see these people because, whether she is alive or not, the whole global television system is now in some way under her control. What you don't want to do, but will have to do sooner or later, is to put these two pieces of information together and see what you get out of it."

The camera closed in on Dexter as he gave one of his impromptu addresses to a crowd of festive shoppers:

"Perpetua has risen! She promised that she would not leave us and she has kept her promise. The world is now the witness of her power as she talks to the world through her humble follower who was a coward, who betrayed her but who was forgiven. She came with a message of hope, a message so perfect that humanity could not bear it and so she was killed; but in a way we do not understand, it had to be. I am no theologian but she said that if I spoke in the power of her Sister the Spirit that I would be truly guided, so now I speak.

"There must be no limit to faith, hope and love; there must be no shackles placed upon them by doctrinal rules. Jesus came to overthrow the Jewish law with love and Perpetua came to overthrow the Christian law with love. She paid for her perfection with her life so that we who are imperfect might more often and more fully choose to love."

"Powerful stuff for somebody who claims not to know any theology." "Yes, very impressive, theologically."

"We live in an age when people want somebody to be blamed for everything; it is all mistrust and enquiries and enquiries into enquiries. About her own death she would not want this. What was done was done. We must look forward in hope. When she caused all records of her degradation to disappear it was not because she was ashamed of what happened to her, she simply wanted us all to move on, to think about what her life meant and what she means now that she is with us. She has overcome death and she is telling us that we can overcome death, too; but it is in our hands; it is in our minds; it is in our consciences."

"It is becoming more difficult not to put the two pieces together, as you rightly said. Her death, the disappearance of all known copies of Poppy's filming and this uncanny control of the television channels are beginning to fit together ominously." "Ominously?" "Well, it's difficult to find the right word but I am now certain of one thing; that no matter what has actually happened, Christianity can never be the same again because there will be a change in perception, and in life it's perception, not reality, that counts. What this means, really, is the end of the Petran authoritarian reaction to its decline and the end of Toran arrogance. Whatever the actual shape of things to come, Hawthorne will come out on top because she has changed the terms of theological trade for at least the next ten years and that's a long time in the twenty-first century. I think I'd better ring him before he goes into his High Mass as they call it over there. Archbishop ... Perhaps I was a little hasty when I rang before but events have been rather unprecedented ... It is impossible to deny the evidence, yes. ... No. Please. This would be precisely the wrong thing to do. Resignation is out of the question. The Church needs you to lead it as it comes to terms with this new direction, this new hope, this new vigour. We can't afford to make the same mistake the Pharisees made when they imprisoned Peter and stoned Stephen. You have to be here with us to hold things together, to work out how we fit this new piece into God's, er, jigsaw ... Well, I know it wasn't very well put but you know what I mean. It's only people like you that can fit things together. People who are narrow and stubborn are just going to fight this new reality and that will be a terrible missed opportunity. ... That's a pity. I think it would be a good time to put out an up-beat statement, to claim the high ground, to put the opposition on the back foot ... I know you don't like cricket metaphors but ... I suppose I expected that. You are right, this isn't a game which we have to win, it isn't about wrong-footing the opposition. I'm sorry, Archbishop, that is the way my instinct works and I must curb it. I know. I have tried my best for you but I know you don't really approve of my working methods. But I know I can change ... I know you believe I can. Thank you. Yes, text me the outline and I will work on it."

As the scene shifted from the market to Grunge Park, the crowds grew until the whole area of the Hollow was packed with thousands of people. "This is powerful," said Smoother. "Dexter is going to preside at a service on the exact spot where she died." "Incarnational praxis," said Damian, apropos of nothing in particular.

"Damian, help me to work this out. There is a God, right? And this God decides to build a bridge with creation so Jesus arrives and dies and rises; and it works for a while but then the effect wears off so Perpetua is sent to do precisely what Jesus did but at a different time in a different place? Have I got it?" "In essence, yes. Whether we are right in all of this or are as wrong as atheists say we are, the idea that a creator creates for a purpose is plausible; and that that purpose is to love and be loved is plausible; and that assisting that love by building a bridge between the divine and the human is plausible; and that the bridge building needs to be iterative is plausible." "'Plausible?' Wouldn't you go any further than that?" "I am just looking at it from outside myself. we keep having fierce and useless arguments about whether God exists. I believe in God, Sneer doesn't, but what we should be doing is to help Sneer to see that it's plausible while we get on with enjoying the relationship and sharing our enjoyment." "So will there be an almighty battle over the Trinity?" "I expect there will. Neither the Petrans nor the Torans will want to give up on it. They will, as usual, put doctrine both above principle and behaviour. They will behave badly in the name of God and while they are behaving badly they will forget love and those they were created to love. Whether they continue to love God is something on which I cannot speculate. I suspect that the row about the doctrine of the Godhead will go on forever but that the Trinitarian aspect will not engage us for the whole of the twenty-first century. I expect settlement to be sooner because, if I am right, the Perpetuan heritage will penetrate society much more globally and deeply than Jesus managed with the resources of the first century." "Here is the Archbishop's statement. He must have written it before going into church. I wonder whether it will form the core of his Easter Sermon; that will give them a shock. Well, for me, the die is cast." He worked with total concentration for ten minutes and then read the text to Damian:

"Archbishop Hawthorn responded to the extraordinary events of Easter

Sunday by announcing a full theological enquiry into the implications of the mission, death and continuing influence of Perpetua.

"In a statement issued from North America where he is attempting to heal the divisions in the Church over gay clergy, the Archbishop said: "There are legitimate questions to be asked about many of Perpetua's statements including: whether the sacrifice of Jesus must be final because it is full; whether the Trinity is an unduly closed way of describing the Godhead; whether our view of the connectivity between choice and imperfection is coherent. She also raises some important issues over the way the Church relates to the world. I look forward to consulting with my fellow Bishops in the House of Bishops and in the wider Anglican Communion and intend, as far as it lies within my power, to give this issue priority over others that have recently exercised the Church. I have no doubt that this statement will cause pain and hardship for many but the road to Calvary—or, might I say, to the Hollow?—must be full of pain. Finally, I wish to emphasise that because the Church is now facing a theological issue of genuine magnitude, I have no intention of resigning."

"Look!" said Damian. There was some kind of ceremony going on, so they turned up the sound: "Dexter has called upon the Grunge Park gang leader to repent and place his weapons at the place where Perpetua died. Here he is, approaching the place where a cross has been made out of all kinds of weapons. There he is, placing his knife at the bottom end of the cross, kneeling in prayer. This is surely a remarkable day for the people of Grunge Park, the place where Perpetua grew up and started her mission."

The camera showed the massive crowds and then came to rest at the cross where Roy had knelt. Dexter said: "Let us begin by remembering, even on this glorious day, how we have done wrong. I don't want the wonder of today to be obscured by my own story but I want to say immediately that I have done wrong. I ran away from Perpetua when she needed me. I was even worse than Roy. I don't want to diminish the importance of seeking forgiveness and wholeness in God but Perpetua said we were never to allow ourselves to drown in guilt. Love was far too important for that."

As the service of thanksgiving proceeded, *god4u* followers distributed bread and small cups of wine to people who had not brought something of their own. "Anything will do," said Kylie, as long as you bring it to her." Dexter, taking some bread, together with some offerings from the crowd, said: "In the name of God Our Parent and Jesus Our Brother and in the memory of our Beloved Sister, God's Sacred Vessel, I call upon Our Sister the Spirit to make these gifts we offer into the very presence of Jesus and Perpetua." "That's going to take a bit of getting used to," said Smoother, "Jesus and Perpetua. It will confuse many people and make others sad; and still more will just walk out of the Church but I am convinced that it will bring us new life and new hope."

As the ceremonies came to an end with dancing, a young black girl came quietly into the office. "Don't bother trying to clean up now," said Smoother. "It can wait." The girl nodded and pulled the bin liner out of the basket under the desk.

"Well," said Damian, "do you think you have finally arrived?" "Yes," said Smoother. "I can't say I will stop being a bit of a bruiser and I sometimes put the institutional interests of the Church above the integrity of its mission— that's why Bishops have press people, to do their dirty work for them while pretending there is no dirty work—but I will stay with Hawthorne and help him to come to terms with the Perpetua phenomenon. What will you do?" "Write my Masters thesis on incarnational praxis." "On what?" "Well, on Perpetua actually. You see, I believe that she was sent by God as a divine messenger, that she stands equal with Jesus. Perpetua really was the Sacred Vessel of God and she died for us to bring new hope to God's Church."

The girl looked round slightly as he approached the door. "Amen!" she said, as she closed it gently behind Her.

PRINCE'S COLLEGE, LONDON

Cover Sheet

Candidate Pseudonym: Damian

Department: Theology & Religious Studies

Course: Systematic Theology

Level: MA

Title: Incarnational Praxis: A Case Study

Lightning Source UK Ltd.
Milton Keynes UK
05 November 2010

162478UK00001B/1/P